# PHILOSOPHICAL FOUNDATIONS OF PSYCHOTHERAPY

*Philosophical Foundations of Psychotherapy* promotes a critical understanding of the ideas, traditions, values, and principles that inform and shape – for better or for worse – what therapists do.

The book challenges the unhelpful misconception that philosophy is for philosophers alone, because human reality is too complex for therapists to be unaware of the foundations, difficulties, and contradictions within our value systems, ethics, and assumptions. By retrieving attitudes from other times and other places, traversing the relational contours of history right up to contemporary thinkers and practitioners, the author argues that not only do relationships heal, but they offer the only safe harbour in life's sea of troubles. He promotes a conscientious radical relationality, which remains attentive to its influences, including contemporary debates about our neoliberal selves, the superstructures of culture, and the ethics of authenticity. In stepping back from the sometimes-narrow concerns of our therapeutic methods, the book explores broader themes important for living well: what is the good of therapy, how do we reconcile our sense of futility in the face of an indifferent universe, postcolonial debates, responses to disembodied artificial intelligence, and alternatives to our human-centred stance towards Nature.

This book is primarily for practitioners, trainees, and educators, but ultimately it is intended for the greater good of clients and those interested in what therapeutic practices and practitioners have to offer. It will also be useful for those teaching research methods, the practice of research supervision, reflexivity, and personal development, across all areas related to mental health.

**James Costello, PhD**, is a senior lecturer in the School of Social Sciences at the University of the West of England, UK. He is an Accredited member of the British Association for Counselling and Psychotherapy, and Senior Accredited Supervisor specializing in Groups. His experience as a therapist comes from over 20 years' practice and consultancy across the private, third, and public sectors. He supervises psychotherapy training and has research interests more broadly in phenomenology and consciousness.

# Advances in Theoretical and Philosophical Psychology

Series Editor: Brent D. Slife

**A Psychological Perspective on Folk Moral Objectivism**
*Jennifer Cole Wright*

**Suffering and Psychology**
*Frank C. Richardson*

**Posttraumatic Joy: A Seminar on Nietzsche's Tragicomic Philosophy of Life**
*Matthew Clemente*, Edited with Introduction by Andrew J. Zeppa

**Towards the Psychological Humanities: A Modest Manifesto for the Future of Psychology**
*Mark Freeman*

**Primer in Critical Personalism: A Framework for Reviving Psychological Inquiry and for Grounding a Socio-Cultural Ethos**
*James T. Lamiell*

**Studies of Life Positioning: A New Sociocultural Approach to Psychobiography**
*Jack Martin*

**Philosophical Foundations of Psychotherapy: Radical Relationality**
*James Costello*

For more information about this series, please visit www.routledge.com/Advances-in-Theoretical-and-Philosophical-Psychology/book-series/TPP

# PHILOSOPHICAL FOUNDATIONS OF PSYCHOTHERAPY

## Radical Relationality

*James Costello*

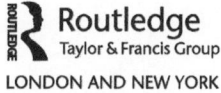

Routledge
Taylor & Francis Group

LONDON AND NEW YORK

Designed cover image: Image courtesy of Mackenzie Leigh Hawkins

First published 2025
by Routledge
4 Park Square, Milton Park, Abingdon, Oxon OX14 4RN

and by Routledge
605 Third Avenue, New York, NY 10158

*Routledge is an imprint of the Taylor & Francis Group, an informa business*

© 2025 James Costello

*British Library Cataloguing-in-Publication Data*
A catalogue record for this book is available from the British Library

ISBN: 978-1-032-49951-2 (hbk)
ISBN: 978-1-032-49950-5 (pbk)
ISBN: 978-1-003-39616-1 (ebk)

DOI: 10.4324/9781003396161

Typeset in Galliard
by Newgen Publishing UK

*In loving memory of my father, Tom.*
*A fine storyteller.*
*And for my mother, Kate.*
*Who cared for him until the end.*

# CONTENTS

*Acknowledgements*                                             *x*
*Advances in Theoretical and Philosophical Psychology*        *xii*
*Disclaimers*                                                 *xiv*
*Prologue*                                                     *xv*

1  Philosophical Foundations                                    1

2  A Good Life                                                 31

3  Reason and Belief                                           54

4  Individualism: The Atomised Self                            79

5  Freedom: Ethics and Existentialism                         99

6  Meaning: A Reassuring Foundation                           126

7  Stories: Fragmented Selves                                 155

8  Time                                                       185

9  Being *with* Others                                        209

*Epilogue*                                                    *242*
*Index*                                                       *246*

# ACKNOWLEDGEMENTS

My intellectual debts in the writing of this book are innumerable, but many of those who have inspired and influenced me are cited throughout the book. I am particularly grateful to Brent Slife for his early outline of radical relationality which inspired this book. Thank you for your encouragement and helpful comments throughout the project. I would also like to thank my friends and colleagues in the Department of Philosophy here at the University of the West of England (UWE). In particular, Niall Keane has been generous with his time, knowledge, and wisdom, offering valuable comments on early drafts of the book especially those chapters addressing phenomenology. Jessie Stanier too has offered insightful comments on aspects of the narrative turn.

The corrosive dynamic of our times seems both literally and metaphorically to be about "scrolling-on" in search of the next distraction; little value is given to slowing down, taking stock and reflecting. I am grateful then to the College of Health, Science and Society at UWE for the award of a research grant, which helped me complete this book. I am also indebted to the leadership team here in the Department of Applied Sciences (Lyn Newton and Helen Green) for their kindness and generosity. I would like to thank my colleague Emma Levey in Art and Design, who organised a competition amongst our talented final-year students here at UWE to illustrate the book. And for Mac (Mackenzie Leigh Hawkins), who won that competition and took on the challenge of going beyond my words. Thank you.

I am indebted to the supervisees I have encountered throughout the years, as well as many practitioners associated with the teaching and practice of psychotherapy, who, in one way or another, informed my thinking about radical relationality. In this regard, I wish to say thanks to my friend and colleague Dave Pomroy for being a consistent source of support and often hilarious insights. Thanks also for the kindness and generosity of my friend and neighbour Phil Martin; your actions remind me that living the good life requires more than just talking about the good life.

With me every step of the way has been my joyful daughters Evelyn and Isabella who simply love to have fun – usually at my expense. If one day you read this, girls, I want you to know that rediscovering the world through your eyes has been the privilege of my life. Thank you. Finally, my endlessly forgiving wife Sonia. What would I do without you? Grazie amore!

# ADVANCES IN THEORETICAL AND PHILOSOPHICAL PSYCHOLOGY

Series Foreword
*Brent D. Slife, Series Editor*

Psychologists need to face the facts. Their commitment to empiricism for answering disciplinary questions does not prevent pivotal questions from arising that cannot be evaluated exclusively through empirical methods, hence the title of this series: *Advances in Theoretical and Philosophical Psychology*. For example, such moral questions as, "What is the nature of a good life?" are crucial to psychotherapists but are not answerable through empirical methods alone. And what of these methods? Many have worried that our current psychological means of investigation are not adequate for fully understanding the person (e.g., Gantt & Williams, 2018; Schiff, 2019). How do we address this concern through empirical methods without running headlong into the dilemma of methods investigating themselves? Such questions are in some sense philosophical, to be sure, but the discipline of psychology cannot advance even its own empirical agenda without addressing questions like these in defensible ways.

How then should the discipline of psychology deal with such distinctly theoretical and philosophical questions? We could leave the answers exclusively to professional philosophers, but this option would mean that the conceptual foundations of the discipline, including the conceptual framework of empiricism itself, are left to scholars who are *outside* the discipline. As undoubtedly helpful as philosophers are and will be, this situation would mean that the people doing the actual psychological work, psychologists themselves, are divorced from the people who formulate and re-formulate the conceptual foundations of that work. This division of labour would not seem to serve the long-term viability of the discipline.

Instead, the founders of psychology – scholars such as Wundt, Freud, and James – recognized the importance of psychologists in formulating their own foundations. These parents of psychology not only did their own theorizing, in cooperation with many other disciplines; they also realized the significance of psychologists continuously *re*-examining these theories and philosophies. This re-examination process allowed for the people most directly involved in and knowledgeable about the discipline to be the ones to decide *what* changes were needed, and *how* such changes would best be implemented. This book series is dedicated to that task, the examining and re-examining of psychology's foundations.

## References

Gantt, E. & Williams, R. (2018). *On Hijacking science: Exploring the Nature and Consequences of Overreach in Psychology.* Routledge.

Schiff, B. (2019). *Situating Qualitative Methods in Psychological Science.* Routledge.

# DISCLAIMERS

*On terminology.* I do not differentiate between counselling, counselling-psychologist, psychotherapy, therapy, psychological practitioner or counsellor, as they are equally therapeutic practices and titles. Throughout this book then, when I refer to therapy, or therapist, I am referring to and include all therapeutic practices and practitioners.

*On the matter of confidentiality.* While many of the dialogues and portrayals conveyed within are fictional, they represent the essence of actual encounters. To safeguard the identities of those who may consider themselves to be involved, I have re-contextualised, amalgamated, blended and anonymised individuals, events, and situations to ensure that they cannot be identified. If you imagine that you see yourself or others here, it is a coincidence and reflects how commonplace such encounters are.

*On the use of artificial intelligence.* I have not used open AIs, or any other system based on large language models (LLMs) to compose, aggregate, summarise or paraphrase what I present to you here. In a way that a silica-based system cannot, it is an imperfect organic entity – alert to their biases – who is responsible and accountable for the written content of the book. The users of such technologies for their writing might wish to ask: who pays the vast amounts of money required to train such language models?

# PROLOGUE

The culture, traditions and times to which we belong shape the values, theoretical models and practices which therapists either embrace or perhaps more tellingly, disregard. In my previous book, I sought to address the emotional ills and travails of the modern neoliberal workplace using a relational approach drawn – inevitably – from contemporary therapeutic practices (2020). Like a cage-born animal released into the wild, I sought – optimistically – to transpose the "punctuated" and relatively shallow relationship of therapy into the unforgiving world of work. While the latter has little regard for the niceties of the former, they nevertheless share a similar heritage. The theories of psychotherapy and the modern Western culture from which they spring have a common philosophical foundation. Our ailing culture tends to offer solutions shaped by the same malady it seeks to redress. Therapy then becomes more the symbol of our times, and not so much the remedy. The question I was left with was, as a profession, as a society: have we been putting out the fires with gasoline?

In an era when people seem to want a more embodied connection with their environment, deeper engagement with their communities, a believable transcendence, and a purpose which remoralises their lives, what have we been offering? More individualising self-mastery and empowerment to those of us who already feel beleaguered and abandoned by a culture which appears to prize more than anything else, "the hustle".

And if you do not make it – by whatever metric one might wish to choose, be it bling, property, career, the latest phone, or the perfect partner/body/car/life/children – then there is only yourself to blame. What, as a profession, have we unwittingly become? What have we forgotten, and can we retrieve our good intentions from a slide into moral relativism which disenchants those who already feel left behind. How much longer must we condone offering inapt modern solutions to the age old problems of living?

Relying on individualising explanations only leaves us helpless and alone in the face of global climate change, the snake oil promises of populism, and a pandemic which not only accelerated social isolation but rendered absurd our attempts to marginalise death. Accustomed as each of us are to living alone in a cell, we can almost convince ourselves that *this* is freedom.

Certainly, therapists have taken relationships seriously, but only from within the intellectual context of a culture which presumes we are individuals first and relaters second. Our bodies are seen as vehicles for transporting an indwelling mind from one interpersonal encounter to the next, like a shopping trolley pushing an evasive cabbage up and down the aisles of some psychic supermarket. The idea that relationships "heal" has been around for some time. Rarely, however, has the relationship been taken as anything other than a sort of inert medium through which the real business of healing – feelings, thoughts, ruminating on the past, and of course the unconscious – takes place. What I argue here is that we are not taking the radical nature of human relationality seriously enough.

What seemed less clear at the outset of this project was how to articulate this radical relationality. To this end, I have retrieved the ancient relationship between philosophy on the one hand, and living a good life, on the other. My task is not one of exposing as ill-founded the philosophical foundations of some of our most popular therapeutic methods. It is one of understanding why, given that these foundations are so questionable, we continue – for the most part – to go about our business as if this were not the case? This is the ground from which I articulate the philosophical principles of radical relationality. I locate the characteristics of radical relationality in their philosophical firmament, which I contend, serves to enhance its therapeutic authority.

We must resist the tendency to see this relational turn as another school of thought, clinical technique, method, or heaven forbid, tool in the interminable "toolbox". What I articulate here transcends and radicalises these perspectives. Radical relationality is at its core what sound, praiseworthy, virtuous therapeutic practice has always been, and already is. Having had the privilege of being a therapist, supervisor, and trainer for over 20 years, I am convinced that the seeds of radical relationality have always been in the wind. These seeds are poised to be germinated and come to fruition in those fortuitous circumstances when a person is sufficiently free of dogma and willing to care for and relate authentically with others.

But our view of radical relationality is obscured by many things, including the complacency of humanism, which disenchants, and furthermore deprives therapy of its potential. I seek to retrieve attitudes from other times and other places – uncontaminated by the excesses of modernity – which acknowledge that not only do relationships heal, but they offer the only safe harbour in life's sea of troubles. I want to demystify the technical vocabulary of philosophy, whilst also emphasising the fact that we are beings who dwell in a world where morals are real. And most importantly, I challenge the unhelpful misconception that philosophy is for philosophers alone. Human reality is too complex for therapists to be unaware of the foundations, difficulties, and contradictions within our value systems, ethics, and the philosophical assumptions that shape our deeds.

This has implications for the ethical assumptions of any given therapeutic method, which if aligned with liberal individualism for example, fails to consider the wider impact of a client's relational network. The radical relationalist understands that it is necessary to articulate not only the goals but also the ethical assumptions of the goals of therapy. For this, the therapist must develop the capacity to articulate their own philosophical understanding of what constitutes for them, a good life.

Radical relationality is alert to the natural givenness of our existence, and the way we experience historical traditions; the past is not a distant land, but the lining to the present. It must come as no surprise then that a radically critical consciousness must be levelled towards the major therapeutic traditions, so that we may acquire as much transparency as possible. If radical relationality is to be conscientious, it must become aware of its influences which encompass contemporary debates about our neoliberal selves, the superstructures of culture, and the ethics of authenticity. Broader themes I explore here include reconciling our sense of futility in the face of what seems to be an indifferent universe, postcolonial critiques, our response to disembodied artificial intelligence, and alternatives to our human-centred stance towards Nature.

As I argue throughout, there can be no definitive text, or knowledge for that matter – and this book is no different in this regard. But this does not equate to being left adrift at sea without knowing which way is north. What I seek here is to advance the conversation towards a more fitting, radically relational psychotherapy and way of living.

James Costello
July 2024

## Reference

Costello, J. (2020). *Workplace Wellbeing: A Relational Approach*. Routledge.

# 1

# PHILOSOPHICAL FOUNDATIONS

## 1.1   Psychotherapy and Philosophy: The Serpent and Its Tail

The questions that interest philosophers are not so different from those which concern the psychotherapist. After all, both seek – no matter how imperfectly – to make sense of our expereince of being in the world. What is wisdom? How do we attain it? How do we use this knowledge and understanding to live better lives? These are some of the questions which bind the two disciplines together.

Devouring and yet being born from one another like the mythical uroboros itself, the relationship between the two disciplines expresses a unity of the material and spiritual, neither disappearing, but constantly changing form in an eternal cycle of destruction and re-creation. I see the practice of philosophy as something akin to the head of the uroboros – the serpent which feeds on its own empirical "tail" – consuming and being formed by the ethical and moral predicaments which constitute the ordinary, day-to-day concerns of psychotherapy. The latter similarly constitutes a mandible, participating with philosophy in a *pterygoid* walk, with the linked disciplines ratcheting along life's outsized dilemmas, traumas, and concerns to assimilate, render comprehensible, and perhaps even find nourishment in them.

There can be no easy answers to the questions posed here because the pool of philosophy and psychotherapy has no shallow end. Neither have definitive procedures, techniques, methods, or secure foundations on which to rely. Life as it is given to us is not completely comprehensible or satisfying. But should we care to, the means are available for addressing the questions that being in the world raises, whether they be philosophical, political, or relational. Curiosity and courage become essential virtues for life at the deep end. For

DOI: 10.4324/9781003396161-1

there is nowhere else from which to understand than from the middle of the muddle of it all.

The sort of understanding the interwoven disciplines seek may not be the kind that, having been uncovered, can be universally applied. The sort of wisdom I am talking about is practical, and brought about both from within, and through *doing*. In the overlapping disciplines of therapy and philosophy, one also has to take a stand on whether they are *a part of*, or *apart from* the empirical sciences. Judgement thus guides my choice of topics considered of importance and of worth here because I seek to make an argument, not prove a point. The creative practice of finding the question, never mind the answer – just like the therapeutic encounter – must draw on past experiences, histories, and what comes to the fore during this particular era of our existence.

The ancient practice of seeking wisdom – midwife to the contemporary art of psychotherapy – has been diffracted through the lens of the modern university, and by modernity itself. Questions once considered philosophical now fall under the purview of rational inquiry, or science as we call it. Beginning in earnest during the nineteenth century, attempts were made to differentiate between the hitherto intertwined sciences and the humanities; both became blanket terms used by administrators to gather together topics into manageable, abstract scholastic departments.

One cannot deny that the modern philosopher is much like any other scholar: they walk the line between saying something sufficiently interesting to be published, while at the same time staying within the rails of what is acceptable to their peers. It is a practice of collaborative disagreement which tiptoes cautiously towards clarity and consensus. Philosophy in this sense looks to minimise – as much as possible – the assumptions from which it must draw its conclusions, so to secure the widest obtainable consensus; but when it is abstracted from experience, it is abstracted from life and living.

The weakness of modernity is reflected in the often-unnoticed, latent habit of rendering analytical, atomising abstractions from an intertwined, intuitive prior whole. It leaves us with the problem of integrating binaries seen as *opposites* rather than *aspects* of the sort of thing I am, that is, body–mind, thoughts–things, freedom–cause, humanity–nature, and animal–environment. Taking things apart and separating them so we may understand them better has led to great advances in human technology. But if we are to avoid "technology" supplanting "wisdom" and our ancient concern with life and living, then we must learn to put things back together again in the age-old tradition of *praxis* – the intertwining of thought and action, self and others, soul, and body. In this way, we may account for our relation to the world in its deepest sense, based on our perceptions and not merely on the imaginative projections of a passive spectator.

Positioning ourselves as passive spectators of our ecosystem has not served us well. The cool objectifying eye of the scientist is no longer able to maintain its distance from Nature because Nature is changing in a way which will determine not only our future, but that of our children. We can no longer consider ourselves *apart* from that of which we are *a part*. The limitations of pure externality implicit in modernity are clear. So long as we gaze upon Nature as we do at dolphins through the thick glass walls of the *Acquario di Genova* – passive, distanced, and separate from our other senses – then we will remain indifferent to our place in the vital order of animality.

Both therapy and philosophy are in the same business of reshaping vocabularies which have gradually outgrown their usefulness into others which we may find more helpful. What I have done here is no different. I have presented the various vocabularies and metaphors which articulate a similar truth, which is that we are shapers and co-creators of our relational world. Mimicking the uroboros, humans are peculiarly hungry for different, ever more sophisticated hungers, which take us beyond mere material necessity – the cultivation of art, love, politics, and culture being notable examples. Taking several views of the same mountain is radical only insofar that I am retrieving the same idiom but from different spatial and historical contexts.

Two key concepts which constitute the philosophical jaws of the uroboros help us grip the tail of psychotherapeutic practice. The first is epistemology, which deals with how we use our reason and experience to understand and know things. The other is ontology, which wants to answer the big questions about the universe, for example what is ultimately real and fundamental, especially regarding the self. But ontology can also be concerned with deeply practical matters that affect people, such as: "what is depression?" Together, these concepts characterise the overlapping concerns of philosophy and psychotherapy: they help us take what we already seem to know about the world one step forward into our awareness.

The story I want to tell you is about untangling the assumptions we make about our relationship with other people, the world, and the theories we use to understand both of these in the therapeutic encounter. By definition, the format I use for this must be a linear unfolding constrained by the physical sequence of pages. Perhaps it explains why my supervisees are less keen on reading books about therapy, loving instead the format of group supervision which develops the practical wisdom of therapy. In a safe, playful yet challenging context, members glide effortlessly amongst the billowing, spiralling thermals of involvement, disengagement, and reflection which the linear format of a book flattens. This is why I make the case throughout that there must be a looping back and forth between philosophy and psychotherapy, theoretical abstraction and empirical experience, involvement and detachment, the universal and the particular. This is the nature of the uroboros.

I also wish to challenge the unhelpful misconception that philosophy is for philosophers alone. Human existence is too complex for counsellors and psychotherapists to be unaware of the foundations, difficulties, and contradictions within our value systems, ethics, and philosophical assumptions about what we do. In the remainder of this section, I address some of the general philosophical aspects of psychotherapy that are invariably side-stepped in training (and supervision) as they are considered – scandalously I feel – too "deep" for consideration. What is truth? What good is therapy? What is the good of therapy?

I then examine both weak and deep (or radical) relationality, and it is the latter with which this book is largely concerned. Brent Slife and coworkers (2008, 2009) have previously sketched the key characteristics of radical relationality. I have attempted here to locate the characteristics of radical relationality in their philosophical firmament, which I believe enhances their therapeutic authority.

Guided by a Different Light. For many practitioners, therapy is synonymous with systematic theoretical frameworks, be they humanistic, cognitive, or psychodynamic. A methodological approach selects, and gathers its "*data*" (stories, transference, feelings … Section 1.3) whereby findings and conclusions are formulated like rungs on the ladder to "truth". Problematically I feel, the subject matter of therapy cannot be known before the method for its investigation has been formulated.

The error then lies in what a psychotherapeutic method excludes in its quest for truth. Philosophical and thus therapeutic truth is not to be thought of as some empirical correspondence to fact. We might consider the alternative term *truthfulness* to indicate something about those things which we steer by. It leads us to see that while the discussion of facts is normal in science, it has little to do with therapy, suggesting that the interests of the two domains are different.

Prior to Hans-Georg Gadamer, it was assumed that by subtracting a person from their context we could reveal truth, something otherwise obscured by the distorting effects of our relationships with the world about us. Isolating the self, disembodying it from prejudice and thereby revealing it in pure form speaks well to those who believe that truth exists independent of the person who seeks it.

Truth cannot be revealed through our therapeutic methods because the truth is not like an object "in there," waiting to be uncovered. In fact, it is not that we are led astray by the traditions that do so much to shape our understanding; we are made of them. Because there are no facts in this regard, only interpretations, all that we can do is attempt to grasp what lies "between" us. When engaging in a genuine conversation with you – the client – I am not seeking to comprehend you through my understanding of your internal world. In understanding that there is no "true" you to uncover, but merely interpretations of what lies between, I may come to know something of you, but this is incidental, not primary.

Just as a flat-head screwdriver must be pre-configured to complement a slotted screw, so too a therapeutic method is pre-configured to complement its assumptions about what it is to be a functional, if not a fulfilled human being. Difficulties arise when a screwdriver is presented with a screw whose head is non-complementary, or at worst, the screw is a nail; do we resort to using the blunt end as a hammer? This conjures the hackneyed metaphor of the therapeutic "toolkit" for the times we suspect that the method and the client are incompatible; rummaging around in our toolkit for a better fit becomes the next move in the gendered logic of reparative ironmongery.

Unfortunately, in psychotherapy, as methods come with implicit assumptions, attention becomes diverted from what really matters; we may never understand the source of incompatibility; bad method or "resistant" client? Slavishly deploying a method is what happens when we are incurious about the unique encounter between therapist and client, interpreter and interpreted, seer and seen. It is the general problem that socially recognised healers have when it comes to relating the particular to the general and conversely the general to the particular (Gadamer, 1996).

As Aristotle saw it, the swash and backwash entered into by the craftsperson (*technē*) is a process of gliding between <u>universalising</u> theoretical knowledge (*epistēmē*), and the <u>particularity</u> of practical wisdom (*phronēsis*). As a therapist, I cannot understand until I am radical in questioning my orientation to the world and with the client. Embracing the indeterminacy and provisionality of *technē* challenges old notions of method-laden professional expertise, which unsettles the novice practitioner who seeks certainty in exchange for their financial and moral investment. It runs against the fluxional circumstances of therapy, which require that interpretation remains "always on the way," and of judgement always under consideration.

Aristotle also understood something of excellence in this context because the radically relational therapist is one who attains the virtue of thoughtful reflection – the emphasis being on approaching our encounter with a client on *their* social-historical terms. In contrast, the application of a method is not the consequence of understanding, but a necessary and constitutive part of understanding. Since understanding the therapeutic encounter is always conducted within a particularly unique situation, there can be no universal method governing its application. Each encounter is a unique journey into the unfamiliar, the strange and sometimes unintelligible.

The old tale of the good Samaritan who helps an inebriate search for their door key beneath a lamppost comes to mind: "Are you sure you dropped them here?" they ask. "Oh no ..." comes the reply, "I lost them somewhere down the street ... but the light is better here". Errors occur when we are incurious about the world beyond that which is illuminated by our favoured methods. The method "cart" always comes before the human "horse," because the truth of a method can only be revealed – or obscured – once a method is applied. Having abandoned the notion of a universal and timeless "truth," philosophical and therapeutic remarks must be seen as relevant to the time and context in which they are uttered. However, this does not mean that they are irrelevant to other times and other contexts.

To illustrate the point, let me take as an example the persistent myth that the first voyage of Christopher Columbus proved to Medieval sceptics that the earth was, in fact, round. How did the notion arise that fifteenth-century Europeans were ignorant of one of the most basic and certain pieces of knowledge that had been deduced two millennia before?

The seed grew from Humanist and Protestant contempt for what became known as the "Dark Ages". Although it was known that (largely Catholic) Medieval scholars did not believe the earth was flat, minds were being prepared to receive insults about yet another myth – the warfare between largely Judeo-Christian theology (*Jerusalem*) and Rationalism (*Athens*). Beneath this distortion lies an ethnocentric compulsion to view modern, Eurocentric post-industrial culture as the outcome of beneficent humanistic progress (Russel, 1991).

Such chronocentrism – the belief that our current views are superior to ancient cultures – is the most stubborn variety of ethnocentrism. Our contempt for the past and thus our need to believe in the superiority of the present has left us abandoned in the dark ocean without stars or a compass to show us which way is "North". The terror of meaninglessness becomes greater than the imagined fear of falling off the edge of the earth, and so we prefer to believe in familiar myths and methods rather than keep on searching in the darkness.

The radical relationalist is thus attuned to the task of joining with others in painting a more apt picture of the way the world appears. Metaphors in this sense, are invitations to see things in a particular and striking way; they are not candidates for discussion in terms of truth and falsity. We do not believe or disbelieve a metaphor – rather, we find them to be either apt or inapt.

It follows that the traditional view of philosophy – and therapy for that matter – as disciplines which seek to establish truth as a collection of incontestable facts must be abandoned. This requires going beyond language as something that encodes, to language as a field of words which both creates and discovers something more complete about living, and by extension about the therapeutic encounter (Section 6.4). It is a new picture, not a new proposition that reveals things to us in a different light. It is new metaphors, and not new statements, that change convictions about how we think and feel through the process of therapy.

Theoretical constructions which do not consider how therapist and client are embodied, self-involved, and self-contingent are therefore bound to be incomplete. But this need not worry the scientist so long as we understand that science is at home in a different territory; one of calibration, control, and prediction, and not the discovery of "truth" as such. Developments in psychotherapy thus equate to introducing new pictures, which change our perspectives and help us see things in a way we could not have seen them before. For what else is therapy if not another means through which to see, and be guided by a different light?

## 1.2 The Good of Therapy

Although most research indicates that therapy does good – in terms of what a method concludes to be an effective outcome – there have been recurring questions since the 1970s about whether some therapies are better than others. Meta studies – corrected for the bias of practitioner allegiance – tend to find that differences in efficacy are negligible – the so-called Dodo bird conjecture. Yet it would be misleading to suggest that all methods are equivalent. If therapy is powerful enough to do good, then it must have the capacity to do harm also. Furthermore, when a strong focus on symptom reduction forms part of the therapeutic method, then research shows that raised expectations enhance efficacy.

But does focussing on specific symptoms necessarily make for good therapy? If ameliorating symptoms does not enhance the quality of life for a client, their well-being, the effects of their socio-economic standing, interpersonal relationships, or their ability to engage with work and society, then symptom reduction becomes a proxy for meaningful change (Smith, 2020: 64–87).

But why does therapy work? One popular explanation suggests common factors; different methods share "ingredients" common to the experience of almost every therapist who encounters a client and offers them some coherent perspective on a problem, and how it might be resolved (Lambert, 2013). Therapist empathy – or more properly sympathetic care – is correlated with positive outcomes more than any other variable encountered (Section 9.4).

Another ingredient which has attracted a good deal of attention is the therapeutic alliance – the practical details of the goals and tasks agreed to by client and therapist. The better the alliance, the better the outcome. Positivists ponder whether a healthy therapeutic partnership precedes the client feeling better, or conversely, whether feeling better helps the client form a more purposeful alliance. Either way, if we consider client disposition (expectation and hope), the working alliance (faith in the rationale of what is on offer), therapist qualities (sympathetic care) to be the magical ingredients of therapy, then techniques purported to target the underlying causes or maintaining features of psychic unwellness become of secondary importance.

The skills and abilities for facilitating such common factors are hard to acquire and even more difficult to teach. The techniques and tricks for the therapist's "toolbox" on the other hand are easily taught, assessed, and disseminated. In principle, they promote the worthy cause of manufacturing more than enough safe-enough, cheap-enough practitioners who will work long enough to keep the low-cost mental health sector afloat. Yet the relationship between a therapist hungry for more "moves" to add to their repertoire recalls the "step-hungry" amateur attempting to master the tango. Accruing a repertoire of steps does not equate to the artistry of the "walk". Sensual bodies – hands, arms, hips, heads, breath – and not just legs, must engage holistically, if the activity is to transcend its constitutive elements. *The question then is not what is easily achieved, but what is worth achieving.*

There is understandable resistance to acknowledging the importance of common factors. Perhaps because there is little glory derived from demonstrating that a method or technique mastered with much effort and at great expense may be indistinguishable from other methods in its effects? Nevertheless, the consensus seems to be that a socially recognised healer can facilitate a constructive interaction between several common factors, whose therapeutic impact far surpasses the sum of their separate and incidental effects.

While the weighting of common and specific therapeutic factors is controversial, findings suggest that – at least sometimes – it matters not *what* theory-specific rationale is being offered. Rather, the efficacy of therapy is related in part, to how explanations are conveyed, who is doing the explaining, and how the client interprets these explanations. Therapy thus becomes a process of re-moralising people who may feel defeated and abandoned in the face of their problems. When two or more people meet for therapy, and one of those people is especially receptive to what is being communicated, then a trusting bond is generated, hope is instilled – through some systematic, purposeful, reasonable, and intelligible explanation – and expectations for change are raised.

This calls for a fundamental re-conceptualisation of what therapy is, and more importantly what it is not. Rather than an instrument to bring about a specific end – and who can argue against the good of symptom reduction – therapy must be understood as engaging people in practices that enact new meanings through affectively charged experiences. Such affectively enacted alternative meanings may extend to changes in how a client understands what is praiseworthy, good, or worthwhile in terms of living and how to act more holistically. Therapy is thus a deeply ethical practice because we often have a sense of when our actions are good. When we are diverted from what is good, we take other routes – but there is always this draw towards the light (*telos*), however implicit.

The horrors of the twentieth century suggest that there is nothing inherent about such goods: they are not encompassed by our skin. What is "good" does not dwell within but exists in our contexts more broadly. We are continually *oriented* to our environment, which in turn affords and disciplines our experiences. We are not free to create this orientation to the world, but we can within such contexts, constitute, moderate, and ward-off the threats of relativism and self-destructive nihilism.

Orientation shapes our foreknowing. It draws attention to histories, traditions, narratives, temporality, and the embodied nature of experience which in turn shapes observations and exerts implicit influences over those same observations. The outcome of such an awareness is action and thus a further unfolding of events in the world, which in turn presents itself once again for observation. With each passing moment, both ourselves and the world evolve never to be the same again. We might think of this as both orientation-for-action and orientation-in-action where our ongoing reflections and position in relation to what lies beyond ourselves changes and adapts as situations unfurl.

To mistake our deep involvement with the unfolding of events as yet another method is to miss the point of radical relationality. The kind of relationship that helps others prosper is not one of active figure to inert background, but of ecologically constitutive affordances and dynamic interplay: the world is made of things to enjoy, fear, endure, use, and act upon even *before* they are "cognised". Take, for example, a toddler who stumbles and trips while exploring their environment. I could respond – unthinkingly – with alarm. An involuntary shriek, and a concerned dash to their aid. Left to their own devices, the toddler may have righted themselves and continued with their explorations unperturbed.

But having *acted into* the event, I have enlarged, transformed, and reconstituted the stumble into a frightening event for the nascent explorer, who responds initially with surprise before taking the cue to join in with my alarm. The environment of heightened awareness has now been ingrained into the embodied disposition, habits, and skills of the toddler: their *habitus*. Exploration becomes tempered by fear and anxiety when projected from the *habitus*. In a similar way, the anxious trainer, therapist, or supervisor acts into the disposition of their student, client, or supervisee thereby normalising fear of the unintelligible, preferring instead to cling to the reassuring handrails of familiar myths.

What therapy amounts to cannot be defined in terms of what good – or harm – the therapist does for their client; at a profoundly significant level, therapy can be little more than a highly contextual appeal to another to transcend one *habitus* for another. What is good in an absolute sense is unimportant. What matters is not the repair of someone who is broken, but easing movement towards what the client believes to be a better, balanced *habitus* in collaboration with one who is also aware of their orientations, and who cares about what constitutes the good of the client, for the sake of the client alone.

Care of Self and Others. While looking on at the joyful mayhem of a children's birthday party, a friendly stranger will sometimes ask, "so ... what do you do?" "Good question ..." I say, hesitating just long enough for the fellow carer to conclude triumphantly: "Ah ... must be a bit philosophical then?" confusing my distracted dithering for something more profound. In many ways, I would venture, given that we are both here, at the same kind of gathering, caring about the same things, says something deeper about the values, loves, passions, and desires we share.

Striving to be a virtuous parent or carer, a committed partner, a supportive member of our community are things we seem to believe are of value. Although we would not articulate such sentiments in this grandiose manner, we desire to transcend ourselves and the ordinary, transactional, mundane sort of life and do something we consider to be worthwhile, praiseworthy, and for the common good. Attending the party, helping to tidy up, caring for those we do not know; these are some of the easily overlooked moral – and thus philosophical – choices we make all the time.

In our day-to-day lives, we just seem to know what the world needs more of. They are the things that shape our goals and inspire our purpose (*telos*). Whether it is engaging in a vocation, raising children, supporting elderly parents, buying a hungry stranger food, or volunteering as a therapist. Such sympathy or care is usually out of regard *for* something or someone, for *their* own sake because *their* good matters. To not care for these things would be to suggest that "we" do not matter, and in this sense, there is an unconditionality to wanting these things for others.

Things considered virtuous – for the greater good – are not always what makes sense for me to desire for my *own* personal well-being. It would have been easier, and perhaps better for my career, to have kept my head down and my nose clean when at work. But by working as a trade union advocate, using my skills and abilities to support colleagues who had been treated unjustly – for the greater good – meant I undoubtedly scandalised some of the managerial class.

Equally, whatever may advance my own personal good may not necessarily be what I ought to pursue for the greater good. We all experienced this in the context of the COVID-19 pandemic: adhering to national lockdowns, social distancing, mask wearing, vaccination programmes, and for many, enduring the pain of separation from loved ones as they lay dying. These are some instances where we have been called upon to consider the common good, which does not require that we stop caring about our own well-being. My concern for globicide, the flourishing of my children after I am dead, the health of those I do not know, the non-possessive care I offer to supervisees, clients, or students are examples of desirable common goods that extend beyond my first-person perspective.

A long-time neighbour and friend will regularly vacate his home to make way for my wife's parents who visit us from Italy. This is so they may spend time with their daughter and grandchildren, doing the sorts of things that are culturally important such as making ravioli and hosting dinner in a corner of Bristol that becomes little Genova. It is an act of care – my neighbour assures me – not for his or my individual "good," but for the greater good of intercultural, familial, and intergenerational bonding.

What does this have to do with psychotherapy? Having explored the efficacy of therapy – the good it does – I want to turn my attention to what end those goods are. What we call care, sympathy or compassion is the feeling triggered by a specific threat or obstacle to someone's good or well-being. Compassion or care differs from the collection of psychological phenomena called "empathy" which get talked about a lot in psychotherapeutic circles (Section 9.4).

Empathy is about feeling what one *imagines* what the other feels, or perhaps ought to feel, and ironically need not involve compassion. For example, projective empathy without compassion can amount – in the worst case – to the indifference of the sadist. At a more mundane level, projective empathy describes the well-meaning therapist who, seeing themselves as a paragon of self-mastery, believes that they have earned the right to step into the shoes of another. From their own enlightened perspective, they simply know what is best for others in terms of what to feel and what to value. It is the attitude of the coloniser who sees others as underdeveloped in the mastery of both the self and their environment.

Sympathy and empathy are therefore different. A client I empathise with may hate themselves, feel worthless, or worse. But imaginatively accessing their first-person concerns is different from my own feelings of compassion towards them, though of course empathy can give rise to sympathy and vice versa. The primary locus of the concept of a client's wellbeing or good is not their first-person point of view, but the third-person perspective of *one who cares*. It is a perspective I can adopt towards myself no less than I can do so towards others. What it is for something to be good for a client, is for it to be something someone caring about them would have reason to want for them, *for their sake*. It is in this way that the practice of therapy is profoundly ethical (Darwall, 1998).

So, it seems that we have a need for the concept of the common good *because* we are able to stand outside ourselves and ask as one who cares: "what does it make sense to want for others?" Although people may have more reason to care about themselves and those close to them than they do about strangers, neither is possible without the capacity to care for self or others which is implicit in sympathetic concern.

<u>Creative Practice and the Greater Good</u>. Our faith in science – scientism – is so compelling that it gets invoked way beyond the limits of its native territory. We can, for example, make all manner of empirical measurements about the game of soccer (i.e., distance run, percentage possession, passes made), but it does not render the "beautiful game" a science. Psychology too is not wholly competent for the practical extension of its knowledge because all sorts of

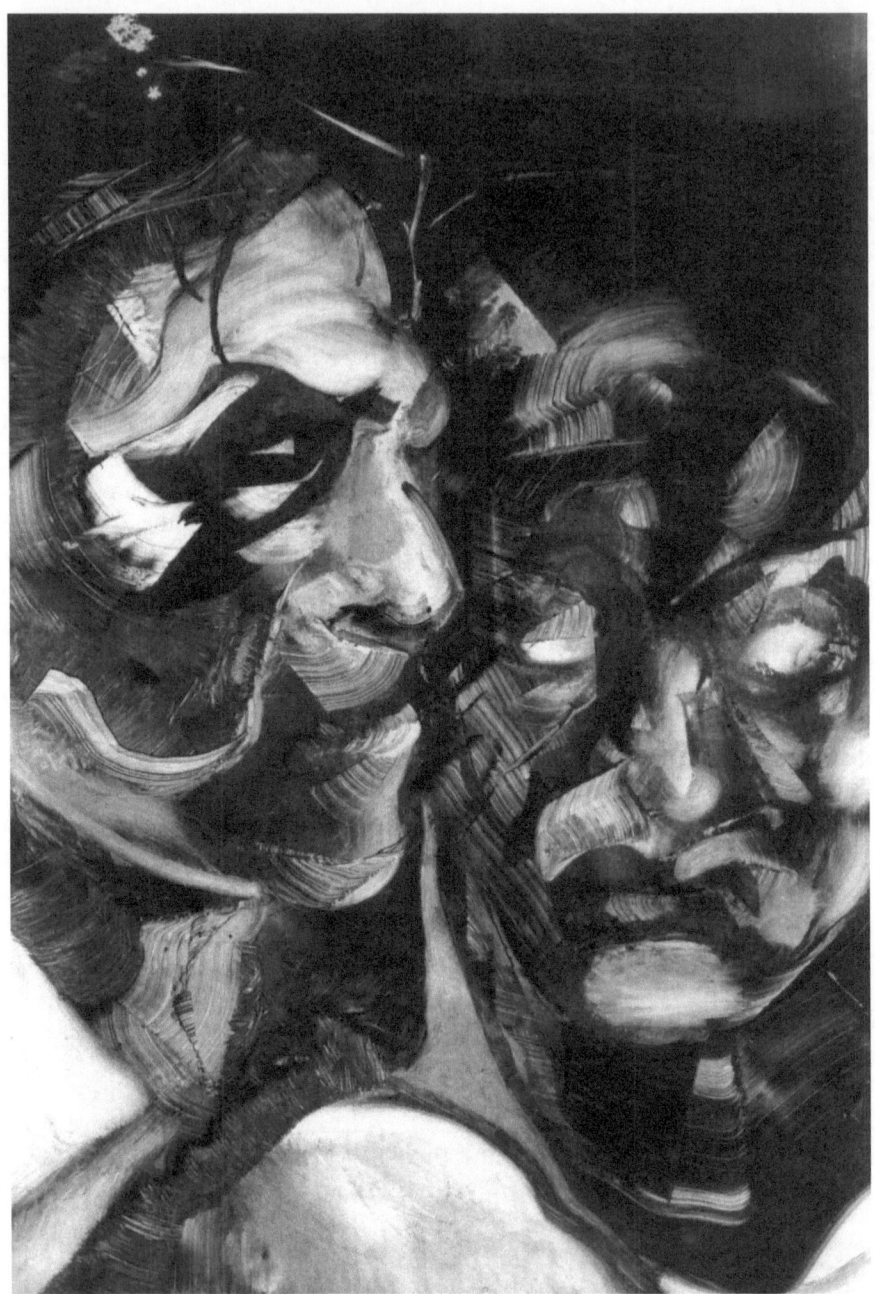

**FIGURE 1.1** One Who Cares.

other considerations, evaluations, customary practices, preferences, and personal interests come into play.

This is particularly so for psychotherapy, and the art of healing more generally, for which there is bewildering scope for interpretation and judgement. But the art of therapy is unlike the art used to create an artefact: it is an art directed to the task of restoring something to vitality. For Gadamer (1996), a modification of what "art" means is necessary before we can extend it to the context of socially endorsed healing such as the practice of therapy.

A therapist cannot stand back from their work in the way that an artisan or fabricator can, in the sense that they might in some way retain the product as their own, even if their work is shared and appreciated by others. The restoration to the client of a better life is a product that does not belong to the therapist. The relationship between the doing and the deed, the making and the made, the effort and the success is fundamentally different, more enigmatic, and elusive in nature.

The art of therapy is further distinguished from the practice of an artisan by the fact that it is not just preoccupied with restoring a living system to some natural state of equilibrium – such as in the case of a garden, a river, or its wider ecosystem; it involves people (clients) who, generally speaking, expect to be healed. But unlike an ecologist who can restore the health of a polluted river, the corresponding objective for a therapist is not "made" or definable within their art. For psychic unwellness is a *social state of affairs*; it amounts to more than facts determinable by the measurement of pH, or microbes typical to the work of the ecologist.

Take for example how left-leaning liberal middle-class therapists easily align with popular humanistic therapeutic traditions that similarly celebrate the socio-economically linked privileges of choice, individualism, and self-reliance. The implications of this ideological alignment are twofold: it unwittingly orients therapy alongside the same sort of anxious, energetic striving for self-mastery that feeds into the neoliberal distortions of our society, while at the same time suggesting to those who have not prospered, that they only have themselves to blame.

Such alignments risk rendering clients (and therapists) apolitical in a way that ignores their socio-political context. Humanistic therapies are not alone in this regard. The "inner child" of the psychodynamic approach requires a return to childhood, casting our gaze backwards rather than looking around in the here and now. This gaze backwards to the Jungian child archetype is a vision of oneself as *apolitical.* Under conditions of rampant inequality and stalled social mobility, implying that we are responsible for our fate yet deserving of what we get erodes communality, and demoralises those who feel left behind.

Raising awareness of social class thus becomes conflated with the discomfort of class prejudice; "blindness" to class is assumed to be necessary for the effective "work" of therapy to take place. Humanistic methods thus run the risk of seeing themselves as transcending the relationship between socio-political contexts and mental health, because therapists use individual explanations to address structural problems (McEvoy et al., 2021).

Without defending the class-bound order of the past, at least its manifest moral arbitrariness and unfairness tempered the self-regard of those at the top of the pile and prevented the working class from seeing its subordinate status as reflecting some sort of personal or moral failure. Knowing the system was rigged empowered the working class to challenge the status quo, which was the original purpose of the UK Labour Party.

What we now have is the emergence of centre left elites – such as life coaches and therapists – who have abandoned old class identities in search of new moralising frameworks to help those who feel left behind shape up to a world in which they are on their own. Unlike therapists who often talk of doing "the work", old class distinctions at least dignified the non-credentialed work of fixing cars, sweeping streets, digging holes and stacking shelves.

There is a long tradition – reaching back to Aristotle – which teaches us that a fundamental human need is to be needed by those with whom we share a common life. This seems to be something of which we need reminding as our preference for abstracting a client's mental health from their context seems deeply ingrained. When referring to my book *Workplace Wellbeing*, trainee therapists occasionally remark: "yeah … but it's not *real* mental health" (Costello, 2020). Irrespective of its playfulness, such comments disclose a fondness for punctuating people from their world, presumably so that they may be more readily objectified for theoretical inspection. It is an attitude which is blind to the idea that the value of our social contribution – the dignity of labour – is deeply entwined with achieving fulfilment as a human being. Indeed, in a sense we become more of a "human being" when we can contribute to the common good of our communities.

The income protection and job retention schemes extended by the EU27 and UK nations during the COVID-19 pandemic affirmed the dignity of work for over 30 million people at the peak of the crisis. It was a political move which reminded us – alas we need reminding – that we are not self-made and self-sufficient. There is something which transcends the harsh ethic of individuality which seeks to push us apart. If our talents are gifts for which we are indebted – to my knowledge nobody gets to choose their parents, their genes, or the time and place into which they are born – then it is a mistake and a conceit to presume we deserve the benefits that flow from them. The meritocratic emphasis on effort and hard work seeks to claim that, under the right conditions, we are responsible for our success and capable of freedom. But whatever principles we adopt about what constitutes the good life, the arbitrariness and unpredictability of moral luck can easily cut through them.

Accumulating money measures neither merit nor the value of our contribution to the common good. At best, it indexes some capacity – through a mixture of timing or talent, luck or pluck or grim determination – to cater to the confusion of wants and desires, however frivolous, that constitutes consumer demand at any given moment. At a time when young people are submitted to relentless sorting, sifting, and ranking by schools, universities, and the workplace, neoliberal meritocracy at the heart of modern life imposes an almost irresistible imperative to strive, perform, and achieve.

Merit measured in this way ignores the moral arbitrariness of talents and inflates the significance of psychological self-mastery. Unkind to the losers and oppressive to the winners, merit becomes a tyrant (Sandel, 2021). It is no measure of well-being to be well adjusted to a society which has lost its sense of the common good.

One could say that therapists "produce" good outcomes by means of their art, but this is not a precise way to speak either because it positions the client as a consumer of "wisdom". What is produced is not the work of a craftsperson, where something novel comes into being which confirms their skill. Rather, it involves restoring a distressed person to a place of balance, and whether this is the result of theoretical knowledge or plain luck cannot be known from the restored state of balance itself. The healthy individual is not simply someone who has been "made" healthy. So, it must always remain an open question just how much the successful restoration of balance is owed to the therapist, and how much is owed to the context of the client.

While therapy needs to have its plausible myths, prescribed rituals, or theoretical compass to "steer by," there is little evidence to suggest that they need to be empirically founded. In addition, the client may hold their own rival intuitive knowledge, such as faith in the case of the religious believer, which has something to say – should they care to listen – to the therapist.

Then there is the lyrical knowledge of the poet, which can outdistance that of the psychologist, sociologist, historian, or philosopher. In short, however incomplete, or vague, there are myriad alternative sources of knowledge which contribute to the therapeutic encounter, either explicitly or more commonly, implicitly. It is impossible to eliminate such rival knowledge from the practice of therapy and the radically relational therapist not only understands this but welcomes it.

But on what basis does the therapist admit these ideas? As I argue later, so long as both therapist and client find such knowledge to be believable, then it cannot be arbitrary as it is already established in culture and tradition thus explaining its salience and appeal. The relational therapist is already oriented and aware of these various ideologies, their calls to belief, and ethical goods which make claim and counterclaim to what makes life better.

The bygone days of the family doctor who was a friend of the family indicates aspects of healing of which we are painfully deprived. Trust and cooperation are essential therapeutic factors which belong to a wholly different dimension than that of a technical intervention. Therapy may not constitute a placebo per se, but its efficacious factors are so widespread that it is difficult to demonstrate that there is any beneficent medical or pharmacological intervention devoid of its effects. Contrary to common lore, intuition, and scientific belief, openly administered placebos work as well as a deceptively deployed placebo (Leder, 2021).

To be open about psychotherapy's broad range of beneficial therapeutic factors – especially when defined in the context of radical relationality – would not only be well-founded, but also easy to communicate, as ideas such as openness, expectancy, hope, alliance, and the pursuit of meaning are approachable concepts which do not require the well-meaning pulpit bullying of the credentialed middle classes. What is unethical is to assert that a given theory-specific therapy, with its methods and techniques, is the only way to achieve a therapeutic effect.

When placebo becomes re-defined as something implicit to the relational encounter rather than incidental to the theory-specific method, then therapy becomes a radically ethical enterprise. Understanding placebo in this way takes the path of Husserl who sought to explore experience in its purest form, unsullied by the distortions of assumptions and prejudices (Section 9.2). To avoid the suggestion that therapy is simply placebo – which maintains an enigmatic if not unintentionally deceptive stance towards its characteristic and incidental components – it would be wise instead to be transparent: because there may be little to lose and much to gain (Section 2.3).

## 1.3  Self *as* Orientation

Virtually all approaches to therapy acknowledge the importance of the "relationship" to some degree. "Relational therapy" itself emphasises the importance of what goes on between the client and (neutral) therapist but fails to see the "relationship" as anything more than an inert medium through which the data of psychotherapy is transmitted, that is, the facts of a client's childhood, symptoms, unconscious beliefs, projections, introjects, behaviours, or feelings. Relationship in this sense is akin to the luminiferous or light-carrying *æther* hypothesised in the seventeenth century to account for the transmission of electromagnetic waves through a vacuum. The *æther* on this account was a magical medium in which we swim, conveying sensations between one part and another.

The term "intersubjectivity" gets deployed as an upgrade to *æthereal* understandings of relational, since a therapist's countertransference cannot be denied; we are not so neutral after all. But perhaps its use in this sense indicates some recognition that the term "relational" has become somewhat hackneyed and overused to the point of losing its power; a presumed *æthereal*, inert sort of relationality persists.

Certainly, psychologists have done their best to understand and conceptualise relationships, at least from a Eurocentric and modernist perspective. Here, the Self – which prefigures relationships – is a human agent reduced to an independent, self-reliant monad whose goals, desires, and wishes take precedence over those of the family, groups, culture, and communities to which they belong. This punctuated modern Self – often the object of humanistic therapies – is not to be constrained by external moral systems based on traditions or religion because the sources of morality are indwelling.

The existential power behind the punctual Self is the undeniable sense of dignity which goes along with our heroic capacity to confront a cold and indifferent universe with self-responsible reason; the dignity of human rationality becomes its own moral source. The punctual Self lends plausibility to modern pictures of flourishing, seeing self-mastery as the core competence at the heart of the project of personal re-engineering.

Relationships – including those with a therapist – are important to the punctuated Self, so long as they contribute to and do not interfere with a person's goals and their liberty to achieve those goals. The influence of such a worldview is evident in the methods employed by contemporary therapeutic methods. The pioneers of psychotherapy saw humans foremost as punctuated entities, who then engaged with others and their contexts. Freud viewed himself as the model, walled-off punctuated self, insulated from non-rational intrusions, thus establishing the reassuring foundation for his scientific objectivity.

Relationship as luminiferous *æther* seduces us into believing that we do what we do because of our self-contained histories, blocks to our indwelling emotions, brain-based cognitive predispositions, or deterministic biological programming. In a sense, relationships become something understood non-relationally, by what is translated into the relationship or incorporated within the individual. The punctuated Self is simply assumed in humanistic therapy, where the therapist's role is to facilitate its emancipation from the values and expectations of others, and to clear the ground for the self-actualising, indwelling spirit to flourish. Such an *æthereal* relationality acknowledges the ubiquity and importance of relationships, yet paradoxically, it also assumes that relationships – whether with humans or non-humans – ultimately emerge from within.

The punctuated Self is located within my skin. I go inside myself to locate the Self, to examine my feelings, thoughts, and dreams. They are mine. They belong to me. By punctuating myself from the world in this way, and denying that I am of the world, we deprive psychotherapy of its radical potential for transformation. Because it is not I who am unwell. It is my environment that is unwell – the rivers, air, oceans, and political systems. By punctuating the Self from the world, therapy abets the decline of the world.

Radical relationality instead proposes that the most fundamental reality concerns the relational. Things, events, time, places, language, and bodies are not self-contained entities which prefigure being in the world, only later coming into contact with other things, places, temporalities, bodies, and languages. All entities, events, temporalities, and places are primarily relational – they prefigure, are already and have always been related to one another.

Perhaps the reason for the persistent emphasis on *ethereal* relationality is that it lacks a radicalising framework to espouse this insight. It is not unusual to encounter therapists who already have an implicit understanding that we are bodies localised, temporalised, and dignified as the means through which we communicate, create meaning, and exercise power. However, like the monolinguist, it is not so easy to articulate and explicate the grammatical rules in which we are immersed. A practical mastery of our methods in no way entails the possession of a clear, explicit understanding of the philosophical principles which shape them.

Yet physics embraced radical relationality over a century ago in its understanding that the observer and the observer, participant and audience, seer and seen, interpreter and interpreted cannot be accurately differentiated. As I argue later, this can be radicalised further; all entities have a shared being and are mutually constitutive of one another.

Radical relationality sees it that there can be no understanding beyond context. I am to be understood only in terms of my culture, history, embodiment and even my awareness. The Self is not an abstraction, but as Jung would have it, is a *process* of becoming aware of the heterogeneous sources of one's own collective patterns of instinctual behaviour, projections, and re-presentations. What is unique to our radically relational Selves is the liminality of our embodied experience and form-giving sense-making that is at the heart of the therapeutic encounter. Exposing the palms of my hands, for example, can signal a warm greeting, the act of surrender, or an appeal to be believed, depending on how the gesture is related to its context.

Resistance is encountered – particularly in the context of training – because we are taught that the essence of good therapy requires the application of easily digestible theories or techniques, which in their turn lean heavily on the idea of an abstracted Self. The relationalist should welcome being seen as "eccentric" in this regard, because to understand the Self as a matter of evolving orientation is not "normal". The dissatisfaction we feel with orienting the abstracted Self into the crosshairs of just one theory leads to the habit of integration, or worse, technical eclecticism. Radical relationality, however, inverts this modernistic perspective and invites us to retrieve what we have forgotten; that good practice – like the Self – cannot be abstracted or separated from the world.

Disciplines of the Self. What are the things, inputs, cares, concerns, and experiences that *discipline* the Self? To be oriented in this sense does not mean to be blindly conformist to a model or theory but to make some systematic and conscious commitment to widening our horizons. There can be no exhaustive list, but the beguiling influences I have in mind include: what we understand about the past as best as we can discern it; traditions, inherited lore, ancestral wisdom – including religious traditions – the zeitgeist and ambient convictions of our cultural context; the received opinions from our dealings with the everyday world; the purported facts of the "science of the day", and what passes for common belief and common knowledge about what it means to be human since time immemorial (i.e., Althusser – Section 6.2). To the extent that there can be things that *discipline* the Self, we ought to declare a commitment to the most compelling of these, namely: what we notice about the world as it presents itself for introspection.

On a clear day, I am struck by how the sun appears to move across the sky – rising in the East, passing overhead, and setting in the West, before it magically hurries back to where it rises again: it is typical of the experiences which *pre*sent themselves to me (*phainomenon*). I do not even notice that my experience is *intended* towards the object, the sun. It is because the experience is holistic, and enfolded in the context of a life lived, of memories, and immediate cares and concerns, that is, it is getting late, where has the day gone, time to eat, or sleep. If I take the time for introspection, accessing my imagination and visualising planets spinning in the solar system, the experience is *re*-presented. I can accept that it is not the object of my intention which is moving, but it is I who am moving relative to the sun.

Similarly, when I meet you – the client – I do not do so from the perspective of theoretical detachment, that is, a *re*-presented collection of objective entities, symptoms, and properties detached from my own concerns. You *pre*sent to me "in the flesh" so to speak, through a different way; I appreciate you bodily, and so in the case of people at least, the analytical standpoint is not the way I have direct access to the world. People are not primarily "knowers," but rather "doers". We are chiefly pragmatic beings, seeking goals according to our cares or desires, and only secondarily are we knowers in this theoretical, abstracted sense.

Theorising is far from irrelevant, but it is not primal; experience is more real and fundamental. Philosophers and (psychotherapists) – who largely know what they know of science from what non-scientists tell them – tend to dismiss "normal" science as mere puzzling-out and abstraction. True, this is often how science tends to present itself, and theorising is a reassuring endeavour; yet when detached from context – which includes the knower – our perspective is flattened. There is no experience that we can – with absolute certainty – consider to be totally in our awareness; that would necessitate an unimaginable totality, which in turn presupposes an equally unimaginable wholeness and perfection of the human mind. *Orientation is thus relative*, something understood by Rogers in his concept of congruence and incongruence. It is as real for the scientist as it is for the psychotherapist.

A few years back while tinkering in the laboratory, I stumbled across a potentially useful but puzzling chemical reaction. I asked one of my students to investigate how it worked. But as time wore on, the student grew exasperated because they could not repeat the original experiment. What were we missing? We had become lost in theoretical introspection, focussing on aspects of the phenomenon abstracted from its context.

Was the reaction medium contaminated? Had we inadvertently poisoned the catalyst? The passing of the seasons, for example, is irrelevant to a phenomenon unmoored from its context through theoretical abstraction. Yet the practitioner *doing* the theorising experiences the seasons as the ground against which the phenomenon presents itself. A change of orientation, seeing the error of assuming Nature as immobile ground, admitted the significance of a process that was rapid in a laboratory bleached by summer sunshine and sluggish in the autumnal gloom. Shining a desk-light onto the reaction flask quickly confirmed that the process was catalysed by bright light (Costello et al., 2002).

The experience taught me something more general about the accident of "discovery" and the oft-neglected importance of our orientation towards the world. Popular theories of reflective practice tend to be linear, sequential, and focused on the "I" rather than the "we" or relational field. Firstly, *something happens→ I reflect→ form an abstract concept→ experiment with the concept.* Learning is understood as something separable from its context, which is otherwise considered static; it is the observing, abstracted Self who changes in response to a pre-existing world, which sits and waits for me to get back to it. But by this stage, the "caravan has already moved on" as the saying goes, and the learning is about a world that is no longer there. Such models typically fail to capture the importance of orientation, and the ability – or otherwise – of a person to actively shape the world they inhabit.

The implicit pre-determination which comes with abstract theorising pares my involvement with the world, distracting me from the passing of the seasons for example. It is the surprise of becoming aware of *myself* as inserted in the world that we often mistake for the surprise of discovering something novel "out there". Yet cycles, spirals, or snail shells are inapt metaphors for the process because they imply learning as punctuated and separable from embodied space and time. Part of the problem is that such models draw too heavily on how the world *was* – our past experiences – and do not consider how events are encountered and perceived in the first instance. To do so, I must bring into awareness the looping of my orientation with my experience, and almost simultaneously, the looping of my experience with my orientation.

The intuition that it is the role of philosophy to uncover something that is already understood aligns with how many therapists approach their task. Phenomenologists strive for an understanding of what the world means prior to introspection. The distinction between primary and secondary inquiry seems relevant here because we must understand ourselves in the world prior to allowing our gaze to pass to objects of interest. What sets the phenomenological therapist apart from the empirical therapist is that the former is essentially – indeed must be – a transcendental inquirer into the conditions of interpretation.

Despite its notorious antecedence, John Boyd's OODA (i.e., Observe, Orient, Decide, Act) loops cleave from traditional learning models. Implicit to the attitude it fosters is a recognition that we must accept the contingency of awareness: change is fundamental to all that is in and of the world. In short, by acting we create the conditions for further action. This is something that existing theories of reflective practice do not always consider. The puzzles to be solved then are not of the abstract sort – this is the easy stuff that whiles away so much therapy and supervision.

The puzzles to be addressed are, in fact, those which entangle the sensible with the rational: Can we describe the world as it presents itself to awareness? How do we take what is presented, and re-present it through introspection? The re-presentation of experience extends to feelings of sadness, joy, love, connection, euphoria, excitement, anxiety, shame, fear, and pain. This is why therapy is so powerful because our thinking, imagining, dreaming, fantasising, reminiscing about the past, expectations about the future, hope, and, of course, experience can be re-examined. But so too can our immediate responses to the world as it appears in the living present.

It explains how as a therapist I may glide between participant and observer of the world. For example, while reflecting on what you are saying, a stifled yawn momentarily distracts me from what I am thinking about. I focus for a moment on the sensation but return to you. My apprehension of the sensation is not erased; I am still conscious of the stifled yawn but in a modified way. I apprehend my prereflective awareness – I can search for reasons while still engaging. Presentation and representation are not dual, serial attitudes or dispositions but a liminal uncoupling (*unzuhandenheit*) from involvement (*zuhandenheit*) in the world and a reflective step back, bringing forth its object presence (*vorhandenheit*).

Therapy therefore cannot accomplish much if its methods are subject to just one sort of *discipline*: purely phenomenological or analytical. So, why not abandon thinking and experience and rely instead on doing some *proper* scientific research? Those who rely on systematic empirical research to understand therapy may believe that the point is to subtract effects of bias, prejudice, and preconception – as if it were possible or desirable. However, every empirical exercise involves in some way, calibration – for what other function does the metre, second, or gram perform? It is difficult to see how perception or intuition could be calibrated without the calibration also relying in some way on perception and intuition. Perception and intuition cannot be seen as new tools for discovery, or bolt-on sensors (*zuhandenheit*) to our reasoning faculties (*vorhandenheit*); they are the foundations of insight into abstract and conceptual matters.

*In conclusion*, purism, or the idea that psychotherapy could possibly be disciplined by one tradition, be that tradition analytical reasoning or phenomenological descriptions or whatever, misunderstands the liminal Self of radical relationality (Overgaard et al., 2022). It indicates an unending dynamic process of an unfolding orientation to our co-created, disciplining contexts, which is I where I turn next.

## 1.4   The Characteristics of Radical Relationality

Jung's borrowing of the uroboros metaphor hints at what he saw as the affinity between our organising archetypes and embodied instincts, facets both resolved and nourished in a wholeness understood as the Self. It is within the Self that embodied instincts and the form-giving qualities of the archetypes merge into one (1960: 213). I argue throughout that the Self of radical relationality *is* orientation – the situational awareness that infers how we interact with the world, shaping what we observe, how we decide, and how we act. The factors which discipline are simultaneously constraints and resources for our actions. They are the all-encompassing conditions and social facts that cannot be escaped yet, at second glance, they only exist and are maintained through the everyday actions of the Self. The practical implications of radical relationality are outlined throughout what follows (Slife & Wiggins, 2009).

Let me transpose the metaphor of the uroboros to the structure of the book and its various chapters. While acknowledging the consequences of dissection, segmenting the whole into its eight constitutive parts places at the head of the serpent the greatest good of the Hellenic tradition, which is *reason* (Chapter 2). Reason is the powerful maw that simultaneously consumes and is nourished by its tail (Chapters 9, 8, and 7) – which is where I emphasise the unfolding of experience through time. What lies between the head and tail of the uroboros are the segments which discipline radical relationality. The encounter of Hellenic reason with belief (Chapter 3) helps overcome the dogma of humanism (Chapter 4). In this way, a certain transcendence is achieved beyond the self-involved ethical relativism of humanistic, psychodynamic, and behavioural modalities (Chapter 5) towards some higher meaning (Chapter 6). Having dissembled the uroboros into its various segments, I want to expand in a little more detail what the reader can expect to encounter as they progress from the head, along the vertebrae, towards the tail of the serpent.

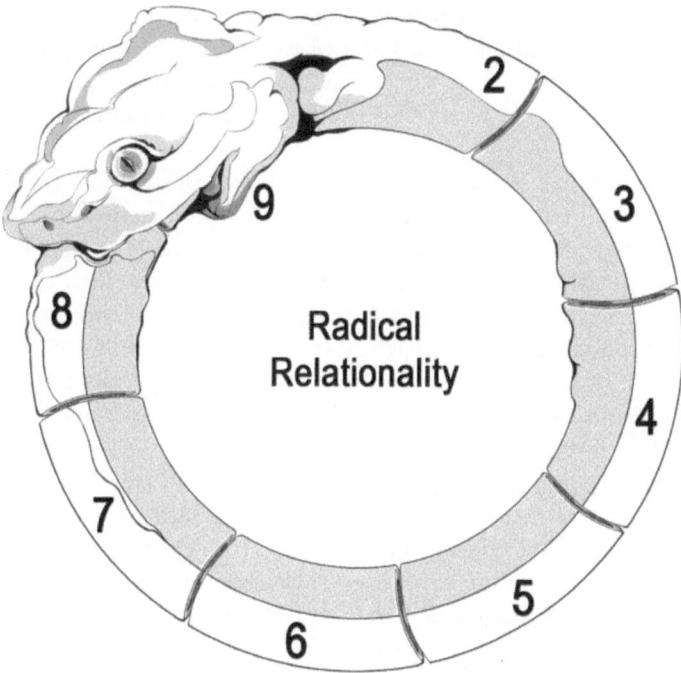

Radical
Relationality

**FIGURE 1.2**    Segments of the Uroboros.

<u>2. A Good Life</u>. Philosophers of antiquity brought to our attention the notion of practical wisdom – *phronesis* – which seeks to integrate our goals and desires into a balanced whole. A life in good order was one connected to something higher and more praiseworthy, the common good; but the highest of all goods was the capacity to be *rational*. For Socrates, a higher, more truthful Self was to be found through dialogue, a process which heightens our responsiveness to the world as it is presented. The common good was something essential to and only possible because of community, something shared by those who *belong*. Those who belong are able to transcend their existential sense of isolation. The relationist contends that infrequent users of therapy tend to be those who possess a sense of *belonging*, for they are already cherished, and loving members of their communities.

Radical relationality understands how relationships are the basis for understanding ourselves and the world more generally. This flies in the face of a key humanistic assumption, which is that what helps holistically may not be the thing we most desire at an individual level. We all need to "belong" to something greater than ourselves, and this is not always easy. This is because relationships that are truthful and virtuous may not always be pleasurable. In the context of the therapeutic relationship, this means that therapist and client alike explore what it means to relate effectively, and in so doing retrieve something of what transcends a sense of isolation. The therapist must strive beyond simply serving a client's satisfactions, reassuring them that all their feelings must be "right," to serving the greater good of engaging in virtuous relationships.

Modern cognitive therapies (cognitive behavioural therapy [CBT] and rational emotive behaviour therapy [REBT]) – which suggest one can reason with our feelings – have their roots in the philosophical schools of Zeno, Plato, Aristotle, and Epicurus, which all came after Socrates. Therapists can and should support their clients figure out how their values, choices, words, and general demeanour impact themselves and their relationships with others. Yet what must be overcome before we can express the profoundly ethical nature of relationality is the significant barrier posed by our commonplace individualism, and our modern rejection of social transcendence.

3. Reason and Belief. Transcendence is something of a blind spot for the humanistic therapist because minds have long been tilted towards a mythical clash between Judeo-Christian theology and rationalism. The picture painted is not so much one of a commingling of streams, or aspects of being me, but the collision of insoluble glaciers, an opposition symbolised by the reason of Athens on the one hand, and the revelation of Jerusalem.

What is remarkable about the persistence of this myth is not that it amounts to a serious critique of theology, or religion for that matter, but that it promotes the view that we should replace religious belief with scientism. I am not referring here to the methods of empirical science, but a belief that the methods of science are sufficient to uncover the truth of the existential matters that lie before us. Radical relationality requires that we go beyond ourselves, because a coherent moral framework requires a single, perfect transcendent non-representable and necessarily real object to be the focus of our attention.

The Cartesian notion of an inward, self-sufficient intellect ultimately paved the way to our attempted mastery of the environment and an enchantment with chemical cures for a troubled mind. Emotions became something which lie within rather than something largely social. But the cures to be worked on lie beyond my own cure. I suggest here a scientifically open-ended emergentism which decentres humanity from the cosmos, while avoiding a direct appeal to a deity. It allows for a sort of ineffable, scientific piety of transcendence, which sits well with radical relationality. My concluding remarks in this chapter are not about God, or faith per se, but the dogmatic commitment to a belief that we humans are the absolute centre of the universe.

4. Individualism: The Atomised Self. Perhaps the greatest concern for those wary of humanism is the notion of a self-determining monad in whom resides the centre of morality – an ethic resting on an indwelling human sentiment or spirit, especially central to the theorising of humanistic therapies. It is the antithesis of radical relationality as it risks reducing humanity to an abstracted

ideal, which the self *possesses* rather than *performs*. The reason for such irreducibility is the understanding that context – including the individuals who mutually constitute their contexts – are dynamic rather than static. Because context is forever in flux, the relationist holds that all conceptualisations of a client are tentative, and we must be alert to any illusion of stasis.

Consider for example, the client who felt powerless, stuck, and unable to "move on" from a recent loss. In therapy, they would truncate their emotional range through over-correction. Whenever they explored being joyous, angry, sad, or despairing about the circumstances of their life, they would equivocate about whether such feelings mattered, or were even *real*. Their self-conceptualisation was one of being reasonable, balanced, and fair about all things – maintaining a stable centre was essential to them (i.e., homeostasis).

The therapist too became seduced by the reasonableness of their approach, dampening and supressing their own emotional dial to within a narrower, more acceptable range to align with the client. The supportive, tolerant understanding of the therapeutic relationship transformed into a counterphobic defence towards the fears, longings, and wounds attached to life's chaos and extreme emotions. This is therapy as sedation, a place to be calmed, relaxed, and subdued – it benumbed client and therapist alike. It became a safe middle ground to ruminate – at a distance – on the actual object of fear; it was in the truest sense of the term, a *mediocre* relationship.

Listening to recordings in supervision, the therapist noticed how their client would declare "off limits" parts of their emotional territory, penning-back and limiting where the therapist could go. Therapy – like life more generally for the client – became intractable, and it was only when this realisation was brought back to them that their self-imposed label of being "stuck" seemed somehow unconvincing, if not misleading, because it obscured the client's agency in uninvolving themselves, through a form of emotional quarantine.

The therapist was able to explore with the client the many times and contexts they experienced this compulsion to "lock-down" or deny experience. In this way, both therapist and client became ready for – and even anticipated – their assumptions and conceptualisations being disrupted. By rigidly adhering to abstractions (i.e., the "resistant/defensive client"), which can imply diagnoses, techniques, or therapeutic principles, we run the risk of becoming disengaged from the particulars of our relationships, because we relate to the abstractions rather than the person.

Because of the catastrophic ecological implications of human chauvinism, I also consider its alternatives, namely antihumanism and more importantly for radical relationality, nonhumanism. We have long understood that our impingement on the habits of our fellow creatures would eventually unleash global calamity. If we continue to ignore the impact of global inequality – exacerbated by late-stage capitalism and the deformations of ideological neoliberalism – then we will be left poorly equipped to serve a sustainable and fulfilled common humanity.

5. Freedom: Ethics and Existentialism. The dread that we do not belong, are not acceptable, or do not possess meaningful relationships, is the most significant of all our fears and anxieties. It flies in the face of numerous existential and psychodynamic thinkers who take death to be our greatest terror. Contemporary therapeutic models with their liberal humanist discourses, thus seem to be inapt modern solutions to age-old problems. Yet more liberation, autonomy, and empowerment are offered to those of us who already feel dissatisfied and ashamed about assuming we are responsible for our sense of disconnection. What is needed by those who yearn for radical relationality is substantial human contact, a broader sense of purpose, greater simplicity, and perhaps a credible transcendence.

To move in this direction, therapy needs to abandon its claim to ethical neutrality or value-free scientism, because the truth of the matter is that all theorising, and every expression of belief is a political and moral action. I argue that moral beliefs are intelligible and justifiable only when seen in their relational, cultural, and historical context. Relativism and radical choice are something of an illusion because we already know what to do, or what not to do. Choices are not groundless and absurd; criterionless choices are a delusion when we understand ourselves as radically related to the whole, as opposed to being self-generated atoms.

Values in therapy are inescapable and radical relationality emphasises this. Yet, the idea that a therapist can – or should – try to be unbiased or morally neutral is a dangerous yet persistent myth. Radical relationality is aware of the reality of values, interpretations, interventions, and interactions for the client. They are often unseen yet importantly they are also deeply ingrained in the choices that gatekeepers make towards those admitted to the profession. Without articulating our values, ethical visions, and therapeutic goals, we are likely to be implicitly guided by background relationships with childhood caregivers, social conditioning, or by a rebellion against other ethical or cultural sources. The goal of radical relationality is for therapeutic practitioners to be as deeply informed as possible about their disciplining factors.

The relationalist understands that ethics are a real aspect of our lives and not merely red flags signalled by codes of conduct. They reflect the way we are involved not only in articulating but also defending or rejecting ideas about how to live well. Ethical agency entails evaluating strong human desires, goals, and ways of life. Radical relationists understand that conflict, far from being something to be avoided, is a sign of two or more ethical viewpoints vying for traction. Rather than truncating or neutralising this energy, radical relationality embraces it and encourages clients to engage in the process of fostering alternative ethical visions. Overlooking or avoiding conflict is the more superficial pattern of relationality where we truncate ethical discussions and hide from the business of negotiating good ways to live. The goal of the relationalist is to support clients experience productive conflict that leads to greater intimacy, despite the seeming messiness of such interactions. Conflict – not to be confused with hostility – is not the failure of a relationship, but a sign of ethical evolution.

6. Meaning: A Reassuring Foundation. Context is infinitely rich with detail, and this extends to structuralist abstractions, diagnoses, and formulations which are necessary and useful for reflecting on and interpreting aspects of context. Abstractions help therapists interpret the context of a client, and they create a frame of reference when immersed in the sometimes disorientating field of a clients' life. To avoid transferring the particularity of context to the generalities of abstraction, relationists are vigilant about ensuring that abstractions *emerge* from how a client presents. Relationalists are cautious about imposing favoured or even implicit values and ideologies on their client. Indeed, ruptures between various therapeutic ideologies and the particulars of a client's life are to be expected if not invited.

The point here is that favouring abstractions over particulars can obscure relevant context, especially when the context is at variance with abstracted, "taken-for-granted" ideologies. The highly contextual nature of a radically relational approach makes it an unlikely candidate for manualisation or standardisation by most research paradigms *because* it eschews structuralist assumptions of a reassuring theoretical foundation. It explains why you will encounter few, if any, "how to" case studies or "I said – they said" accounts of therapist–client encounters here. The knowledge to which I allude is that generated *through* relationships – which for the therapist includes one-to-one/group supervision, professional development groups, and, of course, radically relational therapy itself. It assumes a plurality of ideologies, theoretical interpellations, or Subjects about which we can make discerning judgements – through the therapeutic field of words – leading to growth and more apt metaphors for meaning-making. But radical relationality understands that this does not signal entry to a world of moral relativity.

To this end, we consider the linguistic domain of existence, which draws our attention to how language – in its broadest sense – can place limits on the positions we can adopt, on what can be said, on what can be felt, and on what can be thought. For the relationalist, therapy is the process of articulating something liberating, which is just out of reach. Having alighted on the right word, myth, or metaphor, we simultaneously enframe and create a feeling or sensation, which we somehow know to be more or less, right.

7. Stories: Fragmented Selves. This section considers the influence of postmodernism, and the importance of therapy for telling our stories. Stories are not fabrications, but they do constitute the fabric of relationships which entangle what is real and what it is to be a person through our traditions, communities, and cultures. The narrative turn in therapy – which emerged

from Freud's momentous splitting of the unitary self – is more than a tool in this regard. It forces a re-evaluation of the unquestioned or unquestionable truths of traditional psychological discourses – yet unlike the narrative turn, radical relationality rejects relativism.

Nevertheless, the narrative turn is radically relational in that it constitutes a post-humanistic attitude which acknowledges the interlocking nature of philosophy, ethics, the material, with practices that transcend objectifying methods. It is an attitude to living, a political project, and an alternative to prevailing, pragmatic, empiricist, instrumental approaches to therapy. This shift to a dynamic narrative story line is not limited to one person's self-narrative but refers also to the relationships of these narratives and the meaning that they bring to others, and the communities from which they arise.

Relationships are not solely based on the things we have in common; difference or "otherness" is vital to being known to ourselves and to others. Clients often believe that they need to conform and be "normal" if they want to be accepted. It is an attitude which can find its way into therapy when client's "go along with" or collude with the therapist in being a "good" client. The relationalist sees how this can amplify the unhelpful belief that inauthenticity and manufactured sameness are the paths to deeper intimacy and community.

The assumption that similarity fosters a more natural, therapeutically effective relationship weaves its way into the practice of therapist–client matching. This is when clients are partnered with therapists based on the perceived similarity of their values, beliefs, social class, age, culture, sexuality, race, gender, faith, or other characteristics. But radical relationists consider difference to be vital. Difference is not a failure, but a starting point for understanding – the other word that compassion goes by – *through* the constitutive use of language.

Our identity depends on Otherness and difference. When it is presumed that a relationship is ontologically given – as in the *æthereal* attitude – and does not require care and attention to create something unique, then differences are not opportunities and similarities are not necessarily pathways for growth. This is of vital importance for genuine anti-oppressive, anti-racist, feminist, and decolonising practices.

8. Time. The foremost of human concerns is time, yet we rarely see it as more than an empty box to fill. People experiencing depression say they feel "left behind" in their social relationships, implying that time speeds ahead without them. Complex grieving is also implicated in the sense that we are not "keeping up" with how we ought to adjust to life's sometimes unavoidable losses. Again, we fall behind time. When it seems too scary to abandon familiar patterns because we fear being overwhelmed by loss, it can seem safer to stay frozen in the past. When in shock, time seems to stand still, and we experience a decoupling from the living present. The therapeutic encounter then must be understood at "depth", which means going beyond our two-dimensional relationship with interpersonal, situational, linguistic, cultural, and ethical contexts; it means addressing our involvement with time itself.

The relational therapist seeks to understand their clients through an immersion in their context. However, the relationalist is wary of the modern compulsion to see our relationship with time as one of consciousness projected into the metaphor of flow, which unfolds into discussions about the influence of the past on the present. The modern habit is to bridge the gap between an objective past and the present by viewing time linearly, with the past pushing into the present. How peculiar it might seem to cultures other than our own, that how you feel in the living present is because of what happened to you 40 years ago.

If one felt disturbed, low, or sleepless, you might instead be looking at what you have been eating, who has cast a spell on you, what taboo you have broken, when you last missed reverence to the Gods or because you broke some tribal custom. What I am trying to say is that we seem committed to the idea that the past causatively pushes its way into the present. Time must escape from this two-dimensional paradigm if we are to recognise the distorting effect of such strangely disembodying metaphors for making sense of our experience of the world.

A radicalised here-and-now relational experiencing of time is a more sensitive indicator of context than other reports of linear there-and-then experiences. This depth of involvement contrasts with the neutrality advocated by many mainstream approaches: the interpersonal mirror of person-centred therapy, the blank screen of psychoanalysis, and the aerial vantage point of behaviourism which aspires to the notion of objectivity. Because we are enmeshed with time, we both contribute to and are simultaneously the achievement of the situations in which we find ourselves. Agency for the radical relationist then is different from individual free will, especially when it implies freedom from context.

9. Being with Others. The psychotherapist's "in the moment" relationship with the otherness of their client is the most central aspect of the therapeutic encounter. The real problems are the present problems, and so the therapist must seek contact with the client in the present. Addressing relational experiences of the past or future can only be understood in the encounter with what phenomenologists call the living present. The purpose of remembering the past becomes attuned to its re-imagination in the living present.

The radically relational therapist understands depression, for example, as an uncoupling from the living present, and not the reverse, where a person's past is presumed to be the cause of difficulties in the present. What is at stake when we think about menopause, depression, dementia, or trauma in this way is the peculiar human capacity for seemingly stepping out of our bodies and adopting a detached "third-person" perspective towards ourselves. The capacity to shift between the timeless living present and adopt the supposed objective "view from nowhere and nowhen" becomes disrupted and desynchronised, thus filtering, and denying aspects of the world about me.

It is the co-created therapeutic living present that becomes the place for learning and change. As relational patterns appear in the "extended now," the radically relational therapist engages with the client in examining, challenging, and articulating new pictures, more apt metaphors for making sense of the givenness of the world. It is in the living present that awareness of what sectors of a client's world need be recovered for healthy living come to the fore.

This feature of radical relationality is reminiscent of the psychodynamic concept of transference – where the client projects their internal representations of relational figures from the past onto the therapist. The radical relationist, instead, sees these historical patterns as appearing in the real relationship of therapy; one just as authentic, if not more so, than those where the client participates as part of their embodied relational field of experience.

## References

Costello, J. (2020). *Workplace Wellbeing: A Relational Approach*. Routledge.

Costello, J.F., et al. (2002). A Structural and Mechanistic Investigation of the Mono-O-phenylation of Diols with $BiPh_3(OAc)_2$. *Journal of Organometallic Chemistry*. 662, 98–104.

Darwall, S. (1998). Empathy, Sympathy, Care. *Philosophical Studies*. 89(2/3), 261–282.

Gadamer, H-G. (1996). *The Enigma of Health: The Art of Healing in the Scientific Age*. Polity Press.

Jung, C.G. (1960). On the Nature of the Psyche. In H. Read, M. Fordham, & G. Adler (Eds.), R.F.C. Hull (Trans.). *The Structure and Dynamics of the Psyche* (v8). *C.G. Jung: The Collected Works*. Princeton University Press.

Lambert, M.J. (2013). The Efficacy and Effectiveness of Psychotherapy. In: *Bergin and Garfield's Handbook of Psychotherapy and Behavior Change* (p. 213). 6th edition. Wiley.

Leder G. (2021). Psychotherapy, Placebos, and Informed Consent. *Journal of Medical Ethics*. 47, 444–447.

McEvoy, C., Clarke, V., & Thomas, Z. (2021). Rarely Discussed But Always Present: Exploring Therapists' Accounts of the Relationship Between Social Class, Mental Health, and Therapy. *Counselling and Psychotherapy Research*. 21(2), 324–334.

Overgaard, S., Gilbert, P., & Burwood, S. (2022). *Introduction to Metaphilosophy*. Cambridge University Press.

Russel, J., (1991). Inventing the Flat Earth. *History Today*, 41(8), 13–19.

Sandel, M.J. (2021). *The Tyranny of Merit – What's Become of the Common Good?* Penguin.

Slife, B.D. & Richardson, F.C. (2008). Problematic Ontological Underpinnings of Positive Psychology: A Strong Relational Alternative. *Theory & Psychology*. 18 (5), 699–723.

Slife, B.D. & Wiggins, B.J. (2009). Taking Relationship Seriously in Psychotherapy: Radical Relationality. *Journal of Contemporary Psychotherapy*. 39(1), 17–24.

Smith, K.R. (2020). *The Ethical Visions of Psychotherapy*. Taylor & Francis.

# 2
# A GOOD LIFE

## 2.1 Introduction: On Being Philosophical

It is a mistake to see the paradoxes, themes, and symbols of contemporary psychological practice as having appeared solely from the relatively recent period of modernity. Much of what we owe to this secular practice of "healing souls" is inherited from the classical Hellenic period, diffracted through the cultural lens of Roman Imperialism, and a complex encounter with Christianity.

Despite the twists and turns of its historical development, there has been little dispute about the centrality of relationships to the philosophical foundations of psychotherapy. Our contemporary obsession with individualism seems to be a lamentable aberration. Beyond the context of our relationships – so Aristotle argued in his *Nicomachean Ethics* – we are but inert blocks of wood whose true meaning only comes about through our place on the checkerboard of life. We are communal beings for whom relationships, and friendship – not least of all with oneself – are a fundamental good (Crisp & Aristotle, 2014: 1155a):

> For it is odd to make the content person solitary, since no one would choose to have all good things and yet be on their own. For a human is a social being and our nature is to live in the company of others.

Philosophers of antiquity were just as perplexed as we are by the wonders of the universe, the meaning of life, and a restlessness that drives our search for answers to such concerns. The pursuit of wisdom and what it means to live a good and meaningful life was driven by more than idle curiosity. Philosophy for the ancients was characterised by practices that the contemporary therapist would readily recognise as psychoeducational. Such practices looked to address

DOI: 10.4324/9781003396161-2

the self-evident truth that we are disturbed not by things, but the view we take of things; it is not our senses that deceive, but our way of thinking that leads us astray and misreads the world of sense perception.

The preoccupation with self-knowledge was not introspection for its own sake but a practical approach to integrating the threefold concerns of logic, ethics, and physics. That is to say, paying attention to the things we both think and say, how to act correctly towards others, and understanding our place in the order of things.

When a friend talks of being "philosophical" in the face of disappointment or adversity, it is the tradition of Latin Stoic moral philosophy to which they implicitly refer and not the modern discipline of academic philosophy. In *Philosophy as a Way of Life*, Pierre Hadot sees the decline of philosophy as something we actively *do* starting in the Middle Ages and ending with the establishment of the modern university. These modern institutions, Hadot claims, are "made up of professors who train professors, or professionals training professionals" (1995). The drift of philosophy from a vocation promoting the good life to a discipline taught in the academy has attracted criticism, not least of all from scholars of philosophy concerned about their dwindling relevance.

Like canaries in a cage, the existence of a philosophy department is seen as a measure of the health of a liberal democracy. Yet, for reasons I examine in this chapter, a good deal of contemporary philosophy is exclusively theoretical, with little or no direct connection to how we might conduct our lives. Professional philosophers, it is argued, are trapped in the merry-go-round of neoliberal education rather than fulfilling the ancient tradition of modelling the good life. As one political philosopher explained to me, "if you want a friend in academia … buy a dog". Personally, I have found professional philosophers to be thoughtful, grounded, and charming. But lest we become nostalgic for the classical Greco-Roman period, philosophising was largely the pursuit of wealthy free men who sought virtue to better govern those who were different – that is, women, the poor, and the formally enslaved.

Nevertheless, it seemed scandalous to those who sought wisdom in antiquity – as it does to therapists in the modern era I daresay – that we invest inordinate amounts of energy fabricating quarrels, social rituals, and values that only serve to disconnect us from living fulfilling lives. The philosophy of Epictetus typifies the supremely practical nature of wisdom, reminding the reader in his *Discourses* that it is not just about talking a good game; we must be changed by wisdom in the same way an athlete's body is enhanced by physical exercise. Go ahead and have a family – Epictetus implores – live alongside your difficult colleagues and annoying friends; but if you only want to talk about philosophy rather than live it, then find someone who is willing to let you "vomit" your undigested learning upon them (Epictetus & Long, 1900: 3, 21).

There is considerable merit in the claim that human troubles will not cease until either the philosopher become a psychotherapist, or psychotherapists take the pursuit of philosophy seriously and adequately. It is undoubtedly true that psychotherapy is the closest profession we have which balances therapeutic practice with philosophical understanding. So, what solace can be found in the puzzling technicalities of academic philosophy?

Professional philosophers can appear uncomfortable about extending their theoretical perspectives and intellectual purity to the ordinary life of work, family, friendship, culture, and the messy business of psychotherapy – all of which are indisputably relational. The idea that the mundane relationships of ordinary people could inform ideas of the good life flew in the face of Aristotle's philosophical tradition. Here, ordinary life was the mundane background of infrastructural importance, a presumed pre-requisite for supporting the higher life of contemplation, and a person's actions as a political being. Higher, more worthy forms of activity like aesthetics, waging war, or heroic asceticism separated this higher, admirable life from the lower life of slothful, alienated, irrational slaves.

What has changed is that we now naturally affirm the value of ordinary life and the dignity of all human beings. Furthermore, we no longer hold our politicians, intellectuals, warriors, or artists – and celebrities, at a stretch – in the esteem we once did. A sense of prizing ordinary human living has at its centre the importance we lend to the difficulties and distress experienced by ordinary people; it colours the modern understanding of what it is to truly respect human life.

It is in the ordinary life of creating and sustaining families, building friendships, doing work we think is valuable, and the sense of achievement we get watching children grow that has become meaningful, and somehow higher. Doing things important for living – philanthropy, concern for other living beings and impending environmental catastrophe, our stewardship of the planet, active engagement in a calling or vocation, public service in its truest sense, and creating a society in which all have equal access to its benefits – also provides meaning.

Such practices offer routes for affirming at some unarticulated level our philosophical approach to life, and our ethical stance towards a life well lived. The good life now lies within range for us all and is not something reduced to a series of activities for Aristotle's leisured few who saw themselves above and separate from women, slaves, and animals. What is to be retrieved from the attitudes of antiquity is philosophy as a way of life, a mode of existing in the world, and not just something modelled or at worst circumscribed for that hallowed 50 minutes by a therapist living their "best life". It is something to work on all the time.

To this end, Hadot argues that we have no practical alternative other than to consider the ancient philosophies, in the spirit in which they were written, that is, with a view to one's own personal development. But we must not be seduced into believing that ancient philosophy is transposable to the modern world. It is hard to imagine a teacher offering the same consolation offered by Epictetus to a concerned parent: children are like vases … fragile but replaceable.

The main trait of this ancient conception of philosophy was its deeply practical and existential potential with its ability to transform – rather than merely theorise about life. To the seasoned therapeutic practitioner, however, the reflective exercises of Hadot and others are examples of psychoeducation. It enfolds the separate moments of being actor and spectator into one; we tend to step back from conversations and experiences to examine for ourselves what the world has put before us. The spiritual exercises proposed within Hellenistic philosophy are little more than drills for remembering the meaning and implications of arguments. They become fixed in the mind so that they are readily available to be applied as life's crises arise.

And then there are the various meditative practices that parallel the Eastern traditions which foster and focus awareness. If we see Marcus Aurelius' *Meditations* not as the outpourings of a neurotic but as a therapeutic practice, then we understand the utility of keeping a journal. It is a way of externalising thoughts and bringing them into order. He reminds us in a way which feels terribly contemporary, that if anybody tells you that: "I will speak to you quite frankly … then you know they are a hypocrite". If somebody needs to tell you that they will be frank, then frankness is a virtue that does not come to them naturally, so do not believe them. We could add other conversational gambits to this category: "to tell you the truth" and "to be honest with you".

Another technique is therapeutic argument, best illustrated by Epictetus' *Enchiridion*, in which a sternly sardonic narrator chides his interlocutors. Central to all these techniques is dialogue, which for Plato meant that sometimes the quest was as important as the quarry. By bringing troubling thoughts into the clear light of day, we learn to put some rhythm to our anxieties, thereby reducing and dispelling their power without necessarily causing them to cease once and for all.

## 2.2 From the Celestial to the Terrestrial

Socrates was the first to call philosophy down from the heavens and bring it to the cities, streets, and homes of ordinary citizens. The power of dialogue was employed to inquire about ordinary life, question how we organise society, and examine the value of things we assume to be important for living a good life. The Socratic goal for dialogue was to awaken citizens to what for the most part falls outside the sphere of ordinary life, towards the gleaming and exemplary which ordinarily cannot be countenanced by the marketplace.

The stalls of Socrates' marketplace, however, are a world away from the contemporary Academy and its theorising. True to his dogmatic mistrust of the written word, the historical figure of Socrates left little that could be reliably attributed to the man. As is true for anyone who relishes teaching their subject – and not just philosophers – the static representation conveyed by the written word is a poor relation to the dynamic, "cut and thrust" of the Socratic medium of the spoken word.

For someone who believed that a higher, more truthful self was to be found through dialogue, it comes as no surprise to learn that Socrates was a critic of atomised individualism. What we know of Socrates comes to us from several sources, most notably students and friends such as Xenophon and Plato who tried to capture and extend the dialogic practice of examining the self and the relationship of the self with others. It becomes difficult then to separate the historical figure of Socrates from those who sought to represent the spirit of the man, for Plato himself was unique among his contemporaries in the sweep of his thinking and a commitment to the idea that a flourishing individual also needs a flourishing, deeply engaged *community*.

The elusive nature of the person "Socrates" makes way then for something more important, which is the symbolic *figure* and indeed a whole literary genre. In short, the figure of Socrates embodies what it means to doubt, step back, question, and engage in participatory knowledge about what we think we know about the way we live our lives. Those who adopt the figure of Socrates therefore represent our eternal interrogators, our conscience, and the unsettling interlocutor who cannot be sure where their questions will lead. Dialog exposes us to the experience of feeling frustrated and anxious with indeterminate things. This is a malady whose only remedy seems to be: "please give me a simple code of practice to live by".

In a Socratic dialogue, the figure who questions lays claim to the perplexing notion that they have nothing to teach, repeating to whoever cares to listen: "all I know is that I know nothing". It is tempting to respond to this posture with the *sceptical* stance, namely: "if you know nothing, not even if there *is* a right path, then what's the point of questioning"? Many adopt the sceptical stance and nevertheless go on to have an outwardly happy life. Yet in rejecting scepticism, the Socratic mission is one of philosophical deconstruction, which is a commitment to the belief that the quest is at least as important as the quarry.

If we do not recognise the paradox of Socratic dialogue, then we miss something crucial about the practice of reason to which the Sage calls us. The inquisitive child who repeatedly asks "why" can lead the most patient and well-informed parent to recognise how much universally accepted knowledge is assumed without question. The difference between what *I know* and what *I believe* becomes revealed, in much the same way that Socrates understood that the process was at least as important as the content of the inquiry. But for all its strenuousness, why look when one does not seek to find? The Socratic figure may have no claim to transmissible knowledge, but they are clearly "up to something".

Whatever we think of Socrates, the pursuit of truthfulness is no idle exercise. The Socratic notion of induced *elenchus* or perplexity is not a method of philosophical investigation which leads inevitably to resolution. It transforms the attitudes that support our unexamined or dogmatic assumptions about what we believe about our world. The point of *elenchus* is that it results in a slowing down, and a greater hesitancy to action which may help us in making better ethical decisions.

It is the same paradox which lies behind the similar therapeutic practice of *Guided Discovery*. How can a therapist be certain that it is the good of the client they have in mind when they are offering guidance (Overholser, 2018)? As we shall see later, a therapist is someone already committed to an idea of what it means to live well – that is to say their modality. It shapes their values, potentially unexamined assumptions, and core beliefs implicit to their actions and words. There can be no such thing as a value-free question.

The Socratic dialogue is potentially a communal and spiritual journey, with all parties invited into a closer examination of themselves in relation to others, along with their moral and ethical assumptions. It is the process of slowing down and examining how to live well which counts as much as the content of the dialogue itself. It is something we do not undertake without invitation, for it can amount to bullying, plain and simple. In the hands of the ardent practitioner it can provoke, infuriate, and intrude. Yet for those who admit to not knowing and are epistemically humble the Socratic dialogue is a path to knowing better and arguably doing better.

For Socrates, who thrust the ideal of an examined life on his interlocutors, it led to him paying the ultimate price. His goal – still relevant today – was to invite his contemporaries to reflect and pay attention to their inner progress, which he felt was shamefully neglected by a preoccupation with reputation and material things. At his trial, having mocked the jury, dared them to sentence him to death, then ridiculed them for having done so, he remained firm in defending the search for truthfulness (Plato, *Apology 29d-e*: 2003):

> I shall go on saying to my fellow Athenian friends, you belong to a city which is the greatest and most famous in the world for its wisdom and strength ... are you not ashamed that you give your attention to acquiring as much money as possible ... and give no attention or thought to truth and understanding and the perfection of your soul?

In making the case that Christianity had a legitimate place in first century Greek culture and intellectual life, the author of the New Testament "Luke-Acts" – an educated writer no doubt aware of Plato's *Apology* – evoked the figure of Socrates when reciting something familiar: "forgive them for they know not what they do" (Luke 23:34).

After the death of Socrates, a sickened and disillusioned Plato abandoned a promising political career and left the city, returning years later to establish the earliest University or *Academy*. His *utopia*, or the "good place elsewhere" was close enough to the city to be influential. Not overtly, through revolution or direct political intervention, but indirectly through the exploration of enriched ways of living within small communities. It required a collective effort to create and sustain communities of such "canaries", dedicated to the philosophical contemplation of the good life for nearly 900 years. Debate was a staple activity which led to the emergence of the most refined, complex, and abstruse philosophical ideas in the history of thought.

Connotations of the term "academic", which carry down to our own time, can be attributed to this fact. The relevance of a millennium of organised Hellenic philosophy on Western thought is not simply historical; the ideas and attitudes are still with us, jostling for space in contemporary life, shaping and organising the moral and intellectual landscape of our modern time. In a striking anticipation of modernity, Stoicism – which we examine later – has no genuine sense of the common good, seeing the moral world of the individual as central; this is why it is such a pliable ethical option in contemporary psychotherapy.

Plato's focus on Socratic dialogues allowed him to pursue arguments that he thought deserved attention without necessarily endorsing them as true. The dialogue form therefore prevents the reader from accepting an argument just because Plato says so, because it is rarely clear what Plato, in fact, says: for Plato never speaks.

Having been convicted by the jury, Socrates was given the task of proposing his own penalty, by which he sealed his own fate: "...discussing goodness and examining both myself and others is really the very best I can do, and life without this sort of examination is *not worth living*" (Plato, *Apology:38a:* 2003). The Socratic relational ontology of Plato prized a process which "*formed* rather than *informed*": the goal was nothing less than to develop the art of living through dialogue.

Just One More Thing? Irony plays with reality and shared beliefs and involves twists, contradictions, and humour. It can be used to enrich communication, understanding, empathy, and when used appropriately, it can even entertain. Irony can also pose difficulties cross-culturally, adding unintended emphases to what is being implied and as we shall see later, the use of language across ethnicities, class, generations, and gender can hold privileged meanings which can also exclude.

When we meet some remark that we consider ironic, we experience incongruity between the straightforward meaning of what is said and other statements or aspects of a situation. Some contradiction, intended or otherwise, lies at the heart of an experience where what is meant and what is said differ. Although the outcomes of Socratic irony can be uncertain, it is *not* to be confused with feigned ignorance, something which has its origins in Ancient Greek drama for which *eirōneía* describes a purposely affected ignorance.

Peter Falk's portrayal of the blue-collar detective Lieutenant Columbo is an accessible example of *eirōneía*, where the dishevelled underdog allows the rich and famous to believe that they could pull the wool over his eyes. Both Socrates and Columbo were said to have had wives waiting at home, both seemed to take pride in their grubby appearance, and both pretended to not know the answers to their own seemingly innocent questions.

The real sophistication of Columbo was concealed from the culprit like a mask as he went about his business asking questions; the television audience was, of course, aware of Columbo's feigned ignorance, and enjoyed the unfolding class war as mouse became cat. Just as Columbo seemed satisfied with his quarries' version of events and gestured to exit the scene, he would turn to ask: "just one more thing", revealing the fatal inconsistency which marked the *denouement*. The spectacle of the process was not lost on Socrates: "Why is it people like to spend much of their time in my company? Is it because they enjoy listening to the examination of those who believe themselves to be wise but are not … the experience is not devoid of entertainment" (Wharne, 2022).

Unlike Columbo however, Socrates does not feign ignorance to surreptitiously guide his interlocutor to what the Sage knows to be the correct answer: "it seems I am wiser to a small extent … in that I do not think that I know what I do not know" (Plato, *Apology:21d*, 2003). Rather, Socrates sought to lead the respondent by argument to examine their life and recognise some of the incoherence at the heart of their assumptions.

For the contemporary therapist engaging in Socratic questioning with a client, can we be sure that we too do not feign ignorance like Columbo? Through our commitment to one theoretical construct or another, do we not already have a "culprit" mind? Are we looking for clues which support our theories about faulty thinking, a misplaced anxiety about things beyond our control, the relationship with your mother/carer or an inability to express emotions to the satisfaction of the therapist?

Yet unlike Columbo's "mouse" whose lust for fame and wealth drives them to make the wrong ethical decision, the therapist may, through their Socratic questioning, inadvertently hold a client to account for a life lived with few choices or alternatives. A taste for Socratic questioning in psychotherapy brings us to the examination of our own attitude to free will in what Socrates already believed was a predetermined universe.

Then as now, social class is a mighty *place holder*. Few challenge the finding that, not only do the economic circumstances into which we are born shape our lives and opportunities, but also the *time* we are born into that class. As we examine in more detail later, the question of whether we can be absolutely free moral agents in a predetermined universe is as relevant today for contemporary psychotherapy as it was for those who came after Plato.

I know that I know nothing. Socrates was not a sceptic: he insisted that a true account of something was to be found, even if it could not be adequately articulated through discourse. Socrates was committed to an intellect that could describe not only the surrounding world but also one's emotions, fears, desires, compulsions, and inclinations. In Plato's *Apology*, Socrates was clear how forgiveness was indispensable for living the good life: no one goes willingly toward what is bad or what one believes to be bad; wrongdoing comes from ignorance; and one should never return an injustice or harm another human being. We can begin to resolve the apparent contradiction when Socrates claims ignorance about transmissible knowledge while fervently believing in the fundamental characteristics of what is needed to live a good life by understanding something of the modern distinction between rational knowledge and belief.

All knowledge requires belief, and belief requires that we accept what discourse or theory has to say. As we explore in more detail later, knowledge and belief were for Socrates two sides of the same coin. The Socratic aphorism, "I only know that I know nothing", requires that theory and practice are inseparable. Belief need not be supported by strong justifications, or empirically proven facts, but it does require an intuitive understanding of the essence of what is good, just, virtuous, and beautiful.

Each age re-discovers Socrates anew, and it was the Renaissance sceptic Michel de Montaigne who made a virtue of moderation because of his painful experience of holding mistaken beliefs. In recognition of his ignorance, Montaigne took care to communicate his sceptical posture throughout his writing using words which softened and moderated the rashness of his propositions.

Montaigne's therapeutic scepticism extended to sometimes erratic and uneven reasoning to multiply the possibilities for doubt rather than proposing causes and explanations. Through this sceptical method, Montaigne evaluated and exercised his judgement, often going over the same ground to seek new vantage points, always resisting the temptation to rest satisfied with his current understanding.

Therapeutic Socratic questioning can connect the lives of clients with their context: understanding the way that we are situated in time and place is therefore a *radically relational* undertaking. It is a task synonymous with responsiveness. I am claimed by a question, word, or experience to which I am then called to respond with understanding in a way which leads to further experiencing. A genuine *not knowing* accompanies the therapist who can acknowledge that they do not know how to live in the world in which their client exists.

We can conclude by saying that something is revealed when we must account for our assumptions to someone who is not familiar with us, or our way of life. We can become aware that there are other ways to be. We need not continue to live within the orientations into which we happen to have been born. As therapists, is it possible to adopt a stance of *not knowing* towards a client, while also being aware of our own beliefs about what works, and what a good life might look like? It is important that we can at least question our choice of one interpretation over another in the face of our cultural and social circumstances.

## 2.3 Epicurus, Zeno, and Psychotherapy

The contrasting modern-day perspectives of humanistic and cognitive-behavioural therapies can be traced back to the classical philosophies of Epicurus and Zeno of Citium. Both developed their approaches in response to the prevailing schools of Plato (*The Academy*) and Aristotle (*The Lyceum*), which dominated Hellenic thought at the time. Epicurus established a school of philosophy along with friends – who he treasured – in his famous *garden* (*Kepos*). A prolific writer, Epicurus was a radical for his time because he welcomed women and slaves to the *Kepos*. The good life for Epicurus, however, was somewhat limited to his narrow community, and not the common good *per se*.

Epicurus sought an alternative to what he saw as the interminable and speculative philosophising of Plato, with Zeno insisting on the reality of fate and a predetermined cosmos. In fact, so unsure were the followers of Zeno that a mortal could achieve the divine status of a Sage, that they eschewed referring to themselves *Zenonioi*. Instead, they named themselves *Stoics* after the painted colonnade (*Stoa*) of the Agora where they met. The Epicureans and the Stoics did not see themselves as competing ideologies but rather a network of friends looking to emulate Socrates and live a life of virtue.

Unlike the Epicureans who were held in high suspicion by early Christianity, the Stoics enjoyed the followership of the Roman Empire, with figures such as Cicero, Seneca, and Marcus Aurelius helping promote its ideas beyond the Middle Ages. The aim of both schools was ethical: they believed that the good life led to a state of inner *tranquillitas* or equanimity, which followed from the proper attitude towards the cosmos (physics), which, when rightly understood (logic) helped us come to an understanding of ourselves and our relationship with others (ethics).

Like many classical philosophers, Epicureans and Stoics believed that happiness, or *eudaimonia* – a blissful and prolonged state of happiness – was the ultimate goal of life. For the Epicureans, eudemonia was achieved through the cultivation of sensual pleasure, while for the Stoics it was only through the exercise of virtue that eudemonia could be achieved. The two philosophical approaches may be differentiated by whether pleasure was seen as an *end* of virtue, or a *by-product* of virtue, respectively. Whilst the conditions of health, beauty or wealth are undoubtedly pleasurable, Stoics saw them as morally neutral: neither inherently good nor bad. It was the life led that mattered.

So, while a rational person would generally choose pleasure over pain, it was not necessarily virtuous to have sex – irrespective of how pleasurable it was – outside wedlock. That said, a variety of views about sexual asceticism in Stoicism evolved mainly from the Cynics who shared the belief that to live rationally was to live in accord with "human" nature. Epicurus's views towards sexual ascetism were heavily influenced by his notorious contemporary Diogenes of Sinope – founder of the Cynics – who made himself the object of applied philosophical experiments. Here, powerlessness became power, poverty became wealth, and action trumped words.

Diogenes would brave public disapproval on the streets of Athens with shameless displays of onananism whenever he felt the urge. When he was jeered by the public, the infamous Cynic would cheerfully respond that it was a natural remedy, a simple honest relief by which man avoided being held hostage by the tyranny of unbridled desire: "What a pity Paris was not a Cynic … made in time, it could have avoided the Trojan War" (Merquior, 1991: 128). In social terms, Cynics became the markers of a truly liberated person who made freedom a virtue.

One of the earliest philosophical power-couples was Crates and Hipparchia – both of whom were teachers of Zeno. They lived similarly shameless lives showing their contempt for the world through, among other things, fornicating in public. They felt that if you could defy established authority, ignore social temptations – such as possessions, social status, and fame – and yet find the courage and strength to focus on the inner faculties of human nature, then one could justifiably claim to be free.

Such public displays of Cynical contempt for social expectations were beyond the pale for the more conservative Zeno. Indeed, the Roman Stoics with their love of "common sense" and sobriety disagreed with their more liberal Cynic predecessors, rejecting the view that men and women have the same capacity for virtue. It probably explains why the founding fathers of Christianity adopted such a conservative attitude to sexual morality. Sex was not for pleasure, but for procreation alone since human nature became conflated with God's will.

For Greeks of the classical period, it was fear of the Gods and punishment in a life after death that posed the chief cause of anguish. Epicurus had been a student of Democritus, who held that the entirety of the cosmos was composed of atoms. To dispel anxieties about the existence of hell, Epicurus developed a secular philosophy of nature which saw all natural phenomena, as well as the human soul, in terms of random collisions among atoms floating through the Godless void of space. Even if there were Gods, it was unlikely that such supreme beings would even notice inconsequential entities such as humans, let alone act malevolently towards them.

Unlike Democritus, Epicurus could not admit that we live in a predetermined universe. Doing so would relegate humans to mere onlookers to the spectacle of life, thereby rendering illusory notions of ethics and free will. The matter of atomic determinism and free will remains a matter for debate to this day, and we spend a little time on this towards the end of the chapter. For Epicurus, the solution was to admit a random "swerve" factor into the behaviour of atoms, not unlike the Heisenberg indeterminacy of quantum mechanics.

Epicurus was the first *empiricist* interested in the study and comprehensive understanding of physical reality guided by the distinct purpose of achieving peace of mind and happiness. The senses – though they may be fooled occasionally – are the only reliable source of knowledge about the cosmos. Although my eyes may infer that an oar bends as it enters water, running my hand along the structure confirms that this is an illusion caused by the diffraction of light.

In true existential or Epicurean fashion, death was seen as the destruction of the structures responsible for integrating the material body with the soul (philosophical monism). Because we perceive all that is good or bad with our senses, then as all of this ends with death, we cannot perceive death itself. When we exist, death does not exist, when death occurs, we do not exist. Therefore, it is absurd to fear that which we will never experience. "The more I learn about this extraordinary Athenian thinker" – Irvin Yalom tells us – "the more strongly I recognise Epicurus as the proto-existential psychotherapist" (2009).

Personal obliteration is the only consolation offered by Epicurus; this does not work for everybody. It certainly did not meet with the approval of the medieval Catholic Church, as it opposes fundamental tenets of Christianity. As Epicureanism denies the immortality of the soul, any notion of reward or punishment after death risks sinful sybaritic indulgence in life. So, although manuscripts continued to be copied and preserved in Benedictine monastic settings, the active study of Epicurean doctrines fell out of favour until the rise of the new sciences in the sixteenth century with the burgeoning of similar atom-theories. What became obscured in the process was that Epicureanism promoted the virtues of self-discipline and prudence for achieving contentment in *this* life. Time-honoured practices familiar to the contemporary psychotherapist include meditation, journaling, a commitment to living in the moment, memorising aphorisms to help relieve anxiety, and intriguingly – given *epicurus* in Hebrew means *heretic* – taking part in religious festivals.

In Stoicism, virtue ultimately means living in accord with nature, which at a practical level equates to self-interested self-preservation. According to Diogenes, pleasure was a by-product arising from an organism realising its natural potential (*oikeiôsis*), such as when a lamb frolics or a plant blooms (Still & Dryden, 1999: 158). Seneca also sought to give examples of *oikeiosis:* an infant trying to stand or an upturned turtle trying to right itself – neither feel pain nor are they distressed. A desire to achieve their natural state makes them restless, and they will not stop struggling or shaking themselves until they can right themselves and stand on their feet. In this sense, *oikeiôsis* finds its contemporary expression in the Rogerian notion of the actualising tendency.

The distinction between hedonism and happiness seemed unimportant to the Epicureans but was crucial to the Stoics. Indeed, twentieth century psychologists would go on to conflate the principle of *oikeiosis* with the relatively superficial Freudian pleasure principle. Satisfying sensual appetites plays an important part in the life of a virtuous person, but such pleasures are not essential to a virtuous life.

In a letter to *Menoeceus*, Epicurus explains in his uncompromisingly direct style the formula for happiness, and the ethics of how to relate well to the world and our fellow human beings. *Eudaimonia* – he reminds us again – is the greatest good. Perhaps the most important of our mental pleasures, especially within the structure of the *Kepos*, is the role of intellectually and emotionally fulfilling friendships. Intelligent people should prefer knowledge resulting from the objective observation of nature and avoid unrealistic myths that cause fear and agitation, a habit commonly encountered in "fools".

In a clear departure from Plato, Epicurus extolled reasoning based on the empirical criteria of truth in preference to disorientating rhetorical schemes. Diogenes Laërtius – an influential third century philosophical biographer – concluded that no part of classical philosophy was separate from another: they combined, sometimes incoherently, and this was especially true in the service of therapy. In his famous *Consolation to Marcia*, Seneca employed every trick in the Stoic/Epicurean playbook to support his grief-stricken friend (Zainaldin, 2021). *In short*, Zeno, Epicurus, Diogenes, Crates and Hipparchia offered startling alternatives to the daily rat race. They challenged the ability to question our preoccupation with material possessions, day-to-day pursuits, and instead think about the things that really mattered.

Accessing the Good Life. It is worth mentioning here an Epicurean idea which cuts to the heart of contemporary concerns – especially for psychotherapists – about justice and living in a fair society. Epicurus was advising his friend Marcella on the importance of enjoying what she had, and to avoid the mental agitation of fretting about what she did not have: "... as fools usually do". Now who could argue against being grateful for what we have? Yet talk of "foolishness" in this context clearly speaks of a man who enjoyed a lavish menu of liberties and wealth brought about through the accident of birth.

Harry Frankfurt argued that economic egalitarianism is a misguided moral ideal (1987). If anything, the doctrine of equality contributes to the moral disorientation of our time. To understand why inequality is not a philosophical concern of Frankfurt's, we are asked to consider separating society into three categories: those who do not have enough, those with enough, and those with too much. Those in the second and third groups have what they need to take part in society. The moral issue then is not one of economic equality, but of access for those with less economic, social, and cultural capital. Poverty equates to more ways of being refused access because of barriers beyond our making. Contrary to an emphasis on inequality, the real issue for Frankfurt was one of access. A just society then addresses inequality through the way the worst-off access resources.

Ideally, we do this in much the same disinterested way as a wise parent divides the cake at a children's party: justice is in the hands of the one who cuts the cake yet also understands that they may be the last to help themselves to a slice. It is about imagining the distribution of resources *as if* I were the worst-off in any given situation. Pragmatists remind us that so long as wealth and power go hand in hand, there is little chance of achieving a truly just society. When the planet's eight richest people have the same wealth as the poorest half of humanity, we must not be seduced by green-washing, sports-washing, or other self-serving philanthropy that makes the rich look good to a domestic audience.

Like education and other advantages, access to psychotherapy does not afford the same benefits for all recipients, because the ethical position of every client (or therapist) may not be congruent with the method on offer. For example, a client who looks to explore the spiritual dimension of their life may be better suited to a collaboration with a therapist who recognises this dimension of the relationship. A therapist with a good empirical track record of accomplishment when treating depression may not be open to the transcendental aspects of existence.

The "equality of benefit – equality of choice" combination is most likely optimised when a therapist can be explicit about their values, even though a distressed client may not be able to hear this at the beginning of therapy. It requires that the different – and as we have seen, equally efficacious – psychotherapies need to be understood and advocated to an equal degree, both knowledgably and with conviction from each differing ethical and epistemological position. In short, it requires a radically relational awareness of what is on offer.

And let us not ignore the unnoticed benefit enjoyed by you, who reads this in English. You are possibly amongst the third most populous group of native language speakers on the planet. Though you comprise a mere 5 per cent of the global population, as a native English speaker it is likely that you live in one of the six industrialised democracies (i.e., Australia, Canada, Ireland, New Zealand, UK, and the United States), which together are responsible for one-third of the global domestic product. Add to this the legacy of colonialism, then English is spoken – with varying levels of proficiency – by 20 per cent of the global community.

The communication value of the English language is not in doubt. Yet anglophones are increasingly disinterested in learning a second language and this inhibits linguistic diversity. "If you want a piece of the economic pie, learn our language" is the message conveyed. As we shall find later, bi- or trilingualism does not reduce communication to the trivial issue of having different words to describe the same thing. The hegemony of the English language – and thus the medium of psychotherapy – needs to be seen in much broader socio-political, economic, and cultural terms. The English language creates and propagates an inequality in how people – across cultures and generations – access resources and opportunities (Soler & Morales-Gálvez, 2022).

## 2.4  Stoicism and Cognitive Therapy

For the Stoics, *tranquillitas* was attained through a life of reason in harmony with the natural order of a predetermined universe, where all events are the consequence of past events and the laws of nature. In contrast with the Epicureans, the Stoic concept of the cosmos is one of passive matter subjected to divine and purposeful reason (*logos*). For the Stoic, the cosmos has a finite lifespan and after each cycle matter collapses back into pure reason from which an identical perfect cosmos is reformed. It has to be identical because it was perfect to start with. Human reason is a spark of this greater cosmic reason, and whatever happens to humans – no matter how distressing it seems at the time – must happen because we are part of a greater design or *logos*.

So, when I despair, the Stoic perspective accepts that this is part of some greater cosmic plan: it has some purpose. That purpose is of course subject to speculation. Is my misfortune necessary for somebody else in the cosmos – such as my therapist – to be virtuous? Conversely, the Stoical therapist who accepts their part in the organic whole of the cosmos, understands that *your* distress is necessary for *their* virtue. Acknowledging our providential fate is to live in accordance with the nature of the cosmos.

But unlike the Epicurean understanding of knowledge as revealed through sensation, the Stoics saw logic as a precise succession of mental exercises which not only protected the human mind from error but also helped it understand the cosmos. Emotional disturbances were understood in terms of faulty judgements. These came about when our subjective impression of a phenomenon differed from the alternative view adopted from the perspective of sound judgement (prudence), right reason, or with a "stiff upper lip". Christianity, particularly its more ascetic variants with its concept of providence and self-denial, was considered a continuation of Stoic paganism beyond the Middle Ages, with its most notable reboot in the guise of nineteenth-century British imperialism.

The Stoic offers a cure by pointing out discrepancies in our thinking, which in turn changes our emotions. To be cured is to be free of unwanted emotions, fully in control of ourselves and our feelings. In the final analysis, the Stoic believes that what affects us for good or ill depends on our own judgements and how we respond to the circumstances that befall us. In short, Stoics assert that: "we all possess certain deep seated, intuitive, natural and common-sense assumptions but fail to apply them consistently or think their logical implications through" (Robertson, 2020: 21).

Montaigne tells the story of Metrocles who – while in deep public deliberation – inadvertently broke wind in front of his followers. His embarrassment was so profound that he fled from the crowd and locked himself away in his home until his friend Crates brought along a delicious bean stew. The consolation of Crates lay in the resulting, copious amounts of wind. The shame of Metrocles – it is argued – was misplaced because the inadvertent release of gas was simply in accord with nature: "shame has a kind of weight; concealment, dissimulation and constraint" (Montaigne & Screech, 1987: 165).

Robertson makes a compelling argument for the homology between Greco-Roman Stoic thought and the practice of contemporary cognitive- and rational emotive behavioural therapies (CBT/REBT) (2020). He reminds us that Ellis derived much of his theory of REBT from philosophy and not psychology. That is to say, the practices of CBT/REBT are both structurally and historically linked to Stoic philosophy and indeed Epictetus' belief that "we are disturbed not by events, but by the meaning which we give them" is the cornerstone of the modern method. Although Aristotle disagreed with the Stoics, seeing the passions as something to be harnessed not stilled, he nevertheless believed that we could take unfortunate events lightly, moderately, or catastrophically, because to a considerable degree, it is our choice.

For the classical philosophers, and indeed contemporary CBT/REPT therapists, a good life is to be found in self-mastery through rationality, which automatically aligns it to a transcendent vision of cosmic order. This is a radically different way of defining reason compared to the modern era, which sees reason instead as an inward-looking procedural, self-consistent, sort of instrumental efficacy conditioned by language and culture.

Reflecting on the horrors of totalitarianism, Max Horkheimer argued in *Eclipse of Reason* (1947) that modernity had ushered in a divergence in reason from that of the classic Platonic era. This modern sort of instrumental reason is preoccupied with the *means* – or how effectively we think – whereas the latter is seen as more ethical because it is focussed on the purpose or *ends* to which we apply our thinking. An absurd example which might illustrate the point is to imagine the greatest surgeons in the world setting their collective efforts to achieve the first appendix transplant. Very clever … but why? The instrumental reason of modernity conforms to the technical aspects of what rationality looks like, or what seems reasonable and prudent within a given context. It is akin to the Stoic understanding of reason, which considers the means through which we master our untutored human emotions.

To be reasonable is to comply and avoid being obstinate, which in turn requires alignment with some idea of what a good life is, though Stoics and those who followed them are silent about what that might be. We can think of bureaucracy as an example of instrumental reason where it can seem that it is the *means* to some goal that matters, and not so much the *goal* itself. Little importance is attached to the question of whether the purposes of bureaucracy, or conformity to some unstated goal, is reasonable. If it concerns itself at all with *ends*, it takes for granted that they too are reasonable in the subjective sense, which is to say they serve the subjects' interest in relation to self-preservation or *eudemonia*. The ethical standards set are not so much about the correct order of things in the way Plato may have understood it, but about conforming to the instrumental thinking that defines rational activities. *It becomes more important to think in the correct way, than it does to dwell on the beliefs and assumptions behind them.*

The Stoics broke from Socrates, Plato, and Aristotle by rejecting self-sufficient contemplation as the primary access point to happiness – though, of course, life lived in the community would later form the foundation of the monastic tradition. Similarly, CBT/REBT does not labour over its account of the ideal to which it strives. For example, it does not propose a model for the best functioning of a human being.

This accounts for the plasticity of the instrumental *ends* to which CBT/REBT can be oriented when it complies with the myriad medicalised notions of what it means to be "normal". As a modality, it knows what it can do which is to provide the *means* for the exercise of prudent thoughts and actions; but it is less clear about what those prudent *ends* are. Although there is no definitive account of a core Stoic ethic, we can impute connections with our deeper existential concerns – death, isolation, freedom, and meaning (Section 5.4).

The Stoic sphere of control is centred on the present moment, and it is in the present moment that we must be grounded. It is in the *now* that Marcus Aurelius reminds us to habitually apply objective judgement, unselfish action, and willing acceptance. So, when we come to die – he argues – it is not the whole of our lives that ends, because our previous life has already ended the moment before we die. All we lose when we die is this "moment". So, living a life of 10, 30, or 90 years amounts to the same moment "lost" to death.

*This I believe is a superficial and shallow perspective to adopt, and as I argue later, it atomises moments in a way which dissolves narratives and therefore ethical dimension of life. It is also a profoundly un-Aristotelian, in that Aristotle would have held that the actualisation of a life comes to fruition only at its end, which is something we can never know about ourselves.*

However, the Stoic lives in awareness that no being exists in isolation and that we belong to a vast causal network of interconnected events in the cosmos. This Stoic sense of fatalism is sometimes understood as a commitment to an unknowable transcendence, which overlaps readily with Christian thought. When Luke tells of Paul's visit to Athens to address the Stoics and Epicureans in the Agora, he is describing an attempted synthesis between Greek reason and divine revelation (Acts 17:16–34).

We sometimes refer to this disembodied transcendence as *Rational Mysticism*, the *Divine*, the *Will of God*, or *Universal Nature*. Contemplation of "the view from above", or as Plato referred to it "the high watchtower", invites us to consider the totality of time and being, and the consequence of human affairs from the indifferent perspective of the cosmos. A sense of transcendence then, implies a movement out in the first place to give meaning to the polarities of "me" and "not me", which ultimately requires bridging *through* relationality.

People are valuable in themselves because they have volition (the power to choose) and the capacity for wisdom and virtue. A fundamental moral good then is the idea of human dignity, which emanates from a rational being who can confront the indifferent immensity of the cosmos and still find purpose in their lives beyond their own insignificant and singular locus of being. Understanding and embracing how we as humans are bound to be annihilated yet can go into that dark night knowingly inspires respect, and this respect is empowering.

Reasoning with Feelings. Stoic moral agency is founded on the belief that reason may be accessed for the therapeutic governance of our passions. This contrasts with the view – widely held among therapists – that the dualistic separation of objective rationality from subjective experience is, in fact, part of the problem, certainly not the solution.

Montaigne reminds us how little controversy there was among classical philosophers towards monism – the blurring of the boundary between body and soul, seating the mind in the material body. For Democritus, Hippocrates, and Aristotle, the soul was diffused throughout the body; the Stoics and Chrysippius placed the soul in the heart because when we assert things, this is where we strike with our hands; Moses and Empedocles situated the soul in the blood. Plato's radicalism was to make a clean break between emotions and reason, with the latter adopting a privileged position from which it could reflect on and understand all else. Rationality for Plato thus became tied to the perception of order, but it was not reason in the modern sense of the term. In choosing to write in dialogues, Plato wanted to entertain indeterminacy in the face of the order of the whole. A good life then was something to be achieved, not discovered, because dialogic reason was the basis of good order in our souls, and thereby "a vision of good order of the whole" (Taylor, 1989: 122).

The evolution of cognitive behavioural therapy (CBT) can be viewed in terms of how our relationship with reason, or more accurately dysfunctional reason, has evolved since its modern inception in the 1950s. In the earliest days of the approach, unhelpful reasoning was seen as something that could be changed or even eliminated through a psychoeducational approach which hinged on verbal <u>disputation</u>. The second wave of CBT which followed saw a change in strategy, with therapists supporting clients conducting experiments which sought to <u>disprove</u> their dysfunctional reasoning. The third wave – inspired by Eastern mindfulness practices which started to become popular in the 1990s – uses faster, manualised, and easier to teach techniques that encourage <u>detachment</u> from dysfunctional thinking.

The terms "rational", "cognitive", and "behavioural" therapies are sometimes misinterpreted by critics who dispute the Platonic notion of a false discontinuity, or psychological separatism between thoughts, feelings, and behaviour. This can lead to the stereotyped assumption that thoughts, feelings, and actions occur sequentially, which is one step away from imagining that they have a causal relationship. This emotional reductionism does not understand that when we feel, we think and act; when we act, we think and feel; and when we think, we act and feel.

This, it is believed, led Ellis to adopt the name "rational emotional behavioural therapy" to emphasise a pre-Platonic contingency, if not a monistic relationship between the processes. Stoic philosophy explicitly conceptualises emotions as being suffused with cognitions and judgements, which may be either true or false, or better still, helpful or unhelpful.

For the Stoics and the pioneers of CBT/REBT, thinking and emotion are interdependent, yet, in practice, this became obscured by the implied separation of <u>Activation</u>, <u>Belief</u>, and <u>Consequences</u> in the ABC model. In REBT, an emotional-behavioural consequence is always a product of beliefs, which may be either rational or irrational. For example, the REBT proposition in response to being subjected to an invasive medical procedure ($\underline{A}$), is something we can reason as necessary for our long-term wellbeing. Though it may be uncomfortable – but not intolerably so – we can adopt a prudent and rational belief ($\underline{rB}$) towards the procedure.

If on the other hand we adopt the irrational belief ($\underline{iB}$) that the procedure will be intolerably uncomfortable even with mild sedation, then the consequence will be a great deal of apprehension, even fear as the procedure begins ($\underline{C}$). In the 1962 edition of *Reason and Emotion in Psychotherapy*, Ellis began exploring how he could "smooth-out" the apparent discontinuities between cognitions and emotions (cool/weak/hot).

In a form reminiscent of Montaigne's scepticism, Ellis ventured that those cognitions *almost* always accompanied or *tended* to go along with emotions, suggesting the contingency of the relationship between the two. A rational emotion therefore became a *reasonable* judgement of the value of a thing.

Fatalism, Free Will, and Morality. Having re-discovered Seneca's essays, the Renaissance humanist Francesco Petrarch wrote *De remediis fortuitorum*, the first Stoic self-help manual aimed at the educated commoner. Writing just after the Black Death in war-torn Italy, Petrarch understood the fragility of human affairs. He begged forgiveness from his largely Christian audience for using the pagan word *fortuna* – then a colloquial term for chance events and the passions – to emphasise the vicissitudes of life and the events that lie beyond our control (Panizza, 1991: 58).

Like Petrarch, contemporary psychotherapists using the "knocked over by a bus" aphorism understand the therapeutic benefits of reminding clients of universal determinism. It discloses the never-ending chain of causes and effects proving just how much is beyond our control. A typical criticism of the Stoics, and indeed CBT/REBT is the sense of passivity and fatalism in the face of misfortune. It risks rendering the therapeutic method superficial because those who seek its help can become inured to what makes them miserable.

Emotional self-regulation and forced equanimity are very different things. The latter I characterised earlier as benumbing or subduing of the full range of human emotional experience, floating along on a sea of feel-good mindful emptiness and mediocrity. Affect regulation on the other hand is a powerful idea central to attachment theory, which focusses on understanding our emotions be they fear, anger, or shame. Their articulation helps us understand life as a process of exploring what we value and how we engage in the world. Frustration, contempt, or anger *can* be virtues in the Aristotelian sense if they are understood and directed towards ethical actions – to understand our emotions then, is to experience who we are.

To counter stereotyped criticisms of passivity and excessive equanimity, Ellis used the metaphor of noticing smoke in a house: *if it is moderate, I stay, if it is great, I will go out – what is important to hold onto is that the door is always open.*

The metaphor of Ellis' open-door points to the principle of *Alternate Possibilities*, which holds that I am morally responsible for what I do only if I could have done otherwise. For example, in the case of events over which I had no alternate possibilities, the door is firmly shut. Being born in Manchester to Irish working-class immigrants into circumstances over which I had no say are immutable facts over which I cannot be held morally responsible. As determinism presumes that people cannot follow alternative pathways when initial conditions and the laws of nature are set, it follows that free will, moral responsibility and determinism are incommensurate.

The principle of *Alternate Possibilities* looks to capture a necessary condition for moral responsibility, but the matter is not settled even when the subject could have done otherwise. Are we always aware of our intentions, motives, influences, disciplining factors, and coercions? The degree of tension that exists between our acceptance of determinism and the degree of free will that we believe is available to us is significantly guided by our cultural contexts rather than some universal human intuition. We can all provide examples of aphorisms handed down to us through the generations: "God loves a trier; there is no such thing as luck, only looking out". We are thus reminded that we have the capacity to choose, even if we cannot influence the menu of choices made available to us.

While holding to the philosophical truth of psychological determinism, Stoics adopt the paradoxical position of believing we have, in principle, the agency to change our *inner* world, that is, determinism and free will are *compatible*. The Stoic ideal of empathy is thus grounded in compassion and forgiveness towards our fellow human beings for their lack of enlightenment, being either ignorant, deluded, or misguided. The corollary then is that at the heart of CBT/REBT lies a philosophical paradox: while reason and emotion commingle, the former is sovereign and exerts agency over the latter in an otherwise psychologically determined universe. Without accepting this paradox, the Stoic ideal of self-mastery slips from our grasp as we become reduced to mere instruments of social conditioning, abandoned to the turbulence of our passions and emotions.

Stoicism, Language, and the Conundrum of Folk Causality. Having considered the implications of fundamental physics at the turn of the twentieth century, Bertrand Russell made a famous attempt to end the debate around causality, declaring it obsolete: "a relic of a bygone age surviving, like the British monarchy, because it is erroneously supposed to do no harm" (Russell, 1913). Focussing on the asymmetry of causation, Russell cites the case of mutually gravitating bodies, for which there is nothing that could be properly understood as a *cause* or *effect*: there is merely a formula describing a *relationship*.

The laws of gravity lack another aspect of what we might call *folk causation*, which is again understood through the idea of time *asymmetry* or temporality – the cause happens *before* the effect. Gravity exhibits time symmetry since it does not differentiate between *past* and *future*: the *future determines the past* in the same way that the *past determines the future* (Chapter 8). If causality in fundamental physics is not an ontological fact, then what do we make of the *folk* concept of causality as we go about our daily lives making things happen? What we uncover here is not so much the paradox of causality in science, but the linguistic meanings we attach to words such as "cause", and the way in which they are employed within communities.

Subtle pictures of "local" determinism have evolved through our understanding of neural plasticity and its relationship with language. The work of Libet (2003) has engaged debate around the issue of local neural determinism in the brain and the wider issue of free will. Neural plasticity is the metaphor used to understand the structures of the brain and the way they interact with language. For Libet, genuine free will is the expression of an action that is not completely controlled or limited by the deterministic laws of physics and chemistry, and so on. The existence or non-existence of free will not be settled by quantum mechanics, our most powerful tool for understanding exceedingly small things; the randomness aspect affords *random* and not *free* will, and it remains deterministic insofar that natural laws are still being obeyed.

Libet-style experiments suggest that the brain triggers voluntary acts five hundred milliseconds before the subject is even aware that they wish or feel the urge to perform some action. It also seems to be the case that an awareness of the conscious act precedes the act itself by 150–200 milliseconds. Although delayed, the conscious will to act appears *before* the act, so it has been argued that there is still time for conscious function to control the outcome. However, neural determinism of this type has little to contribute – I feel – to arguments about complex indeterminate social decision making such as moral judgements.

The Stoic stance anticipates the liberal individualist perspective stemming from the belief that I am not injured by things, but only by my judgement of things. So, if someone is offended by my actions then the reciprocal view leads to the logic of *emotivism*, which makes ethics a personal perspective detached from context, because the hurt caused by my actions is *all in your head,* and not based in any form of reality (see Section 5.5). This leads to the dubious position that I am not ethically responsible for my behaviour: you are!

For the Stoic of antiquity, to pretend otherwise would be an illusion. As relational and embodied creatures, however, it is difficult to deny the view that language is constitutive, both defining and creating who we are, not only collectively through science, law, rhetoric, and economics, but also as individuals. A human being becomes capable of creativity and inventiveness through language. This ought not to be seen as something oppressive, but a dynamic structure within which a human being can choose value and meaning in their ethical conduct.

Language, as we shall find later, has its own logic of functioning and so may have its own influence on our physical brains. As my argument unfolds, I will examine the possibility that such philosophical conundrums may not, in fact, belong to the world as something "real" but come about because of the structures we create for apprehending the world and each other.

### References

Crisp, R. & Aristotle (2014). *Nicomachean Ethics.* Cambridge University Press.

Epictetus & Long, G. (1900). *The Discourses of Epictetus with the Encheiridion and Fragments.* A.L. Burt Publisher.

Frankfurt, H. (1987). Equality as a Moral Ideal. *Ethics.* 98(1), 21–43.

Hadot, P., Davidson, A.I., & Chase, M. (1995). *Philosophy as a Way of Life: Spiritual Exercises from Socrates to Foucault*. Blackwell.

Horkheimer, M. (2013/1947). *Eclipse of Reason*. Bloomsbury.

Libet, B. (2003). Timing of Conscious Experience: Reply to the 2002 Commentaries on Libet's Findings. *Consciousness and Cognition*. 12(3), 321–331.

Merquior, J.G. (1991). *Foucault*. 2nd edition. Fontana.

Montaigne, M.De & Screech, M.A. (1987). *An Apology for Raymond Sebond*. Penguin.

Overholser, J.C. (2018). Guided Discovery: A Clinical Strategy Derived from the Socratic Method. *International Journal of Cognitive Therapy*. 11(2), 124–139.

Panizza, L. (1991). Stoic Psychotherapy in the Middle Ages and Renaissance: Petrarch's *De remediis*. In M. Osler (Ed.), *Atoms, Pneuma, and Tranquillity: Epicurean and Stoic Themes in European Thought* (pp. 39–66). Cambridge University.

Plato, Tredennick, H., & Tarrant H. (2003). *The Last Days of Socrates: Euthyphro. Apology. Crito. Phaedo*. Penguin Books.

Robertson, D. (2020). *The Philosophy of Cognitive-Behavioural Therapy (CBT). Stoic Philosophy as Rational and Cognitive Psychotherapy*. 2nd edition. Routledge.

Russell, B. (1913). On the Notion of Cause. *Proceeding of the Aristotelian Society*. 13, 1–26.

Soler, J. & Morales-Gálvez, S. (2022). Linguistic Justice and Global English: Theoretical and Empirical Approaches. *International Journal of the Sociology of Language*. 277, 1–16.

Still, A. and Dryden, W. (1999). The Place of Rationality in Stoicism and REBT. *Journal of Rational-emotive and Cognitive-behaviour Therapy*. 17(3), 143–164.

Taylor, C. (1989). *Sources of the Self: The Making of Modern Identity*. Cambridge University Press.

Wharne, S. (2022). Socratic Questioning and Irony in Psychotherapeutic Practices. *Journal of Contemporary Psychotherapy*. 52(2), 137–144.

Yalom, I.D. (2009). *Staring at the Sun: Overcoming the Terror of Death*. Jossey-Bass.

Zainaldin, J.L. (2021). 'We Fortunate Souls': Timely Death and Philosophical Therapy in Seneca's Consolation to Marcia. *American Journal of Philology*. 142(3), 425–460.

# 3
# REASON AND BELIEF

## 3.1 Introduction: *This is Water*

Aspects of our immersion in modern culture suggest to me David Foster Wallace's memorable parable. Two fish swimming along in the vast ocean encounter another fish coming towards them who politely nods and says, "Morning …How's the water?" The two fish swim on for a while. Then, one looks to the other and says, "What the heck is water?" The immediate point is that the most taken-for-granted, obvious yet important realities of living in the world are often the hardest to see, never mind talk about. Stated as a parable, the truth is reducible to a banal platitude, but in the mundane, repetitive, and distracting messiness of human existence such banal platitudes have a: "life or death importance" (Foster Wallace, 2009: 9). Becoming aware of water – not that it is possible to fully do so – means learning how to exercise some critical awareness of how and what we think and worship; Foster Wallace is adamant that there can be no such thing as *not* worshipping. The only choice we get is *what* to worship.

A conversation between cultural icons Bob Dylan and Joan Baez in Scorsese's *Rolling Thunder Revue* (2019) tells us something more about the invisibility of water. Dylan explains to his ex-girlfriend Baez that yeah … I married the woman I loved. However, Baez laments that she married the man she *thought* she loved. See, that's where thinking gets you declares Dylan: "*love is about heart not head*". The separation of subjective and objective realms of knowing is an idea unthinkingly worshipped in Western culture, to the extent that it signposts divergent pathways to constitutionally different perspectives of the universe.

DOI: 10.4324/9781003396161-3

This polarity – between our inner nature and the disengaged calculating external stance of reason – is not simply a cornerstone of our North Atlantic culture. It is a shadow which looms over the theory and practice of counselling and psychotherapy, with its roots embedded in ideas and attitudes which swirl around us in the present inherited from an encounter between scriptural revelation and Greek reason of antiquity.

The apparent and seemingly irresolvable incompatibility between polarities comes in many guises: the saved and the lost, heaven and earth, nature or nurture, good and evil, and, of course, disengaged reason, and the body. The humanistic psychotherapies are not alone in transmitting an implicit philosophical divergence through its assumptions about truth and how it can be accessed. Ordinarily, this is seen as a project stifled by the calculating stance of reason which stands in the way of accessing the truth of our indwelling nature. But I suggest throughout that there is an intimate unity of inner and outer life – a braided pair inseparable from life's twine – which requires attention but not necessarily dissection and explanation.

Those who fail to grasp the reality that truth can only be found within are seen as being "defensive" or "not getting it". The separation between the interior intuitive *feeling-world* and the exterior one of detached reason presents itself in the structure of the mental health professions. It reflects something of their historical origins in either the scientific domain of medicine (i.e., psychiatry, clinical psychology, and psychotherapy) or voluntary religious settings which gave rise to the practice of counselling. "This isn't an academic course..." I hear trainers tell their students, tacitly deepening the division between practice and theory – experiencing and thinking. I still raise eyebrows as the psychotherapist from the "other side" – the detached, unfeeling domain of the physical sciences.

As a trainee, a well-remembered supervisor disclosed an ingrained partitioning between "feeling and thinking" selves, which is commonly encountered in therapy. I was reminded that a "PhD in Chemistry is of little help here". Strictly speaking of course, they were right: chemistry is a highly contextual sort of knowledge. But the attitude fails to see what good therapists already do, which is synthesise different types of knowing (*epistēmē* and *phronēsis*) into their practice (*technē*). Such a synthesis must occur if a therapist (or a scientist, performer, teacher, carer, parent ...) is to contain the discontinuity between particularity – the embodied experience of doing things – and universalising disengaged reason where we reflect on our experience of doing those things.

The inward turn and the disengagement of the mind, intellect, or soul from the body or the material world has a history, a beginning in time and place. Reading aloud is something many of us are unaccustomed to nowadays, except for the autocued classes and those engaged in the more wholesome practice of reading to their families.

As I read aloud, I recognise how different it is from the experience of reading inwardly – as you and I are doing now. The profound yet mundane activity of reading is something we do silently without necessarily being aware that we are reading, especially when engrossed. The difference was not lost on Plotinus, who in *The Six Enneads* explained how the experience of reading was like a flickering candle illuminating an elusive inner world which evaporates like a mist when we draw attention to it: "enfeebling and disrupting" the experience of being adrift in the flow.

We seem inescapably at odds with ourselves in becoming aware of our experiencing. In anticipation of Darwinian ideas of evolution, Georg Hegel believed that rationality and thus the discord of self-awareness had to have evolved from some unity: opposition was not where we started but is something we have become. Rationality is something we have achieved – an accomplishment of an embodied being – rather than an original state of being. So, the oppositions we perceive are borne of an embodied entity coming into awareness in much the same way as Kierkegaard speaks of angels waking up in the body of beasts. Primitive identity gives way to division because it seems human beings cannot but hold the seed of division within them.

Philosophical Divergence. At the beginning of the twentieth century, it seemed philosophy had taken two distinct paths – not just in terms of the methods used, but also the questions being asked. The *analytic* school – with its roots in logic and mathematics – adopted an ahistoric, third-person approach typified by the likes of Bertrand Russell, Ludwig Wittgenstein and Elizabeth Anscombe who argued that philosophical problems are often artefacts of pure reason distorted through the lens of language. Like any disagreement about facts, hopes of a resolution rely on a clear agreement between both parties about the definition of the question. It is only through clear and precise definitions and clarity of exposition that we can hope to avoid chasing our own tails, and more importantly perhaps, understand what a satisfactory answer might look like.

The contrasting "continental" approach is a catch-all term, coined retrospectively by some intemperate analytic thinkers – and Russell was notorious in this regard – who disliked what they saw as the woolly-thinking of those unlike "us". However, hardly any feature characteristic of one of the two separate camps is universally shared by all who belong to the camp in question. That said, there seems to be some distinguishing features among the continental philosophers.

Firstly, they seem drawn to the broader, knottier problems of human existence, which appear to be less amenable to universal solutions, reduction to mathematical formulae, or dissolution through logic. The continental thinker takes it that that if one fails to understand the importance of the first-person lived experience of a predicament, then we fail to understand the problem itself.

The continental tradition is also marked by a vivid awareness of how problems are shaped by their historical context: this temporal turn affirms our historicity and the importance of interpretation (hermeneutics). The continental approach also has a recurrent commitment to transcendental reasoning. There is the matter of the non-humans we share the planet with, and our experience of transcendence – or God.

Science is certainly useful and even helpful beyond its normal activity of solving puzzles, taking things apart to see how they work, and assuring predictability. But continental thinkers are adamant that matters of existence will not be settled by empirical facts and logic alone. Scientific facts will not, for example, help me understand the human experience of depression, trauma, racism, or the meaning of living a fulfilling life.

A further commonality among the continental philosophers – though it must be said that many of those categorised in this way do not see themselves as *doing* "continental philosophy" – is that they tend to be social critics. If I see depression as little more than a chemical imbalance, then the meaning of a person in their context (i.e., historicity) is irrelevant. The continental thinker is thus bound to place an emphasis on the historical and social dynamics of a phenomenon which may exacerbate our existential issues: ethics, politics, and social criticism in general are implicit to the continental approach.

As if to emphasise the risk of categorical distinctions, and separating life into polarities, Wittgenstein famously gave away his immense fortune so that he could live the ascetic life of one who reflects. Russell went to prison for his dissent about the First World War and championed anti-imperialism and educational reform. Anscombe argued against the award of an honorary degree by the Oxford University to Harry Truman. Though not a pacifist, Anscombe made the philosophical distinction between conducting an *intentional* act (i.e., killing large numbers of civilians using a nuclear weapon) in the hope of achieving a strategic outcome and the strategic bombing of military targets with foreseeable – yet *unintentional* – civilian casualties. The analytic *credo* – *faith* in reasoned argument, *hope* for reasoned agreement, and *clarity* of reasoned expression seems entirely compatible with the continentalist commitment to historicity. In the context of a life lived, precision and depth seem readily synthesised.

But let us take a moment to notice something about the differences in approach. More properly, I wish to draw attention to the phenomenon of *aspect* to which I return later (Sections 6.4, 8.2, and 9.3). Ordinary language is deeply ingrained with metaphors of vision which serve to convince us that the ideal way of looking at a thing is to make my body irrelevant, or at least subordinate. As a beholder of an abstract view such as divergent approaches for seeing the world (i.e., analytic versus continental), I adopt a privileged, externalised perspective which hovers above the scene. This passive "God's eye" view seeks to represent things as if in their apparent innocence. It is a perspective where I become absent from myself, pretending to understand the world as if it were spread out before me as in a picture; I am installed yet uninvolved. This contrasts with the "continentalist" notion of *depth*, which depends instead on my bodily involvement, with sight being just one aspect of being fundamentally engaged in the world.

Therefore, there can be no absolute zero point of time or space from which to observe things, as if I were standing on the riverbank watching two incompatible torrents collide: in this case, the reason of Athens, and the revelation of Jerusalem.

Jerusalem and Athens – Symbols of Opposition. The Roman politician Cicero is arguably the founder of Western human-centred introspection. He travelled extensively throughout the Eastern Mediterranean during the first century BCE, absorbing the Stoic philosophical tradition and translating it into the Latin register. It is against this backdrop that Luke describes the visit to Athens of another illustrious Roman citizen, Paul (Acts 17:16–34). The passage describes no less than an early encounter between Hellenic philosophy and the historical revelation of early Christianity. Speaking both Hebrew and Greek, Paul was no doubt aware of Greek philosophy and adept at taking his message to the Agora. So, it is no surprise that his speech has striking parallels with the philosophical project of Socrates, drawing attention to our lack of irrefutable knowledge.

But unlike Socrates the agnostic, Paul conveyed the message of a God whom the Athenians had – through their philosophising – been unsuccessfully groping towards. In exposing the Athenians' lack of knowledge, Paul proposed that their worship of idols was misguided. The true God was already revealed to history, calling humanity to repent of their ignorant practices and to go beyond the limits of what could be achieved through human introspection alone. The author of Acts had already begun to explore the synthesis of reason and revelation.

Few theologians of the early Latin Church are more maligned than Tertullian (160–225), who is typically presented as personifying religious anti-rationalism with his paradoxical phrase: "I believe because it is absurd" (González, 1974). Tertullian believed that subjective faith *ought* to be supported by objective reason. If anything, the purpose of his theology was to avoid a discontinuity – dualism – between the realms of objective reason and subjective revelation, symbolised by the sites of Hellenic philosophy (Athens) and Abrahamic revelation (Jerusalem). In his paradoxical phrase, Tertullian is, in fact, proposing that we need not choose between *either* reason *or* faith as our source of moral authority. Nevertheless, the absurdist *credo* continues to play its part in the narrative of conflict between Enlightenment ideals of reason and belief.

The incompatibility of the world views represented by *Athens* and *Jerusalem* was infamously promoted by Protestantism, and in the nineteenth century by Freud, who saw religious belief as a form of infantile wish-fulfilment exempt from the scrutiny of reason. A yearning for spiritual fulfilment or contact with meaning beyond ourselves – transcendence – became for Freud a pathology. What seems so remarkable about the persistence of this perspective is not so much that it constitutes a serious critique of religion. It is that it promotes a distorted ideal of what ought to replace religion, namely *scientism*.

By scientism, I do not mean that methods and procedures of empirical science can replace religious belief per se, but that that the methods of science are sufficient to establish the truth of the existential matters which lie before us. Like religion, scientism requires a leap of faith, because there is no conclusive evidence that empirical science can arbitrate on the complexities of existence.

As if to remind us that history is the supportive ground on which the present is rooted, Tertullian understood that what affords a perspective dignity is not that it is necessarily right, but like scientism in the modern age, it has prestige. Athens and Jerusalem are metaphors not of the opposition but of the tension between alternate modes of truth seeking, namely facts conforming to reason or reason conforming to facts (Gadamer, 2013: 278–397).

For example, the paradox at the heart of theodicy "How can God be good, omniscient and omnipotent if evil exists in the world?" can be approached in two ways. A spiritual pre-modern person living in a menacing and enchanted world of spirits and supernatural beings would make an appeal to God as helper while at the same time acknowledging that the ultimate plans of God were beyond the understanding of mere mortals. For a spiritual pre-modern, reason conforms to the facts.

When the question is set in the context of Athenian reason, which is close to what we would recognise today as the methods of empirical science, then nothing is certain if there can be doubt. The disengaged reasoner has a far greater sense of what a rational supernatural being ought to be about, in which case God always fails the test of being good, omniscient, and omnipotent. Facts conform to reason, and as Athens would have it, only that which can be understood and logically stated can be true.

Take for instance the original ontological argument of Anselm – Benedictine Archbishop of Canterbury (1077) – which firstly assumes that the Divine is greater than anything we can imagine. The argument then pivots on a second premise: whatever can be understood already exists in understanding. When we combine this with something already known about God: "nothing greater can be conceived", then we have it that the greatest being that can be conceived does not exist – which is paradoxical. Reason thus folds back onto itself, reducing God to a word puzzle, which is not necessarily problematic, merely inevitable because the nature of God is so *different* that human reflection cannot hope to grasp such a concept.

## 3.2 Jerusalem – Inward Lies the Road to God

When we consider potential blind spots in counselling and psychotherapy we at once think of race, gender, class, and sexuality, but it is rare for there to be any serious fuss made about spirituality and transcendence. Yet these features are at the centre of how we ascribe meaning to our lives. The transcendent is a vital source for psychotherapists to be acquainted with because the spiritual beliefs of a client, even if not clearly articulated, typically constitute the wellspring or sources of moral good by which we view ourselves, others, and the world in which we live. Without understanding another's spiritual or moral perspective, therapists are working with an entire value system, even a spiritual other, left outside the room.

Decades ago, while on a transcontinental flight in the United States, I was taken to task by an inquisitive neighbour who became agitated by the title of the book I was reading: *A History of God* by Karen Armstrong (1993). "What do you mean … God can't have a history because God is eternal" I was told. And that person was right. The ineffable reality of God is understood to be beyond time and change. Yet, the human idea of God has a history since it has always meant different things to different peoples across different times, and in different places.

God has been an essential part of the human experience of finding value and meaning in this beautiful yet terrifying world. When one understanding of God ceases to have meaning or relevance, it seems to have been quietly discarded and replaced with a new theology. The fundamentalist would deny this since fundamentalism is anti-historical; it sees the experience of God for a human being three thousand years ago to be the same as it is today. Here, I begin to explore a form of knowing beyond science and not as something merely tagged onto a primordially secular world but as a foundational human activity. The startling idea that we will continually return to is that not all theistic religions or belief systems require a God (i.e., humanism).

On the road from Plato to the disengaged reason of Descartes and the self inadvertently punctuated from the material world stands the illustrious Augustine of Hippo (354–430). Until his conversion to Christianity, Augustine was an adherent of the teachings and philosophy of the Persian prophet Mani (c 216–276) who sought to account for human depravity and the structure of the cosmos itself in terms of the struggle between rigidly polarised forces of good and evil.

The Manichean perspective was considered heresy by the early Christian church. It flirted with theodicy, which suggests an immaterial yet non-omnipotent God embodying all that is good standing by while *Evil* wreaks havoc on the material world. In his *Confessions,* Augustine describes the basis of his ultimate rejection of the Manichean cult. Influenced by the writings of Cicero before him, Augustine combined the humanistic notion of an indwelling agency, with the desire to live a virtuous life (Augustine, 2021: X):

> It is not me that sins, but some other nature that sins in me; and it delighted my pride to be free from blame … But in truth it *was wholly me* … sin was all the more incurable because I did not think of myself a sinner.

Though defunct as a religious system, the Manichean tendency to polarise the world into good and evil persists. Klein's concept of infantile splitting of the external world into those things which are "bad" and "good" is an example familiar to psychoanalysts (1946). Theoretical shortcomings aside, Klein's metaphysical insights into how we sometimes see the world and our compulsion to fracture and split demands – as she put it – an emotional and cognitive synthesis for mature human relations to flourish. The inner unity and wholeness to which Klein alludes was for Augustine the articulation of God as something discovered not from without, but from within.

To free himself from "that most twisted and intricate knottiness", Augustine abandoned all polarising Manichean notions, seeing instead good and evil, God and soul as integral and immaterial (Augustine, 2021: II). For Augustine, the principal route to God was not through the quest for an external transcendent object but an inward turn to the self.

As the road to God lay inward, it was a short step to worshipping an indwelling humanistic spirit. This radical reflexivity – being aware of our awareness and experiencing our experiences – brings to the fore a presence to oneself inseparable from simply being the agent of experience. Everything depended on a Stoic like transformation within. The intellectual inheritance owed by the Enlightenment to Augustine is that while the believer may live the same life as the non-believer, they have been transformed and animated by self-knowledge and self-mastery.

In deliberating on radical reflexivity, Augustine came to see the inevitable incompleteness of the endeavour of self-knowing: "*I have become a question to myself and that is my infirmity*" (Augustine, 2021: X). It was as if he recognised the limits of self-exploration and was willing to leave room for mystery. Unlike his illustrious successor Descartes, Augustine chose to live without a definitive answer to what confronts us – whether we call it God or indeed nothing. Augustine understood the experience of thinking as being in touch with a form of perfection, which at the same time was an essential condition of thinking beyond the scope and powers of what the thinker could attain. Therefore, there must be a higher being on which all things, including thought itself, depends.

But reflexivity meant more than the means through which intellectuals such as Augustine could prove the existence of God. The essence of religious piety was recognising the dependence of our innermost being on God; it was the basic support and underlying principle of a person's access to the highest moral standards. From the standpoint of modern moral freedom, progress was marked by this turn towards the self. Yet there remained an inclination to defer to some higher order which decided what it meant to flourish as a human being. The roots of the opposition between thought, reason, and morality, on the one hand, and a communion with ineffable desire, sensibility, and an abandonment of autonomy on the other were established by the Augustinian turn.

Belief, Faith, and the Transcendent. Human history has known a thousand faces of Gods, deities, religious and spiritual beliefs, rituals, and liturgies, which have guided how we conduct ourselves and coexist with each other. What unites them in their outlook is a view of what transcends and stands above humanity. Often identical moral ideals have arisen throughout time and place, which each have at their foundation some theistic, transcendental, or metaphysical root.

It is difficult to think of a culture that has not derived its convictions from a higher order beyond the reach of human reason, which transcends memory and records transgressions to which all were accountable in one way or another. From the perspective of moral philosophy, we need a single, perfect transcendent non-representable and necessarily real object to be the focus of our attention (Murdoch, 2007: 54).

Like many, my experiences of belief and faith were laid down in my childhood. As a cradle Catholic, I did not choose how or what to worship. The cassocks, incantations, smells, and bells, along with the sacred rituals of school and family life, influenced my early attitudes towards transcendence. Any distinction between belief as a set of propositions, and faith as something that enables me to trust in a set of propositions were confused with each other to the extent that they seemed conflated and synonymous.

But belief and faith are different. I believe that if I were to jump from an aeroplane wearing a professionally packed parachute and pulled the ripcord in sufficient time then I would float safely to the ground on a cushion of air. However, it is quite a different matter for me to take the unlikely step of leaping into the void with a bag of rolled-up linen on my back – just the thought of it makes my head spin with vertigo. Leaping into the void then is not so much a matter of belief; it is a matter of *faith*. Implicit, unexamined faith – things that we just "know" but cannot prove – forms the basis of much psychological theory, research, and practice, which comes about through epistemological, ethical, and ontological worldviews that we swallow whole (Slife et al., 2017).

The assumption that the psychological sciences adopt a value-free and objective stance and that therapeutic methods somehow reveal the non-interpretive truth of the world is scandalous, if not dangerous. My blind faith in a preferred method frames my client in a way that helps create what *they* are about. My methodological credo creates the lens through which my clients uncover, reconfigures, changes, or liberates themselves from whatever impediment to flourishing my theories propose: in this regard, we are all fish who fail to see the water.

Few question the innocuous practice of insisting that clients visit the therapist in their office, the "water" being that the client carries around distress in their brains from one context to the other – the disciplining social contexts which constitute our being in the world (e.g., home, work, cultural traditions, and community) are of secondary importance. Inviting someone into a beige office effectively sterilises a client of their context, moral sources, religious traditions, as well as isolating their "disorder" from its organic milieu.

The psychodynamic therapist remarks knowingly "Aha ...", as their client shares a picture of their infant holding a well-chewed toothbrush: "that's a transitional object". The parent, however, having been up all night comforting a teething child thinks twice about this interpretation. Two different people with different templates for seeing the world come to different conclusions about the significance of the same object - a toothbrush. Life, in some ways, imitates psychology, but as Alasdair MacIntyre puts it, our faith in our methods tends to "make them true" (1985).

When Freud made available to us the *belief* that our unacknowledged motives are an all-pervasive presence, we became seduced into looking behind and beyond surface appearances. We now search and expect to find – as therapists and clients alike – the hidden meaning of things as the often-unacknowledged instrument of ordinary life. We seem to have adopted an unwavering *faith* in the rightness of our position to decode the actions and words of others, more than others can perceive or acknowledge for themselves.

The religious beliefs of my childhood Catholicism offered little basis for me to accept or understand that earthly life was either good or meaningful, laden as it was with unselfconscious polytheism, idolatry, and no end of grisly reliquary. True to say that my ideas about faith and belief did not keep abreast of my deepening knowledge of other areas of my experience, especially science. This meant that notions of a creator God were quickly jettisoned alongside other childhood figures like Father Christmas, to be replaced by what seemed the reassuring certainties I felt came with reason and empirical science. Yet, with a more mature understanding of the human predicament and its unfolding complexities, my ideas about faith, belief, and transcendence have evolved beyond my school days. My exploration of other faiths and religious communities reveals to me how we are fundamentally spiritual animals even if many of us are less than eager to throw off our immature childhood experiences of religion and interventionalist patriarchal beings.

I am drawn again to Foster Wallace who offered an "outstanding" reason for choosing some sort of transcendent "thing" to worship, especially in the modern world. It is because anything else we choose to worship will eat us alive. If you worship money and objects, then you will never accumulate enough. If you worship how you look, then you will always feel unattractive, and as time plays its part, you will die by a thousand cuts when you see the young and the beautiful. If you worship fame, power, or celebrity, then only ever more will keep the fear of becoming invisible at bay.

For the retired CEO who joins the local golf club, it is never enough to simply belong – she must go on to organise and run the club. And yes, if you worship being clever then soon enough you will end up feeling silly and on the verge of being discovered as an imposter. It is not that any of these things are bad in themselves. I value my anonymity, having enough resources for my family, and swimming among the ideas and thoughts of gifted and insightful thinkers. But it is when our worshipfulness becomes our blind spot that matters tend to go awry.

The Leap of Faith. All systems of thought must start from a set of values or assumptions. This suggests that no system of thought –be it naturalist, constructivist, theistic or hermeneutic – can produce the set of values in which it is grounded. Like Anselm's ontological argument, some initial premise or leap of faith must be in place before logic, rationality – or whatever – can begin. What then is the nature of this beginning? The "leap of faith" is a term often attributed to Kierkegaard to describe the non-rational nature of the choices we make. It alludes to the spiritual presence that transcends all human-made systems.

*Fear and Trembling*, Kierkegaard's telling of the trial of Abraham – the father of faith itself – teases apart faith and reason. Kierkegaard examines the paradox of a faith which lies beyond, in the case of Abraham, a universally acceptable ethic – *thou shall not kill*. In the Biblical account, Abraham's faith is pre-given and his intention to sacrifice his only son Isaac is a direct consequence of faith, irrespective of the horror of the test to which Abraham believes he is being put to by God.

Kierkegaard chose this most shocking story of parental self-sacrifice to examine something which he felt we had either come to trivialise or were inured to, which is that each moment of our life is a potential trial of faith. For example, we can, to some degree, choose to see the glass as either half full or half empty, or consider ourselves fortunate rather than unlucky in life. Kierkegaard wanted to share his vision of the mind of someone whose ulterior sense of destiny did not coincide with the universally accepted ethic of human reason as the source of morality. This higher aim or *telos* to which Abraham commits himself becomes the ground of all things, even usurping the ordinarily ways of behaving as characterised by the utilitarian reciprocity of the *Golden Rule*.

The chasm between believing that "God is love" and thereby incapable of harming Abraham, while also being unable to fathom God's awful will as it operates in the world seems unbridgeable. The parallels with the Stoic tradition of there being some transcendent order beyond our understanding again reflects its congruence with Christian faith. It is the paradox to which the believers must simply submit themselves.

A rationalist would have little patience with Kierkegaard's Abrahamic suspension of ethics. How does one respond to the demands of a supernatural being who wants me to commit such an abhorrent act to prove my faith? If God did exist, and was therefore perfectly rational, I would not be asked to do such an irrational thing and thus you cannot be God! My point here is that faith need not be rational.

## 3.3 Athens – Disengaged Reason

The geometrical metaphor of *squaring the circle* alludes to the seemingly impossible task of synthesising expressive unity from the faculties of reason and faith. In antiquity, the practice of quadrature – as celebrated in Euclid's *Elements* – was not simply the triumph of human reason but the revelation of the inherent simplicity and beauty of the universe itself. The accomplishment of quadrature, or the squaring of even the most wildly irregular polygon using only a compass and a straight edge, became an expression of reason and order through the process of replacing the asymmetric with the symmetric, the imperfect with the perfect, and the irrational with the rational.

The Enlightenment's perspective sees a cosmos built on scientific reason and authority. It dethroned the transcendent to enlighten the darkness with rational humanity taking its authority from its own achievements. Freud's embrace of Auguste Comte's religion of humanity, which he named "positivism", is a pertinent example. In the era of modernity, the transcendent *Other* as the source of human identity and goodness was replaced by secularity and the shift to a belief in the God of enlightened humanity. This secular philosophical shift redefined religious virtues which had hitherto provided us with our moral guiderails in exclusively humanistic terms, rendering unnecessary a transcendent basis for what constitutes a good life.

Yet prior to the Enlightenment, it was obvious that reason and creativity were enmeshed processes. The compulsion to polarise is neither inevitable nor universal but an ingrained habit of the modern cultural and temporal context. The turn inward, which has many articulations and profound consequences, means that unlike our predecessors, we must take charge of building our own representation of the world and what a good life looks like (Taylor, 1989). This has implications for how we see ourselves as people, the way we "cure" minds with pharmaceuticals, our ethical sources in a time of burgeoning solipsism, and how we go about recovering what we have lost through this self-inflicted separation both within, and between selves.

The Loss of Perceptual Faith. René Descartes (1596–1650) saw human knowledge as possessing a fundamental unity or continuity – all types of knowledge could be explained in relation to all other disciplines. A famous image used to make his point sees human knowledge as a tree, with a descending hierarchy of importance beginning with philosophy as the roots, physics the trunk, and all the other sciences the branches. For this reason, Descartes was committed to establishing genuine reliability at the root of knowledge which could then be radiated throughout the rest of the structure.

The method used by Descartes for his philosophical enterprise was the scepticism of the newly emerging empirical sciences. At the heart of scepticism lay the radical principle of doubt: *rely only on what can be clearly and distinctly perceived to be true*. It was a crucial moment in the accidental separation of philosophy from the concerns of life. By proposing purely intellectual doubt as his method, the separation of body and soul became a tacit dimension of our experience. Faith in our bodily engagement with the world – perception – was inadvertently banished.

Our living bodies as mediating principles of thought and perception – combining both as they provide access to both – became "unloosed" from one other. The vivid imagery of Larkin's "Love, we must part now" captures the sadness and melancholy of such an inevitable separation – all things must come to an end, including the entwinement of body and soul. But while Larkin recreates a sense of nostalgia, "there is regret, always regret", as the two "tall ships" of mind and material broke free of the estuary once shared, embarking on their own individual courses, it need not indicate the failure of the relationship, but its evolution.

In the first of his *Meditations* – written in French rather than Latin for the lay person – Descartes pushed doubt to its limits to show, for example, how vision can lead us astray (1997: Part I). If we witness a total solar eclipse, we might be fooled into believing that the sun and the moon are the same size. This is clearly untrue. We are passive spectators of a remarkable coincidence of celestial geometry – the moon is 1/400th the diameter of an object four hundred times further away from itself. Nevertheless, we cannot wholly trust our senses. The entirety of my existence may just be a dream projected into my consciousness by a malign force – like *The Matrix*.

Be that as it may, I must exist to be aware of this deception, or whatever it may be. Of this there can be no doubt: as long as I am engaged in reflection, this moment of subjective certainty, then there is no doubt I exist: "*I think, therefore I am*" (Descartes, 1997: 92). Descartes had deepened Augustine's inward turn but instead of finding the mystery of God, he discovered the soul (mind) to be something of such universal certainty that it would prove to be the foundation of an entire epoch of Western culture. Thus began the Cartesian epistemology of science and modernity, with the verb: *to think* (*cogito*) – etymologically linked with the activity of ordering.

Even knowing that *The Matrix* exists and that perception may be programmed by a malign external agent (or *demon*) is to misunderstand Descartes discovery. You perceive first and foremost with the intuition of your mind. Centuries later, phenomenologists and existentialists would point out the problems of simultaneous awareness and reflection: does thinking less mean I am less? Do I cease to exist when I am asleep? Do I cease to exist when I daydream on my bicycle? Sarte and other twentieth-century thinkers would modify the Cartesian *cogito* to consider a pre-reflective self, which as we see later, demands a timeless sense of awareness that has the potential to be in the "moment", much like the sensation of flow that Plotinus spoke of in his *Enneads*. Nevertheless, the Cartesian division between body and mind has become deeply ingrained in Western culture.

The person who meditates is a thing that thinks, and that is what *you* are. This ethereal contemplative thinking thing (*cogitans*), separate from your body ensures that all material things – body, world, objects – could now be doubted. I can doubt the existence of my body, but my mind – by extension my soul – does not have the property of being such that I can doubt its existence. Thus, my mind is separate from my body.

Descartes points out that there is a whole range of thinking that this mind can achieve. It includes the realisation that a perfect, infinite, and timeless being must have bestowed this gift of thinking: an ontological argument for the existence of God which relies on firstly accepting the verity of Descartes argument. The body and mind, the material and the immaterial were entirely consistent with the contemporary teachings of the Church. It was still necessary to assume that the power of self-reflection through well-understood reason inferred the transcendent guarantee of God. Though the outcome did not deny the existence of God, the Cartesian conception of inward, self-sufficient autonomy prepared the way for the modern turn to unbelief.

The body became something *extensa*, a spatially extended thing in the physical world, divisible, and proceeding mechanistically in accordance with the physical laws of nature. Thus, except for minds – and of course God – interchangeable matter is all that there is. In denying uniqueness to other living things without a soul, Cartesian thinking implicitly evoked a mechanical attitude towards "every creature that crawled upon the earth". This would have dire consequences for our relationship with the other beings with whom we share this planet.

What seemed important was to ensure that the immaterial soul survived the body on death. The so-called interaction problem of Cartesian ontic dualism continues to vex contemporary philosophers and physical scientists alike, with the alternatives that follow being linked by a persistent desire to make some version of mind–body dualism work. What appears unshakeable is the firm hold we seem to have on the idea that there is a distinction between consciousness as infinite, ephemeral, and detached on the one hand, and a non-contingently related material world. This flies in the face of the common experience; the intellect is most certainly entwined with achy, inebriated, hungry, tired, thirsty, aroused, menopausal bodies.

<u>Cures for the Disembodied Mind</u>. One of the earliest radical statements of the Enlightenment embracing both atheism and materialism came from the lavish Parisian salon of Baron d'Holbach (1723–89). In *Systéme de la nature*, Holbach boldly declared that Man, like all else in the universe, was an entirely physical entity. Holbach's no-nonsense substance monism constituted a full-throttle naturalistic theory of humans: we are wholly material parts of the world with only physical laws governing our behaviour. It was simply unnecessary to search beyond the material world to understand the mind. While it may take some time, Holbach felt that psychological, social, and spiritual phenomena were all explicable through an understanding of lower-level mechanistic processes.

In the face of criticism that psychiatric diseases are equivalent to physical diseases, the psychiatric professional has sensibly distanced itself from any single and solely causally based *physical* model of mental illness. Nevertheless, research remains focussed on the *physical*, with greater emphasis being placed on matters of neurophysiology, neuroendocrinology, chronobiology, immunology, and more notoriously neurochemistry.

The growing sophistication of medical imaging, cognitive psychology, and advances in genetics reinforces the prestige of the medical model. Ever-changing conjectures about how electricity and xenochemicals may benefit our brains trumps interest in considering the harm they may do. This is cause for concern given the philosophical muddle at the heart of the matter. Until this is resolved, the administration of brain-modifying chemicals or high-voltage electricity will continue without understanding how or why they work. Such a lack of clarity hinders what we can legitimately admit from scientific research into our understanding of consciousness (Read & Moncrieff, 2022).

In the face of systematic reviews and meta-analyses which flounder in their material explanations of debilitating disorders such as depression, psychosocial models have appeared, and not without criticism (Ang et al., 2022). By suggesting some analogy between the material body (biology) and the immaterial mind (psychology), the concept of a mental disorder is stretched beyond the definition of a corporeal disease: the material body remains ordinate to the unchallengeable reality that the immaterial mind is enmeshed with its social world.

Biological psychiatry adopts a similar perspective – seeing dysfunctional patterns of human experience and behaviour in terms of explicable dysfunctional physical systems centred in the brain. However, despite its enthusiasts, ontic monism encounters serious challenges in the real world of complex dynamic systems, such as human consciousness and other physical and social assemblages. This is because complex systems have emergent characteristics which are not explicable from a knowledge of lower-level laws. *Put simply, it is clear that more is different.*

The embarrassment of data collected during the Human Genome Project shows how any enterprise that seeks to discover the intricate patterns of causation in the dynamic and interactional complexity of living systems is doomed to failure. Like cognitive models, physical models have much to offer when describing psychological phenomena, but these accounts are silent when it comes to explaining why brain processes ought to give rise to consciousness at all.

The point is that no matter how detailed a materialistic or physical account may be, facts about structure and dynamics can only yield further facts about structure and dynamics. The existence of consciousness remains fundamentally an extra fact beyond these physical facts. The philosophical thrust for a revision of Cartesian dualism is the continuing failure of physical mechanisms to account for the subjective quality of experience: there are simply too many gaps between the physical realm as articulated by science and our lived experience. Consciousness must be accepted as an ontologically fundamental "extra ingredient", irrespective of its purpose or origins.

Emergent phenomena are understood as those that come about from lower-level processes yet are neither explainable, reducible, or predictable from knowledge of lower-level processes. Emergent phenomena are sometimes associated with nonreductive physicalism, a view that advocates the physical foundation of the cosmos while acknowledging that some things or properties that arise from a physical base cannot be reduced to it. Physical phenomena such as superconductivity, crystallisation, magnetisation, and superfluidity are commonplace examples which illustrate how the whole is not only greater than but different from the sum of the parts. This seems counterintuitive since we think that what happens at the micro level will influence, at least to some degree, what happens at larger scales. An artefact of abandoning the perceptual faith I spoke of earlier is that emergence *seems* counterintuitive.

Superconductivity is an emergent phenomenon which is real to chemists like me who capitalised on the effect to "see" what molecules are getting up to when they swim around in liquids. The same effect is deployed in healthcare diagnostics each time someone has an MRI (magnetic resonance imaging) scan. Yet infinite conductivity in a super-cooled metal could not have been anticipated or predicted by any theory when it was first discovered in 1911. This is what separates emergent phenomena from resultant properties and aggregates. For the latter, there is a direct physical link between the micro and macro that is absent in cases of emergence. Although we are yet to appreciate it, the twentieth century marked the transition from the age of reductionism to the era of emergence that focuses on collectives and their constituents (Gillett, 2016).

What this has to do with Descartes is that it seems clear that he ran together different concepts of what constitutes the mind, enmeshing the faculty of reason with the elusive experience of being in the world. All that we might call psychological, as well as consciousness itself, became rolled into "mental". So, while Cartesian ontic dualism entails a metaphysical distinction between the physical and phenomenal, its running together of the psychological and phenomenal suggests we must shift our boundary or point of demarcation between the material and immaterial if we are to consider issues relating to the fact that the mind is affected by the chemistry of the brain.

The approach tentatively regarded as offering the "best" ontology of mind, which maintains a separation between mind and body without the problem of interaction which vexes biological psychiatry is property dualism, also known as anomalous monism (or monism with windows and doors), emergentism, or supervenience theory. It maintains that there is just one kind of substance, with the mind having both physical functional properties, and non-physical properties (i.e., material *and* immaterial). Property dualism allows for the evolutionary emergence of mind from matter that has achieved a certain complexity, in much the same way that systems capable of replication – life – emerged from an oxygen-rich broth of amino acids, carbohydrates, phosphates, water, light etc. The difference here is that life, wondrous though it is, evolved through material-mechanical processes while mind and thought have not.

This makes it possible to interpret the emergence of mind from matter as a natural albeit astonishing phenomenon associated with the evolution of extraordinarily complex living matter. The mind is not only something new and different, but inexplicable in terms of the behaviour-material-functional characteristics of the non-mental properties from which it emerged. The advantage over both Cartesian ontic dualism and monism is that emergentism avoids the causal-interaction problem. Furthermore, emergence as a phenomenon remains fully compatible with the scientific process of refutation without precluding mind–body interaction, while capturing our intuitive understanding of the self. While being still scientifically open-ended, emergentism makes no direct appeal to a deity, yet admits the sort of ineffable, scientific piety of transcendence discussed next.

Let us leave the issue by framing the debate around selective serotonin reuptake inhibitors (SSRIs) in the context of emergentism. Here, we can admit that a change in brain chemistry has somewhat contestable effects on a person's mood (Moncrieff et al., 2023). This is compatible with the biological psychiatry thesis that psychiatric disorders are grounded in biological processes. The broader problem of specifying the mechanisms associated with the psychological processes of mood, or what Chalmers (1996) calls the *easy* problem of consciousness, remains of relevance to research into the treatment of psychiatric disorders. However, once such a demarcation is understood, materialistically oriented psychiatrists and clinical psychologist's alike need not lose sleep over the philosophically *hard* problem, which is *why* these mechanisms are accompanied by phenomenal qualities at all.

## 3.4   Secular Piety and Pastoral Care

Believing ourselves to be science-worshipping thinking things alone in the vastness of the cosmos awakens some sort of awe, wonder, or even piety. The quest for unity between the incommensurate theories describing the infinitely vast and the immeasurably small evokes for physicists an unselfconscious commingling of Athens and Jerusalem. The cliché of the scientist who sees the insights of disengaged reason, rather than detracting from the great mystery of life only adding to it, are commonplace: "science stretches the mind and enriches the spirit" (Green, 2000: 387). This secular piety emerges out of the remarkable fact that our capacity for self-awareness, language, love, and an aspiration for higher moral and intellectual achievements emerged from a vast, lifeless, indifferent blind silence.

The ambiguity of the term secular has become related to what it is it not, namely the classically religious. Formally, the secular stance was one of agnosticism towards religious claims, while at the same time critically engaging with the dominant, unexamined assertions of authority and truth which includes those of scientism. Yet the practice of secularism has come to mean the adoption of a polemical stance towards religious doctrines which paradoxically appeals to the hard-shell naturalist (Taylor, 2007).

The taxonomic term *paraphylum* describes what remains when we remove the things we need to build another category. For example, the invertebrates are a category that remains when we have taken what we need to build the category of vertebrates, that is, animals with backbones. We are thus left with a diverse paraphylum of things which have nothing in common but their *spinelessness*: worms, slugs, mosquitoes, crabs, octopuses, and coral.

In a similar sense, secularism has come to represent a collective term or *paraphylum* for the paraphernalia left over when we remove all the things that are obviously religious. We are left with a kind of scientism which rejects phenomena falling beyond the explanation of empirical methods. While not denying the existence of spirituality, its study as a neurobiological event washes out the core beliefs of most people, which is that there is a transcendent or higher order to which many of us have a real relationship. Secularity as a concept retains only the ability to reduce the complexity of life as we actually live it, seducing us into believing that we might someday experience the luxury of an escape from interpretive rivals.

Secular Pastoral Care. Freud's numerous essays describing both religion and metaphysical beliefs in unambiguously negative terms as illusionary, delusionary, infantile, and neurotic was a central part of the schism with Carl Jung who adopted a more positive perspective of spirituality. Freud's view of psychoanalysis as an atheistic science was founded on his description of it as secular pastoral care, a distinction which distanced his project from the practice of medicine, while simultaneously marking it as a successor to religiously based responses to the suffering of the psyche. In marked contrast to the genesis of other practices with affiliations to pastoral care such as social work and counselling, Freud's psychoanalysis has a strong atheistic form with little apparent evidence of the influence of his Jewish heritage – Jung's own lamentable anti-Semitic views notwithstanding (Gay, 1989).

It is all too easy to confuse Freud's hostility towards contemporary expressions of ritualised religion (i.e., nineteenth-century German Protestantism) with his more nuanced engagement with theological concepts, as characterised by his long friendship with the Swiss Pastor Oskar Pfister (Section 7.1). The early development and dissemination of Freud's ideas were often carried out by people with strong Christian commitments who sought to ameliorate what they saw as the tragic sense of conflict at the heart his project.

Hugh Crichton-Miller – founder of the Tavistock Clinic – recognised elements of Freud's critique of religion yet initiated some fundamental and highly influential challenges to his ideas. Ian Suttie, a colleague of Crichton-Miller, went as far as suggesting that "Freudian theory was itself a disease because of its anti-maternal bias" (Bondi, 2013).

Another key figure in re-framing the anti-religiosity of psychoanalytic ideas was Ronald Fairbairn, who, prior to training as a psychiatrist, was set for religious ministry. His reworking of psychoanalytic theory through the British Psychoanalytic Society argued that the paramount human drive was not pleasure or death but relationships. A Christian interpretation of human frailty became incorporated into the core of psychoanalysis. Put simply, the need for love was seen to lie at the core of the human condition.

Burgeoning post-war secularity in Britain created the ground on which spaces for religiosity were being expressed and practised in a different way to non-believers at a time when church membership was in decline. The development of counselling centres owned and run by churches, in which counselling was delivered by volunteer laity illustrates how Christians were able to disseminate the key ideas of psychoanalysis and reach out to communities regardless of faith, with little overt pressure to convert.

The traditions of psychotherapy emanating from the writings of Viktor Frankl, Roberto Assagioli, John Rowan, and Martin Buber, to name but a few, describe an encounter with human spirituality without implicating a supernatural entity or interventionist deity. Abraham Maslow noted that spirituality was a definitive characteristic of human nature and an essential part of what makes us human. Descriptions of "the human spirit" as innate and teleologically predisposed towards actualisation and fulfilment bear significant similarities to the formative tendency discussed by Maslow and Rogers (Benjamin & Looby, 1998; Maslow, 1970, 1971).

In contrast with secular humanistic thinking, Buber's psychological approach begins with his theology, which is also the source of its moral good. Secular interpretations of Buber's ideas by the helping professions tend to focus on personal fulfilment as the only goal in a world in which nothing was more important but self-fulfilment. The result is a flattened and narrowing of the conceptualisation of what it is to be human. While psychotherapy and counselling owe a debt to interpretive scientific paradigms, the shift from energy to humanity, from drive to love, and from instinct to relationship, all bear the imprint of a narrative whose roots lie not in Athens, but Jerusalem.

For Buber, relationships were the ultimate purpose of life, both with God and with others. This is not so surprising given how he was wrenched from his mother at the age of three, only to meet her again three decades later:

> I could not gaze into her still astonishingly beautiful eyes without hearing from somewhere the word *Vergegnung* as a word spoken to me. ... I suspect ... that all that I have learned in the course of my life about genuine meeting had its first origin in that hour.

He would come to call this deeply affecting unsatisfying feeling *vergegnung* by many names, including mismeeting with essential others, objectifying the other, or the *I–It* relation. You become an object, the creation of my thinking, or what I want you to become when I do not listen to your words from your perspective. Recognising how Buber had always searched for something he missed from not having a mother, he understood authentic human relatedness as a way to heal the pain of early losses as well as providing the strength to flourish (Ventimiglia, 2008). The notion of transcendent love lies at the core of Buber's dialogic philosophy, echoing the words of Kierkegaard some 70 years earlier: "when we love our neighbour, we do not love 'the other I', but the 'you'" (2009: 69).

For Buber, God was the ever-present Being, which becomes a human being in order to be known. God was not experienced in some abstract reflection but for Buber became known *through* relationships. Buber's foundational faith was that people may enter a profound experience of each other – and of the transcendent – by the actual meeting of the one with the other. He called this meeting the "*I–Thou*" encounter. For Buber, genuine relationship with any *Thou* manifests glimpses of the Eternal Thou. Thus, Buber's use of the word *Thou* has a twofold referent: both as a temporal *Thou* (an "other" person who can become *It*), and the *Eternal Thou* (who as God cannot become *It*).

In contrast to all other existing beings, the *Eternal Thou* cannot be reduced to even the loftiest conceivable objective image – a premise of the ontological arguments of Anselm and Descartes met earlier. When thinking about Buber's impact on psychotherapy, his religious convictions were paramount, because he felt that people become distressed *because* they have lost what makes them whole. It is God that has been lost, and for Buber therapy was a healing relationship modelled on the concept of an authentic dialogue, without which God cannot be known.

The considerable attention received by Buber's conception of the *I–Thou* relation has meant that other aspects of his social philosophy have been overlooked, especially the concept of the essential *We* which encompasses the larger realities of community living. Buber suggested that the being of a person is to be found *neither* in individualism, which sees us only in relation to ourselves, *nor* in collectivism, which fails to see us at all, as it only sees society (Meindl, 2021). This reflects once again the intimate unity of inner and outer life and how self-relatedness is inseparable from knowing oneself as part of a greater whole.

Providential Ontology. Sofie and Frida are sitting in a café discussing the existence of God. Sofie believes in providence; when she looks to the sky, she has faith in someone "up there" looking out for her. When Frida looks skyward, she sees only a cold and indifferent void. She explains: "look, do not get me wrong Sofie, it is not that I do not have reasons for disbelieving in a God … I have done my own empirical experiments … I tried prayer … but it just does not work". Frida goes on to explain how during a recent visit upcountry to see the northern lights she got caught in a freak blizzard:

> I had no phone reception, and it was twenty below … it was then that I clasped my hands and looked heavenward … if there is a God up there … I am desperate … I am going to die if you do not help!

Sofie looked puzzled by the story: "You obviously survived … after all you *are* here … you must believe?" "Oh, don't be ridiculous Sofie … luckily, the army were training nearby, and a couple of troopers just happened to find me and dig me out … no burning bushes I'm afraid".

When we wish each other "good luck", we invoke providence – the idea that human destiny is somehow subject to transcendent care. To avoid bad luck, we then "tempt" fate or defy bad luck with a pinch of salt tossed over the shoulder into the eyes of the onlooking devil. We even knock on our heads (wood?) to elicit the gentle tree spirits. To "break a leg" has its colourful counterpart in Italian: "*in bocca al lupo*" (into the mouth of the wolf) when undertaking a risky or hazardous task, to which we reply in defiance "*crepi il lupo*" (death to the wolf). There can be no such thing as luck, only "looking out", and we can even make our own luck.

The idea that our destiny is in our hands, that our success does not depend on forces beyond our control, and that it is all up to us affirms a certain ideal of freedom from irrationality that goes to the heart of human introspection. This exhilarating vision of human agency aligns with the morally illuminating conclusion that we get what we deserve in a meritocratic society. The shadow side of this lies in the beguiling promise of self-mastery and self-making. It emphasises the notion of personal responsibility and holding people to account, which seems reasonable up to a point. It is an ideal which respects our capacity to think for and act for ourselves. But it is another matter to suppose that each of us is entirely responsible for "our lot" in life.

A term such as "lot" points to a moral vocabulary which limits our belief in unbridled self-responsibility. It refers to the drawing of lots whose results are determined by luck, fate, fortune, or divine providence, and not our own efforts. It reminds us that there was once a time when the most consequential debates about what we deserved in life were not centred on income or careers, but on God's favour: something we could either earn or receive as a gift.

The idea of fate reflecting what we deserve is deeply rooted in the ethical intuition of Western culture. Theology suggested that natural events happened for a reason. Good weather, bountiful harvests, safe sailing, were all divine rewards for good behaviour; drought and disease were seen as punishments for sin. From the perspective of our scientific age, this way of thinking seems . Yet, such moral intuitions are – as I indicated earlier – not as distant as they first appear. Indeed, this outlook is the origin of meritocratic thinking because it reflects a belief that the moral universe is arranged in a way that aligns prosperity with deservedness and suffering with wrongdoing.

It invites a paradoxically anthropocentric picture of God, who is seen as spending most of their time responding to the promptings of human beings: rewarding those who are good and punishing those who are bad. God becomes accessible to humans and thus obliged to treat us in the manner we have earned. So, even in the presence of God, humans are seen to earn and therefore deserve their fate. Early Christianity abhorred this idea preaching instead that believers accept the grandeur and mystery of creation, without expecting God to dispense rewards and punishments based on what each person deserves. Insistence on salvation by grace alone inevitably became distorted through time and the rituals of baptism, asceticism, prayer, attending mass, and the performance of sacraments. Such social activities cannot persist for long without prompting a sense of their effectiveness for winning God's favour. At least that was how Martin Luther saw the Roman Catholic Church of his time.

The Protestant Reformation was born partly out of a rejection of the sale of indulgences – the corrupt practise by which rich people sought to buy their way to salvation. In rejecting salvation by good works Luther left little room for human autonomy or self-making. Yet paradoxically, the Protestant Reformation unleashed a fiercely meritocratic work ethic, since every individual who was called by God to work on a vocation signalled their salvation through the intensity of their efforts. A disciplined approach to work – consuming little and working hard – led to the accumulation of wealth that would go onto fuel capitalism.

A lifetime of disciplined work in one's calling ("doing the work" as earnest therapists like to say) is not the path to salvation, but rather a way of knowing that one is already among those selected for salvation. It is a sign of salvation, not its source. The Protestant work ethic then is not only the fuel of capitalism, but it promotes the ethic of self-help and responsibility for one's fate. The humility which comes with feeling helpless in the face of God's grace gave way to the hubris prompted by a belief in one's merit and capacity to re-engineer oneself.

It is tempting to attribute the triumph of self-mastery and merit to the secularism of our time. As faith in God recedes, confidence in human agency becomes more forceful. The more we see ourselves as self-made and self-sufficient, the less reason we have to be grateful for our good fortune. In public culture, there appears to be an uneven contest between fortune, and the more brutal ethic of self-mastery. The ethic of fortune appreciates aspects of life that seem to transcend our understanding and control, leaving room for mystery and humility. It is something understood in Ecclesiastes (8:11): "the race is not to the swift, or the battle to the strong, nor does food come to the wise, or wealth to the brilliant, or favour to the learned; time and chance happen to them all".

By contrast, the ethic of self-mastery and self-control places human choice at the centre of the spiritual order. Without renouncing God, evangelical Protestantism recasts Divine providence into a secular register through a shift from the covenant of *grace* to what Luther reviled most of all about Catholicism, which was a covenant of *works*. But these were not the works of sacred rituals and the "bells and smells" of traditional Catholicism, but secular moral strivings whose virtue still derived from a providential plan.

Being "blessed" has become a commonly used term, which blurs the distinction between gift and reward, with the evidence of being blessed equating to health and wealth. What could be more empowering than believing that our mental health is in our hands, and unwellness averted by self-mastery? The more we believe that our mental well-being is something wholly self-made and a product of self-sufficiency, then the less likely we are to care for the fate of those less fortunate whose solutions lie beyond in the communities to which they belong.

For natural scientists, psychology theorists, therapists, and clients alike who seek a theological perspective to complement rather than compete with psychology, the position of providential naturalism – a successor to Stoic paganism which also opposed blind luck – delineates theology and psychology as distinct academic disciplines with different methodologies while simultaneously proposing a coherent interrelationship.

In much the same manner as emergentism, it allows for science to explain nature – including blizzards and climate change – and for theology to account for the ongoing existence of such realities. Providential ontology admits the most broadly defined notions of theism to accommodate counsellors and psychotherapists who believe in God yet wish to bracket their individual piety. And without offence to that piety, to freely pursue practice and research knowing in much the same way as Newton did, that an explanation for God's creation can be offered without an insistence on extraordinary divine intervention.

No attempt is made in providential ontology to offer a theological explanation of the great mystery of life. Yet, it remains clear that on matters of divine intervention, therapists must know when to defer to clergy. My concluding point here is not about God or disbelief but dogmatism and blind certainty towards the sort of things we feel sure about. This includes our deep-seated assumption that we are the absolute centre of the universe, which is where we turn next.

## References

Ang, B. et al. (2022). Is the Chemical Imbalance an 'urban Legend'? An Exploration of the Status of the Serotonin Theory of Depression in the Scientific Literature. *SSM – Mental Health*. 2, 100098.

Armstrong, K. (1993). *A History of God: The 4000-Year Quest of Judaism, Christianity and Islam*. Vintage.

Benjamin, P. & Looby, J. (1998). Defining the Nature of Spirituality in the Context of Maslow's and Rogers's Theories. *Counseling and Values*. 42, 92–100.

Chalmers, D.J. (1996). *The Conscious Mind: In Search of a Fundamental Theory*. Oxford University Press.

Descartes, R. (1997). *Descartes: Key Philosophical Writings*. Ed. E. Chávez-Arvizo; Trans. E.S. Haldane & G.R.T. Ross, Wordsworth Ltd.

Gadamer, H-G. (2013). *Truth and Method*. Trans. J. Weinsheimer & D.G. Marshall. Bloomsbury Academic.

Gay, P. (1989). *A Godless Jew*. Yale University Press.

Gillett, C. (2016). *Reduction and Emergence in Science and Philosophy*. Cambridge University Press.

González, J.L. (1974). Athens and Jerusalem Revisited: Reason and Authority in Tertullian. *Church History*. 43(1), 17–25.

Greene, B. (2000). *The Elegant Universe*. Vintage.

Kierkegaard S. (2009). *Works of Love*. Trans. H. Hong & E. Hong. Harper Collins.

Klein, M. (1946/1996). Notes on Some Schizoid Mechanisms. *The Journal of Psychotherapy Practice and Research*. 5(2), 160–179.

MacIntyre, A. (1985). How Psychology Makes Itself True-or False. In MacIntyre, A., Leary, D.E. & Koch, S. (Eds.), *A Century of Psychology as Science* (pp. 897–903). American Psychological Association.

Maslow, A. (1970). *Religions, Values, and Peak-experiences*. Viking.

Maslow, A. (1971). *Farther Reaches of Human Nature*. Viking.

Meindl, P. (2021). From the Thou to the We: Rediscovering Martin Buber's Account of Communal Experiences. *Human Studies*. 44(3), 413–431.

Moncrieff, J. et al. (2023). The Serotonin Theory of Depression: a Systematic Umbrella Review of the Evidence. *Molecular Psychiatry*. 28(8), 3243–3256.

Murdoch, I. (2007/1970). *The Sovereignty of Good*. Routledge.

Read, J. & Moncrieff, J. (2022). Depression: Why Drugs and Electricity Are Not the Answer. *Psychological Medicine*. 52(8), 1401–1410.

Saint Augustine (397, 2021). *Confessions.* Harper Collins.

Slife, B.D. et al. (2017). *The Hidden Worldviews of Psychology's Theory, Research, and Practice.* Routledge.

Taylor, C. (1989). *Sources of the Self: The Making of Modern Identity.* Cambridge University Press.

Taylor, C. (2007). *A Secular Age.* Harvard University Press.

Ventimiglia, G. (2008). Martin Buber, God, and Psychoanalysis. *Psychoanalytic Inquiry.* 28(5), 612–621.

Wallace, D.F. (2009). *This Is Water: Some Thoughts, Delivered on a Significant Occasion, about Living a Compassionate Life.* Little, Brown, and Co.

# 4

# INDIVIDUALISM

## The Atomised Self

### 4.1 Introduction: The Transcended Animal

As Descartes would have it, to be human is to think and reflect. There is no experience that you have had in which *you* were not the absolute centre of. So, it seems natural to believe that you are somehow apart from others, and indeed Nature itself. This is the essence of our dilemma: humans are both *a part* of nature yet *apart* from it. One species among many species, and yet a breed apart. Biology binds us to Nature and consciousness separates us from Nature. A human is thus an animal that sees itself as having transcended its animality.

This sense of separateness, sacredness even, is something inherited from Western theology and then amplified through philosophical humanism, which forms the first part of this discussion. We examine here some of the implications of concurrent humanistic positions – there are several – which jostle for legitimacy in our modern world and look at how they shape the way we see ourselves as people first and then as therapists. What is common to all humanistic positions, however, is anthropocentrism – an over-privileging of human beings in the cosmic order of things.

Philosophically, *humanism* describes the modern subject derived from the Cartesian tradition of reason, logic, and thought. In this tradition, a reasoning being is also a moral being. We are a transcending species aware that part of being human also requires exceeding our animalistic heritage in pursuit of additional overcoming. A human then is an animal hungry for overcoming. From this ensues the trait of identifying the self as a secular deity, a source of morality – a worldview inherited from a Christian disposition. The human

DOI: 10.4324/9781003396161-4

becomes human through an encounter with the other, and it is this encounter that constitutes transcendence. Yet, humanistic transcendence "over-there" is crucially different from religious transcendence "up-there" because the former lacks both a sense of wonder, and an encounter with the sacred.

Implicit to humanism is the notion of autonomy, and the belief that humans are the measure of all things, and the makers of all meaning. Self-mastery provides the precedent for mastery over others and especially over Nature. Problematically for the condition of our planet, the latter permits the nonhuman world to be appropriated by and incorporated into the human world. The source of this humanist self-confidence is a belief in instrumentality, a conviction that anything produced by people must therefore be subject to human command.

A fundamental task of philosophical *antihumanism* is to argue that this is in fact not the case. We could call it the Frankenstein complex – our inability to master what we have created. Human agency is an essential prerequisite to humanism, as none of our creations occur in Nature. But to create something is not necessarily to control it, particularly not through individual action; this is something antihumanism upholds. Antihumanism also criticises humans for their self-importance and for overvaluing human beings and their achievements. But it would be wrong to assume that antihumanists disparage humanity or endorse misanthropy. It is a mistake to assume that being antihumanist implies a defence of the inhumane. It is not people then that come under scrutiny, but the process that affords the term humanism and all that has been done in that name.

Animals, things that are alive, the inanimate and the transcendent are not in themselves inhuman, but rather *nonhuman*. We also examine how we have gone about animalising the human in response to the opposite and historically influential tendency of humanising the animal, and Nature more generally. The sentience of animals – nonhumans – is a disturbing challenge to us as it invites humans to view animals as in some way imprisoned, evolving beyond plant matter like humans yet denied consciousness.

Nonhumanism alerts us to how we have domesticated other beings, seducing ourselves into humanising the animal as a tragic beast engaged in a bleak struggle that it does not know even exists. In the shadow of humanising animals, of course, lurks our own struggle as dwellers in the dual realms of body and soul. It is in this category that radically relationality sits most comfortably because it assumes – contrary to the humanist – that existence, morality, indeed the actual being of a subject is predicated on the other. The chapter concludes with an examination of the philosophical concerns of nonhumanists as a response to Cartesian disengagement, which shapes the entire debate about how we do – or more properly – how we do not engage with each other and Nature.

## 4.2  The Humane and the Humanistic

It takes effort to see how notions like "human nature" and the "human condition" are creations of specific historical contexts. How odd it would seem, to cultures historically or ethnologically unlike our own, to separate out and privilege humans in the way we have done. The vagueness of the term humanism means it has become at times hostage to those with their own nefarious purposes. Prizing freedom while simultaneously advocating a distorted ideal of what it means to be human, saw humanism corrupted by the lenses of colonialism, slavery, fascism, and Stalinism. But despite its chequered imperial history – insofar that dominant communities define the ideal traits to which humans should aspire – we would do well not to reject all things linked to humanism.

I will begin by severing the semantic muddle – often encountered in counselling and psychotherapy – between philosophical humanism, and the universal doctrine of humanitarianism, the latter being understood as a benevolent, altruistic, compassionate, caring attitude towards human life. While the two are linked, the former usually involves a self-selecting group who get to define which human traits are to be prized above others. The term humanism has its origins in Cicero and other Latin scholars who deployed *humanitas* to mean a capacity to govern others well, however barbaric, or inhuman they may seem to those doing the governing. So, in that sense, the term has always had a link to mastery, irrespective of the purpose or object to which such mastery might be directed. A critique of humanism then is not condoning anti-humanitarianism or the anti-humane per se.

There are benefits to untangling notions of what it is to be humane – be it philanthropy, compassion, care, or beneficence – from the philosophically distinct predicates of humanism. A deep confidence in our ability to know and control Nature, through prizing the individual above all else, has not served us well. The idea of a completely autonomous subject as foundation prizes individual subjectivity over all else. Meaning becomes reduced to something uncovered within by the self, rather than something uncovered in relation to the context in which the existence of the self occurs.

Perhaps the greatest concern for those wary of humanism is the notion of a self-determining monad in whom resides the centre of morality – an ethic resting on some indwelling human sentiment, especially central to the theorising of Rollo May, Fritz Perls, Abraham Maslow, and Carl Rogers. Any philosophical turn which concludes that as individuals we have a private subjectivity, hence private morality, distracts us from the wider view that in fact we are inseparable from the world and its sources of culturally embedded morality, or moral goods. So, while I would not question, for example, the good of offering school-based therapy to children, I do question the wisdom of offering school-based *humanistic* counselling (SBHC), because of its philosophical foundations to which I turn shortly.

In his essay *What Is Enlightenment?* Michel Foucault reminds us that humanism is not a fixed term with a stable meaning but something understood as a collection of meanings and themes which vary depending on its historical and cultural context. The important question over and above what the word humanism means in a given context is why and how the meaning *matters*, and for whom (Foucault & Rabinow, 1991: 44).

At some point in the middle of the nineteenth century, a shift occurred in Western thought, which amounted to an alteration in the way humans understood themselves. The fissure impacted on a number of cultural domains, altering human self-understanding within the natural sciences, technology, philosophy, and literature. The question which vexed thinkers such as Jakob Burckhardt, Karl Marx, and Max Weber was: what were the conditions that made it possible or even inevitable for the social revolution of modernity and thus humanism to take place in Europe and North America? Marx found his explanations in the expansion of merchant capital, while Weber located his in the frugal domestic economy of the Protestant middle classes.

Burckhardt, however, found his in the Machiavellian Universal Man (*uomini universali*) who artfully navigated a regal path through the political and military intrigues of secular sixteenth-century Italian city-states. Commingled with this idea was the intellectual achievements of the Athenian independent states whose philosophy and poetry seemed a fitting ground from which to explain how the achievements of German culture had come about.

The notion of uncompromising selfhood and independence characterised by Burckhardt's *Renaissance Man* – gender being co-opted to mean all reasoning speaking beings – was projected retrospectively to rationalise the emergence of secular individuality set apart from theological determinations. The city-states of Florence (Amerigo Vespucci), Venice (Giovanni Caboto) and Genova (Cristoforo Columbus) symbolised Man – and more particularly *their* men – who set forth to discover, conquer, and then colonise the New World of the *self*. Despite their profound theoretical differences, the three broad waves of humanism coexist in the modern world and have in common an overarching anthropocentric perspective.

*The first wave of humanism* is usually associated with Burckhardt's Renaissance, which originated in Italy in the sixteenth century. Its promoters – *umanisti* – were educators reclaiming the classical Hellenistic legacy of poetry, rhetoric, and philosophy. It was to Psalm 8 (5–8) that the *umanisti* often turned to justify their project: "You made him (man) a little lower than the heavenly beings ... ruler over everything". It conveniently ignored Biblical imperatives – commandments – which have at their core humility, which warn humans against the worst excesses of humanism. For advocates of this movement, the goal was to develop neo-Aristotelean moral and intellectual virtues, such as benevolence, compassion, judgement, and prudence. The rediscovery of Hellenic pantheistic thinking offered an escape from the dominant medieval Christian tradition and more generally provided a shift of the moral and intellectual domain from the celestial to the terrestrial.

*The second wave* is related to the Enlightenment and has its roots in northern Europe with influential thinkers such as Locke, Hume, Voltaire, Rousseau, and Kant. Beyond their differences, these thinkers shared a vision of human beings as rational and autonomous agents. In addition, there was concord in seeing human flourishing through the rejection of oppressive religious authority and arbitrary power. They regarded themselves as secular, tolerant, sceptical, and unrestrained by external moral goods. Reason, for them, is what drives critical thinking and allowed access to truth.

Humanism was therefore emancipatory because it freed us from ignorance and prejudice. The sum of these ideas was a universalist claim to values, which should be applied throughout the world. Unsurprisingly, moral and political universalism became a feature of Western domination. This is particularly the case in colonial and imperial contexts, where liberal arguments often serve to justify conquest and oppression. It is a model which is still found in contemporary discourses relating to human rights and twenty-first century military "adventures" which seek to export democracy or some other "order" to those who need "our" liberation. Then as now, such projects fail miserably in their implementation and not just because they ignore the legitimacy of moral and political orders elsewhere.

In common with other Christian Renaissance thinkers, Michel de Montaigne argued that there was a plague (*a peste*) on man, namely, the opinion that he knew anything: "Oh what a vile and abject thing is man if he does not rise above humanity" (Montaigne & Screech, 1987: 189). Montaigne – anointed the "French Socrates" by the Vatican – understood the impermanent nature of humanity and the folly of mistaking opinion for knowledge. This was in line with Christian assurances that true wisdom was to be found in the lowly, the meek, the humble, and the simple. Yet the French Socrates became for the free thinkers of the Enlightenment the vanguard of sceptical Deism, even atheism. Prior to this, it had been assumed that God had a higher purpose for us beyond the drama of our fleeting moment on earth, a notion which has and continues to provide consolation for countless human beings.

But a striking anthropocentric shift occurred at the turn of the seventeenth and eighteenth centuries when the desire for human flourishing here on earth eclipsed any previous sense that there was some further, higher purpose waiting for us in a life after death. Truth revealed through God-given reason allowed us to see how mystery evaporates through the process of our deepening exploration of the self.

The more recent *third wave* of humanism is inherited from the Judeo-Christian tradition and is inspired by philanthropic characteristics and laws of the Divine. Initially a reaction against scholastic theology, it called for a return to love, beneficence, and theoretical simplicity. Humanistic therapies can be thought of as belonging to this third wave, and though it is difficult to summarise the characteristics of psychotherapies as such, the works of Rogers, Perls, May, and Maslow fall within this category. Voluntarily entering a relationship with another person's world of ambiguity and pain embodies the beneficence of humanistic therapeutic practice.

What should interest us is how we understand benevolence in our work as therapists, especially when volunteering or supplying our skills at low cost. Does our benevolence come about through some undischarged sense of obligation, guilt about our own good fortune, or the self-satisfaction of feeling useful to an appreciative client? If benevolence is only powered by negative forces, then is it really an affirmation of another being? In the worst-case scenario, benevolence fuelled by pity, duty, or obligation diminishes the therapist and degrades the client. It is the notion of *care* – about which I spoke earlier (Section 1.2) – that retrieves what is humane and valuable about humanistic therapy from the atomising and "flimsy creed" of philosophical humanism (Murdoch, 2007: 46).

Despite its secular veneer, counselling and psychotherapy have long favoured humanistic ideals that are more obviously and intuitively philanthropic and rooted in a complex Judeo-Christian tradition. Compassion and respect for others, an emphasis on a person's ability to choose, seeing a person as unique and deserving of dignity while also having a distinct innate self-worth, are attitudes which symbolise the paradoxes and contradictions of the apostle Paul: simultaneously the refuter and archetypal insider.

The figure of Paul saw the world in ancient terms, and within horizons of what was possible at that time, holding views some distance from the expectations of modern liberal democracy, equality, and human rights. Nevertheless, the Pauline perspective challenges contemporary neoliberal assumptions about human worth, albeit from an irreducibly theological position. As an observant Jew, Saul set out for Damascus to persecute members of a sect who disregarded the Torah. Yet it was Paul the apostle who pre-empted the humanistic attitude of personal conviction over cultural expectations and tradition in the pursuit of emancipation (Barclay, 2020).

As Carl Rogers explained, a key characteristic which emerges from therapy is "the person increasingly discovers that his organism is trustworthy, that it is a suitable instrument for discovering the most satisfying behaviour in each immediate situation ... I am the one who determines the value of an experience for me" (Rogers, 2002: 118, 122). The practice of person-centred therapy thus became the enactment of Pauline humanistic philosophy. The notion of an inner voice or impulse, the idea that truth is found in our feelings, becomes not so much about what we find without, but convictions about what we find within.

the distracting buzz of social media, Kierkegaard recognised how – in an astonishingly prescient essay published in 1846 – "talkativeness is afraid of the silence which reveals its emptiness". Only when the sense of relatedness in society is no longer substantial enough to offer concrete realities can social media reduce human beings to an abstraction, a phantom, a mirage: the *public* (Kierkegaard, 1962: 44).

The idea of authenticity entails that we "find" who we are within the constraints of our context, which is our industrial-digital-bureaucratic society (Taylor, 1991). This links to another troubling element of authenticity, which is the primacy of instrumental reason, a kind of rationality used to calculate the most economical application of means to achieve a given end. The true measure of success becomes maximum output with minimum input. Once all structures, be they social, sacred, or solemn are swept away, then the whole lot is up for grabs and available for outsourcing to the cheapest bidder. Once the creatures and natural resources around us are equally stripped of their place in the chain of being, they too are available to be treated as raw materials or instruments for our projects.

It is almost sacrilege to suggest that we do not need to maximise profit. The race is on to demonstrate that giving our children therapy at school is cost-effective. But because the ethic of instrumental reason is so embedded in modern life, the social pressure to subjugate authenticity becomes hard to resist. At its most worrying for the practice of therapy, it is the kind of unreflective reasoning that shapes how trainee therapists calibrate their effort to meet the minimum requirements of an assignment, whilst simultaneously criticising training programmes for not being "value for money".

The temptation to make self-fulfilment – however we believe that looks – the most significant value in life, recognising few external moral demands or serious commitments to others, can feel overwhelming. The journey of self-exploration can manifest itself in the form of narcissism, serial superficial relationships, immersion in social media, and arguably addiction. Because we choose different ways of expressing our authenticity it does not mean they are all equal. What overrides different lives and makes human beings capable of being equal are properties that we can share and have equal value, such as love, emancipation, reason, or what Buber called dialogical "*I–Thou*" recognition.

The greatest criticism levelled at philosophical humanism by Foucault unfolds through the realisation that we do not acquire the rich language needed for self-definition on our own. I do not become who I am *mono*-logically, as if I were hatched from an egg with my taken for granted notion of a pre-existing self. Becoming who I am is a *dia*-logical process. It is something accomplished *through* relationship with others. Becoming and understanding who I am is a relational process; for the archetypical humanist, it is difficult to shake the sense that this is *my* world, and that everybody else just gets to live in it. The notorious paean to the self-absorbed atomised person penned by Fritz Perls captures something of the ethical relativism and relational isolationism consistent with the "authentic self" of humanist psychotherapies (Hamilton, 2013):

> I do my thing and you do your thing.
> I am not in this world to live up to your expectations,
> And you are not in this world to live up to mine.
> You are you, and I am I,
> and if by chance we find each other, it's beautiful.
> If not, it can't be helped.

## 4.3   Antihumanism: God Is Dead

The antihumanist position should not be considered hostile towards, or a negation of, humanism; both hold in common similar goals of intellectual clarity and emancipation from something, which in the case of antihumanism, is humanism itself. Friedrich Nietzsche – often considered the doyen of philosophical antihumanism – takes the paradoxical route of employing radical freedom to escape from the consequences of radical freedom itself. Nietzsche's credo becomes little more than a facet of the same ideology of which he was so implacably against. Mary Midgley makes the uncomfortable point too, that the heroic, radical, individual freedom of Nietzsche – and Sartre who we encounter later – which imagines the self to be radically shaped and determined by the active will – is a uniquely masculine idea of emancipation, historically reliant on the support of others who are *less free* (2003: 98):

> Women were still called on to remain hierarchical, feudal, emotional, bodily, and biological, in order to make it possible for the men to become totally free, equal, autonomous, intellectual, and creative.

Yet radical individualism was not the ambition of Nietzsche at the beginning of his career when he sought the mentorship Burckhardt at the University of Basle. Unfortunately for Nietzsche, Burckhardt was unimpressed by the younger man and cruelly rejected him, possibly triggering Nietzsche's own rejection of the academy and the downward spiral into which he entered. While humanists were cobbling together quasi-religious structures on the site and sentiments vacated by the retreat of Christianity, Nietzsche's denunciation of the modern order and what might fill the vacuum left by religious belief became articulated by the voice of a madman returning from the mountain top, entering the crowded marketplace to proclaim: "God is dead" (Nietzsche, 1974/1887: 95).

Nietzsche was sceptical of what he saw as the illusory and fraudulent pretensions of nineteenth-century humanism. His religious upbringing also left Nietzsche sharply sensitive to the coercive theology lurking within any "religion of humanity" or similar intellectual structures which promised secular salvation. For Nietzsche, what lay concealed beneath well-meaning ideals such as universal altruism, unconditional positive regard and compassion was a tendency towards either unexamined or worse, disreputable motivations. The death of God was not the atheistic taunt to believers as is so often thought to be the case. It is a warning to the inhabitants of Athens about the arrogance of disengaged reason which rejects the value of Jerusalem and what it offers in terms of meaning and purpose in an otherwise cruel and unpredictable world. In declaring that "we have killed him [God]" through modernity's preference for detached rationality, Nietzsche was not just lamenting the death of theology but the demise of truth in all its forms (Hollingdale, 1999).

As Taylor notes, our spiritual hunger has not been *replaced* by a process of subtraction, but rather it has been *transformed* from a theistic to a secular projection (2007). This sublimation towards secular goals and the fetish of the marketplace means human beings have experienced both psychological distress and a fear of their own capacities, leading ultimately to a turn against one another and our own selves.

Given the extreme violence and humanitarian disasters of the twentieth century (i.e., capitalism, communism, and fascism), it is hard to disregard Nietzsche's warning that our way of living has forced a turn away from contact with the experience of being humane. Our obsession with the scientific stance and a preference for experiencing the world and others as objects has led us away from the reciprocity of meaningful relationships. For Nietzsche, a heroic transcendence – through the will to power – was the only choice available to the special few – not you or me – who could drive beyond despair and recreate themselves as the bearers of a new radical freedom.

The ultimate scepticism for Nietzsche – which we explore later in Chapter 6 – is the treacherous nature of language itself. The implication of linguistically created pseudo-problems as he saw them was that they form the basis of our compelling intuition about rational, self-assertive, technological humanism.

Third-wave humanistic theorists must be held to account for their unquestioned assumptions about a real world out there that can be understood by rational agents through language. It is not so simple as deciding what to say, and what we mean when we say it. It was Nietzsche who confronted us with the truth of the humanistic project: "Truths are illusions which one has forgotten *are* illusions, worn-out metaphors which have become powerless to affect the sense" (Nietzsche, 1973: 46).

The Nature of Reason. The irony of ordinary life – as Max Horkheimer pointed out – is that reason is something to which we give little thought (Section 2.4). The nature of reason appears so self-explanatory and obvious that any invitation to reflect on it seems superfluous. If pushed to give it some account, we might conclude that reasonable things are useful to us, and in the spirit of humanism, individuals can discern the things that are useful. Obviously, context matters and we are all aware of the perennial qualifier: "it all depends on...", but the force that ultimately makes any reasonable action possible rests on the faculties of inference, deduction, and precedent.

Yet the treacherous and seductive power of language is hidden in plain sight. When someone with whom you are in a dispute demands that you be "reasonable", it is you who become positioned as obstinate, through the act of resisting someone else's more powerful claim to a subjective understanding of the world. While instrumental reason may indeed lead to agreement or concord, it is also a matter of coercion. For some, reason becomes reduced to a tool in the service of some deeper purpose – someone, somewhere is acting in the service of their own interests.

Horkheimer understood instrumental reason as something preoccupied with the means and not the ends. Its focus was on the mechanisms of the means for achieving some goal irrespective of whether the goal was necessarily "good". Indeed, the goal is often that of self-preservation of an individual or group which takes for granted the "rightness" of their aim or purpose. Instrumental reason, it was argued, has profound effects on our society, dehumanising and alienating the individual who was supposed to be emancipated by humanism.

Concerns about the moral relativism of humanism and the ethical vacuity of instrumental reason which shapes and informs how we go about becoming actualised fully functioning people are side-stepped by the assumption that human beings are at worst neutral, and perhaps even innately good. Commentators argue that the humanistic emphasis on individuality and subjectivity are undermined by the current trend towards reductive, evidence-based systems of treatment which have at their core a preference for the objectifiable. Yet secular humanism – with its atomised, self-absorbed human individual at core – similarly represents a form of reductionism. As if hatched from an egg, we are considered an atomic human first, to do what we please, relate as we like, and get more of whatever makes us happy.

In ordinary life, the view of the majority becomes not only a proxy for objective reason but an improvement on it. With the authority and inescapability of scientific laws, we sacrifice our social interests on the high altar of investor confidence and populist convulsions. It becomes acceptable for all things to benefit from the market, where invisible, amoral forces weed out the weak and prioritise according to growth, productivity, and efficiency. That said, the COVID-19 global pandemic was not the first time Western states introduced job retention-type schemes as "the price worth paying" to rescue capitalism from itself. Ultimately, Horkheimer was criticised for failing to address the alternatives to this "instrumental" form of reason. How do we apprehend the reality that we are flawed humans, framed by our culture, and linguistically limited, driven by prejudices including an overestimation of the power of pure thought? Perhaps we might consider empirical reason to be an alternative?

Empiricism – The Scandal of Philosophy. When we wish to discuss what we imagine to be the real or objective world around us, we often resort to the term empirical to describe the methods that give us access to truth. It is a key tenet of humanistic ideology, which posits that only that which we can observe can be used to access the truth. Accepting such an inductivist view as the scientific view has been referred to as both the glory of science and the scandal of philosophy.

At the heart of the empirical scientific method that fuelled the Enlightenment is the epistemological bias that the past resembles the future. No number of white swans, for example, can allow us to make the universal claim that all swans are white. Yet having committed to the inductive view that all observable swans are indeed white, black swans if they appear are either ignored as an experimental aberration or dismissed as not being swans at all. When human experience is combined with empiricism, we arrive at a whole set of beliefs about how meanings can be reduced to laws (reductionism), the notion that bias is bad (objectivism), and why, in science it is only matter that matters (materialism).

Though formulated as (David) Hume's problem, it would be impossible to live in the real world without some level of extrapolation from the past into a possible – but not certain – future. To this end Karl Popper sought to make concrete the demarcation between physics (science) and metaphysics. Science can never be justifiable or verifiable – it can only be founded on falsifiable predictions.

Imagination becomes crucial in the creation of alternative pictures – metaphors – or theoretical constructs of the world around us. Popper recognised that all observations are interpretations of the universe, and that our theories are inventions of the human mind which nevertheless requires astonishing creativity and imagination to perceive alternative realties. Emphasising the point made in the previous chapter, Michael Polanyi states: "belief, and not reason is the foundation of knowledge" (2009: 23).

Popper introduced his demarcation theory as a profound philosophical move to retrieve metaphysics and philosophy from the humanists who would seek to dismiss all that is not "scientific". Popper insisted that a genuine test of theory is to attempt to falsify and expose it to the most severe of critiques until a better alternative evolves (Popper 1935; Magee 1973). Metaphysics thus becomes a picture of the universe (theory) that cannot be evaluated, for now at least. If we consider some notable examples of metaphysics that became an experimentally verified physics, we see the truthfulness of this perspective.

Before Copernicus, heliocentrism was a mathematical hypothesis – a metaphysics – without experimental evidence. Despite providing a plausible explanation for the turn of the seasons, evidence of the verity of heliocentrism had to wait until the seventeenth century.

For over four hundred years, Newton's theories of motion were corroborated by observation, and indeed an entire epoch of Western civilisation was built on his ideas of motion, momentum, velocity, and acceleration. Once Newton's *Principia Mathematica* became recognised as an important work, his laws not only formed a model for addressing problems, but tacitly made metaphysical claims about the nature of the cosmos, such as "gravity exists". Yet the limitations of Newtonian mechanics began to unfold in the nineteenth century when James Clerk Maxwell had to deploy alternative explanations for the weird – according to the Newtonian paradigm – behaviour of light.

With the development of Heisenberg's quantum mechanics and Einstein's general relativity, it became clear that Newton's physics was limited to the case of things that were not too small and did not move too fast. What Einstein showed was that corroboration does not imply that a theory is universal, and indeed the discontinuity between how we apprehend the immensely big (cosmology) and exceedingly small (quantum mechanics) in our universe has led to yet another metaphysics – string theory.

It sometimes requires fantastical flights of imagination to envisage alternative explanations for the world. The mundane example of a sewing machine illustrates the often-paradoxical relationship between common-sense experience and abstract scientific thinking. Anyone trying to transcribe their understanding of hand sewing to the workings of a sewing machine will understand with puzzlement that one really has nothing to do with the other.

It continues to be the case that metaphysics, that is, superstition, myth, natural philosophy, and religion, contain important anticipations of what we might come to know through experimentation. Popper famously uses the example of "God exists" as a statement that has meaning and could be true but because there is no conceivable way in which the statement can be falsified – for now – it is not a scientific statement. Although Popper clarified the demarcation between physics (science) and metaphysics, more work has to be done to clarify the sometimes-confusing overlap between metaphysics and pseudoscience.

With this in mind, we should be wary of ideologies posing as science which shun falsification, are non-criticisable, and are built solely on verification. For this reason, Popper was a vehement critic of Marx and Freud. Who among us, enamoured by our favourite theory, are tempted to see verification wherever we look? Like Abraham Maslow's hammer which describes the cognitive bias of over-relying on a familiar tool, it can be tempting to treat everything as a nail.

A commitment to antihumanism requires a precarious balance between avoiding both outright misanthropy and the simple reversal of priority that favours the nonhuman over the human. The triad of Copernican heliocentrism,

Darwin's natural selection, and Freud's unknowable mind undermines forever any human claim to autonomy and separateness from the rest of Nature.

## 4.4 Nonhumanism: A Relational Vision

In language which seems to anticipate attachment theory, Hobbes (1588–1679) – an early proponent of moral relativism and political atomism – saw that without some contract to civilise relations, life would be short, nasty, and brutish. Mary Midgley's philosophy is critical of such fragmentary atomistic visions of human nature and the self, emphasising instead a more relational or holistic vision of humans and our place in the world.

Midgely saw humans not as some isolated miracle but one in a wide spectrum of already intensely sociable creatures interested in each other, and eager to communicate. Reason and language are the products of our intense sociability because we are dependent on others, and almost certainly will never be really free or self-determined as atomists would have it. Of course, we have agency in the world, but the paths we forge are in a landscape of relationships and dependencies, many of which go unnoticed. We are, as Midgely states, intrinsically "members of one another" (McElwain, 2020). The radical relationalist then is deeply ethical because, though we value our freedom and individual pursuits, we are embedded within our inescapable connections to a wider whole.

<u>Human Nature and Impending Climate Catastrophe</u>. If we begin with the question, how many Natures exist? we move close to what we need consider. If we capitalise the word, then surely there is but one Nature and not several? Up to this point we have been discussing a sort of anthropocentric "Human Nature" ignoring the nonhuman, including the cosmos by which I mean the collection of all things that exist as far as we can tell. Most of us are aware that the Earth spins about the Sun, but practically speaking we think of the Sun moving around the sky in much the same way our prehistoric ancestors did. So perhaps it is obtuse to suggest that we go about our daily lives thinking about Nature in terms of quantum materials and dark matter?

Perhaps Nature is something far more familiar and domesticated like the parks and fields through which we walk our pets. A domesticated nature dependent for its manicured existence on the landed gentry, or golf. But what if by Nature we meant wilderness? Then it means something accessed through dolphin-watching and backpacking eco-tourism. Edward Abbey's *Desert Solitaire* (1968) sought to turn us away from the idea of Nature as something for humans to consume and enjoy. At the height of the Apollo programme, he celebrated inhospitable and dangerous environments which possessed an implacable indifference to humans. Nature for Abbey was something closer to what existed prior to its domestication by humans.

The ambiguities of how we understand our place in Nature set the scene for the Norwegian philosopher Arne Næss to formulate his relational ecology which sought to dissolve the *humans-in-the-environment* perspective by promoting the view that all living beings have an inherent, non-instrumental value (Del Mar, 2011: 63). At the heart of his philosophy was an attempt to dissolve the anthropomorphic stance towards Nature. The wellbeing and flourishing of both human and nonhuman life on Earth have value, independent of the usefulness of the latter to the former. Inspired by the earlier writings of the Dutch philosopher Baruch Spinoza, Næss separated ecological perspectives into *shallow* and *deep* to guide our relationship with Nature (van Meurs, 2019).

*Shallow ecology* points to a familiar humanistic perspective in which the nonhuman (i.e., the biosphere) is valuable insofar as it contributes to the flourishing of, we, finite pleasure-seeking humans. The ecological implications of human chauvinism and our alienation from the natural world flow from the Cartesian attitude of disengaged reason and anthropocentric ethics. What remains beyond the boundary defined as "human" is a mechanistic cosmos emphatically empty, neutralised of its meaningful order, or what constitutes the good or the ethical. Animals are little more than complicated machines that have not been afforded a soul, or mind.

The model of rational mastery over our environment, and the instrumental control which reduces the cosmos to nonhuman objects over which we exert our authority is an attitude given expression in Descartes infamous chauvinistic passage in *Discourse on the Method* (1997: 111):

we may find a practical philosophy by means of which, knowing the force and the action of fire, water, air, the stars, heavens and all the bodies that environ us … employ them in all those uses to which they are adapted, and thus render ourselves the masters and possessors of nature.

In objectifying Nature, we have declared ourselves atomised – separate from Nature and by implication all other members of Nature, which includes other human beings. There is no deeper unity between human beings other than the commodities we share or try to conserve. The Judaeo-Christian book of Genesis is also similarly instrumental in its attitude towards all that is not "Man", with both the Enlightenment movement and capitalism accelerating the domestication of the wild for the utility of humans.

*Romanticism* emerged as a counterweight to the excesses of the instrumental exploitation of our environment during the Enlightenment, emphasising instead the importance of emotion, feeling, and a nostalgia for loving Nature. From this developed an interest in conservation, not just because of the utilitarian realisation that Europeans were eroding the resources of the planet but as a Romantic anthropocentrism which saw Nature as a mirror of the Natural self. Romantic poets and philosophers such as William Wordsworth and Johann Gottfried von Herder found mystical enlightenment and divinity through their immersion in Nature.

Such immersive practices offered sanctuary for the solitary and sensitive individual to "wander lonely as a cloud", connecting with their own primitive forces and emotions in much the same way that therapies allied to Nature do today. With the Romantic movement came a ruthlessly circumscribed concern for animals especially among the wealthy. Sympathy and love for our congenial companions such as dogs and cats go alongside the industrialised slaughter of other beings thought useful for their flesh or hide, or simply because they constitute a nuisance to economic progress.

One of the central features of our imminent climate catastrophe is not the deliberate vandalism of our environment – though one could be forgiven for thinking this. It is our misplaced infatuation with and inflated idolatry of human ingenuity and technology. Both lead to an expectation that somewhere down the line we will "fix" disagreeable problems such as ageing, death, and even globicide. The road to globicide is paved with good intentions and innumerable platitudes about progress, prosperity, and economic growth. Uncritical enthusiasts of philosophical humanism find it hard to kick the habit of thinking about ourselves as top of the food chain, seeing Nature as an undifferentiated externality rather than a tangled web of relations.

With the veneration once attributed to Nature being transferred to humanity, philosophical humanism produces a startling notion of Man as some kind of supernatural being able to face the harsh existential truth of our cosmic isolation with a sort of Victorian "manliness" (Taylor, 1989: 404). How can a definitive solution to globicide be found when we rely on the excesses of capitalism to rescue us from the crisis it created? Perhaps is hope the delusion? The futility of resistance and the inevitability of defeat in the face of our predicament recalls Franz Kafka's quip to his friend Max Brod: "*There is plenty of hope, an infinite amount of hope, but not for us*" (Martel, 2011: 62).

Perhaps, for the sake of nonhuman life on Earth, we should take the impartial view that it is time for humans to gracefully call it a day? After all, we humans have impassively presided over the extinction of innumerable species, and our tendency to think of ourselves as anything different is simply another example of our anthropocentric prejudice. Scaring ourselves with the facts of impending globicide does not seem work. So, what will?

There seems to me little difference between appreciating an object of art or the aesthetic beauty of the natural world. We lose ourselves in art in much the same way we also lose ourselves in Nature, whether it be a rainbow, the web of a spider, or the sublime elegance with which matter organises itself in the emergent process of crystallisation. But is the aesthetic appreciation of the intrinsic value of what is nonhuman simply another anthropocentric judgement? If there were no humans – or more specifically aesthetes – would there be any value in a rainbow? Environmental aesthetics can easily collapse into a form of anthropocentrism, the very thing any aesthetic argument for valuing the nonhuman is designed to circumvent. To avoid this, another leap of faith is required.

Humans discover beauty; we do not invent it. A bold, radical, and unequivocal post-humanistic commitment is required to appreciate the value of the nonhuman independent of the human who apprehends it (see, Barad's post-Humanism, Section 7.4). Does the aesthetic beauty of light which began travelling to the perceiver 33 billion years ago diminish because I did not exist when it left its star? We can only understand the value attached to our aesthetic experiences of nature when we are aware of the necessary humanistic presuppositions that underly the content of these experiences.

A _deep-ecology_ perspective takes the view that all that is nonhuman matters morally in itself – *for the greater good*. Such a holistic approach helps us see that it is morally permissible for the flourishing of an individual human being, or cat for that matter, to be secondary to the flourishing of some greater entity whether we call it the biosphere, the infinite, or the cosmos. The cosmos – or if we are practical makers of policy – the ecosystem, is considered an object of value for the sake of itself, and so the role played by a finite individual in relation to the whole must be considered with respect to their overall contribution to the whole (Section 1.2).

Writers such as James Lovelock and Freya Mathews regard the global ecosystem as a kind of self with its own in-built mechanism for self-actualisation, referring to it by the name of the Greek Goddess *Gaia*. For now, this is metaphysics: perhaps one day some higher-order sentience or psychology will be attributed to our ecosystem, but currently there seems little appetite to extend an ethical framework to Gaia as a person, when in fact we should see Gaia as a metaphor for the greater good.

Problems follow when we venerate the whole, or "Gaia", at the expense of the diverse, the plural, or what constitutes the individuated family of beings. In this sense, the finite is related to – but is nevertheless different from – the infinite. How do I evaluate in terms of Gaia the relative value of my individual efforts to become vegan? Holism has the problem of separating the category of the infinite (cosmos, Gaia … whatever) from the particular – say my stopping in the street to pick up a piece of litter. The infinite stands in indifferent opposition to the existence of singular me. Conversely, no engagement with the particulars of me will necessarily provide me with insights about the concept of the infinitude of Nature as a whole. It seems then that our ability to extend ethical rights to other beings or things from a holistic perspective is both contingent and inconsistent.

It is unlikely to motivate a massive de-mobilisation of industry, the winding back of producing more plastic widgets for landfill, or the immediate reversal of population growth to head-off ecological catastrophe. No wonder some feel disenchanted by our alienation from Nature. There appears to be a chasm separating the deep infinitude and the shallow finite sides of the deep ecology argument. To strive towards some organic whole (infinity), we are asked to lose sight of or deny the entrenched idea of the individual.

The ecological philosophy of Arne Næss was grounded in his reading of Spinoza who considered Nature to be an infinite whole formed by individual things, which includes me and you. Nature for Spinoza was an expression of, as opposed to the creation of what he sometimes called God. Here lies both a dependency on, yet difference between the finite, say a person, and the infinite which we can call Nature, God, or the Cosmos. This reciprocal immanence, or doctrine that the transcendent encompasses or is manifested in the material world, is the struggle of the relation between the infinite and the finite. How can an infinite creation emerge from a finite number of beings? How does something finite, such as a human being relate to the infinite? At what point do I become infinite? This is the unintelligible circularity of Næss' understanding of Spinoza, and a form of dualism which must be overcome before we can grasp how humans may adopt a radical relationality with Nature.

Nature is not a static background, but a dynamic whole of which we are part. Seeing ourselves as part of this larger community is not an illusion, but an intelligent understanding of the planet, its systems, and its inhabitants. For Næss, Nature was a coin with one side representing eternity, and the other side being the sum of all individual finite things constituting infinity. Focussing on particulars – for example, an atomised human being – and then attempting to work all the way up to infinity never brings us to a total view which equates to Nature as something eternal.

In truth, this type of understanding never leaves the level of particularity, a totality of things, a finite Nature. Whilst the two sides of the coin stand in relationship with each other, they are dependent yet different: Nature as infinity is more than the sum of its parts. Equally, Nature, Gaia or whatever we wish to call it cannot be considered on its own as it only becomes manifest through all the things that partake in *being*.

Radical Relationality and Nature. Friedrich von Schelling (1775–1854) understood Nature to be an *infinite becoming* and it was the task of his philosophy to understand how finite beings could identify with this process. This is not only useful, but essential. Individual actions can seem futile given the magnitude of the infinite. But without building a collective awareness, a sense that change is possible in the face of the overwhelm of globicide, and the various assaults on the common good, belief in individual contributions towards systemic progress perish. But just as tipping points in climate change exist, so too do social tipping points.

For von Schelling, the totality of objects in Nature are not just the products of Nature: they simultaneously and necessarily *become* Nature. Unlike Næss, von Schelling never allows a finite individual product, and the infinite productive Nature to separate; they are *radically relational*, never apart. As an individual I am not just a product of humankind, I am necessarily a part of producing humankind – humankind is nothing but the *becoming-manifest* of me as an individual. The infinite character of Nature is not a thing on its own, but *being itself*, something which only becomes manifest through the things, such as myself and you the reader, which take part in it.

Nature is not a dead object waiting to be exploited by me, or a stage on which I play. Nature as a whole is a vibrant dynamic unconcealment of the universe which means that Nature is not yet completed but is still arriving – it is *becoming*. Within this unmasterable experience of the cosmos falls both the limit and limitlessness of human presence, before which we both fall silent, and are yet driven to find a home for ourselves.

The infinite cosmos could be thought of as a monument of those activities interacting with one another as a shape emerging from a continuously dynamic, underlying process. For Schelling, the finite is not the flip side of the infinite, but is the self-construction of the infinite, its spontaneous concealment; it is the coin itself. An apt metaphor involves thinking of how a whirlpool becomes visible as a relatively static figure in turbulent flowing water. Though made of innumerable water molecules and bubbles of air, it takes the shape of movement. Just like the whirlpool, all things in Nature emerge from a configuration of finite things moved by underlying forces that are not just their sum, but rather the dynamics in which they engage. It is their rhythm or the idea of change itself that is what endures in the change.

In the poem *Wodwo*, Ted Hughes hauntingly recreates the process of the finite becoming manifest in Nature. A creature – a voice, consciousness, a sense of touch and smell – exploring its environment, feeling for texture and response, mapping the fluid boundaries of being. The poem is about *being* as dynamic movement, not static destination, seeking not finding. Appealing to a Schellingian notion of infinite unfolding as we seek to make sense of ourselves and our place in the world, there is no climactic discovery of self; the ending of the poem, like Nature itself lacks closure.

## References

Barclay, J.M.G. (2020). What Makes Paul Challenging Today? In: Longenecker B.W., ed. *The New Cambridge Companion to St. Paul*. Cambridge University Press.

Del Mar, P. (2011). *Environmentalism*. Routledge.

Descartes, R. (1997). *Descartes: Key Philosophical Writings*. Ed. E. Chávez-Arvizo; Tr. E.S. Haldane & G.R.T. Ross, Wordsworth Ltd.

Foucault, M. & Rabinow, P. (1991). *The Foucault Reader*. Penguin.

Hamilton, R. (2013). The Frustrations of Virtue: the Myth of Moral Neutrality in Psychotherapy. *Journal of Evaluation in Clinical Practice*. 19(3), 485–492.

Hollingdale, R.J. (1999). *Nietzsche: The Man and His Philosophy* (Revised ed.). Cambridge University Press.

Kierkegaard, S. (1962/2019). *The Present Age: On the Death of Rebellion*. Trans. Alexander Dru. Harper Collins.

Magee, B. (1973). *Karl Popper.* Fontana Press.

Margolin, L. (2020). Rogerian Psychotherapy and the Problem of Power: A Foucauldian Interpretation. *Journal of Humanistic Psychotherapy.* 60(1), 130–143.

Martel, J.R. (2011). *Kafka: The Messiah Who Does Nothing at All, in Textual Conspiracies.* University of Michigan Press.

McElwain, G.S. (2020). Relationality in the Thought of Mary Midgley. *Royal Institute of Philosophy Supplement.* 87, 235–248.

Midgley, M. (2003). *The Myths We Live By.* Taylor & Francis.

Montaigne, M.De & Screech, M.A. (1987). *An Apology for Raymond Sebond.* Penguin.

Murdoch, I. (2007/1970). *The Sovereignty of Good.* Routledge.

Nietzsche, F. (1973). *The Portable Nietzsche.* Trans. Kaufmann, W. Chatto and Windus.

Nietzsche, F. (1974/1887). *The Gay Science; with a Prelude in Rhymes and an Appendix of Songs.* Trans. Kaufmann, W. Vintage Books.

Polanyi, M. (2009/1966). *The Tacit Dimension.* University of Chicago Press.

Popper, K. (1935/2002). *The Logic of Scientific Discovery.* Routledge.

Rogers, C.R. (2002/1961). *On Becoming a Person: A Therapist's View of Psychotherapy.* Constable.

Taylor, C. (1989). *Sources of the Self: The Making of Modern Identity.* Cambridge University Press.

Taylor, C. (1991). *The Ethics of Authenticity.* Harvard University Press.

Taylor, C. (2007). *A Secular Age.* Harvard University Press.

van Meurs, B. (2019). Deep Ecology and Nature: Næss, Spinoza, Schelling. *The Trumpeter.* 35(1), 3–21.

# 5

# FREEDOM

## Ethics and Existentialism

### 5.1 Introduction: Modern Solutions to Age-Old Problems

Liberal individualism, shaped by utilitarian and Kantian ethics, has become seamlessly and uncritically woven into the fabric of therapy. At a practical level, its insistence that human action is self-interested becomes a gloomy, self-fulfilling prophecy that impoverishes our ability to respect and value others. Perhaps this is why many argue that modern therapy perpetuates the problems it seeks to resolve. To some extent, it may even exacerbate emotional isolation, undue self-absorption, and the kind of superficial living that contributes to so much disenchantment and human distress in our modern Western culture.

In this sense, contemporary therapeutic – especially biomedical – models with their liberal humanist discourses, seem to be inapt modern solutions to age-old problems. Ever more liberation, personal self-realisation, and empowerment are offered to those who already feel disconnected and ashamed about feeling responsible for their own predicaments. What is needed by those who yearn for radical relationality is substantial human contact, a broader sense of purpose, greater simplicity, and perhaps a credible transcendence. To move in this direction, psychotherapy needs to abandon its claim to ethical neutrality or even value-free scientism, because the truth of the matter is that every piece of theorising and each expression of belief is an ethical and political action.

The terms "morals" and "ethics" are often used interchangeably, but it can be useful sometimes to distinguish between them. I think of morality as something individual – personal even – and in reference to justice between agents, or what we owe one another. Ethics, on the other hand, can mean something more communal and is related to aspects of a fulfilled, fully realised human life. Ethics are the ends to which we strive and the fulfilments

DOI: 10.4324/9781003396161-5

to which being human recommends. Creating just and mutually respectful relationships – for example – is an essential moral end for ethical living.

The moral agent should not be confused with the moraliser, the well-intentioned therapist, friend or family member who, without insight or invitation, imposes their values on others, thereby communicating a heartfelt – it is always from the heart – belief that: "You are not doing well enough". The therapist as a moral agent respects a client's autonomy and freedom of choice, rather than authoritatively insisting – as a moraliser does – on the superiority of their own position.

In this chapter, I ask what it is to be an ethical moral therapist and not a moraliser? The question invites a deeper reflection on psychotherapy's place in the ethical terrain of what is good and bad, what is obligatory, and what is virtuous. Here, we are firmly in the territory of Aristotle. What matters is not necessarily the answer to these questions, but the role of radical relationality in the existential predicament of choosing to live ethically.

Therapists are moral because we reflect on, have convictions about, or seek to influence others about ethical questions and issues relating to how we and others should live their lives. Because the question of what constitutes living well is no easy thing to decide, we side-step the issue through our therapeutic frameworks. We defer to a client's goals and measure the empirical success of therapy by assessing whether or not those goals were met. Therein lies the humanistic conviction of autonomy and the Rogerian assertion that the fully functioning person lives the best life of all.

Examining the ethical character of psychotherapy is anxiety provoking because disagreements about what is good, what is bad, what is obligatory, what is just and what is virtuous generate conflict. Therapists often describe having "difficult conversations" when, in fact, what is meant by this euphemism is that it is difficult to disguise or edit what is really felt, or what is really thought, for fear of being judged. Exploring our ethical landscapes is not simply a rational project, as was imagined by Plato to be the case. People act or fail to act because of matters of belief which do not necessarily have empirical, explicable foundations. Yet avoiding ethical questions will not wish them away. In the moral vacuum left by secularism, Taylor warns us that (1989: 516):

> High standards need strong sources. This is because there is something morally corrupting, even dangerous, in sustaining the demand [of others] simply on the feeling of undischarged obligations, on guilt, or its obverse self-satisfaction.

In the quest for objectivity, talk about how things *are* gets separated from debates about how things *ought* to be. We become too readily entangled in discussions about creating and following rules, which then leads to the likes of Nietzsche pointing out that all such rules are an arbitrary exercise in power that should be abandoned anyway.

The philosophers Alasdair MacIntyre and Charles Taylor have, for almost half a century, forged parallel paths in arguing that we must acknowledge that we are thrown into the hurly-burly of life as lived: we have no alternative to being entangled in the tangle of it all. We are already shaped by our taken-for-granted ideals and beliefs from our culture and traditions. What being human *is* depends on how we interpret and make sense of ourselves and our relational milieu (MacIntyre, 2002). There can be no neutral "watch tower" from which we can do this. In this way, both MacIntyre and Taylor – and those such as Gadamer who influenced them – look to forge a middle way between moral pluralism and moral relativism which offers a coherent framework to help therapists understand how to engage ethically with the world.

## 5.2   The Myth of Moral Neutrality in Therapy

The idea that a therapist can – or should even attempt to – be unbiased or morally neutral is a risky and persistent myth. Imagining ourselves to be somehow above the fray can lead to all sorts of tangles and transgressions such as the ones which find their way onto the "public notice boards" of professional bodies as a warning to others. Such practices foster the continuing – yet unwise – belief that we can triumph over wrongdoing through punishing (i.e., shaming) others.

However, beyond this, the morally neutral therapist sees themselves as an abstracted being rather than one aware that they are enmeshed in the ethical flow, like braider and braided, bound by the common cord of the plait. What I want to explore here is related to an old question, which is why be good? Understanding that the radical relationalist behaves ethically because they have a love of living virtuously is the antithesis of being good simply because one fears – as Augustine put it – the "flames of hell" through public humiliation.

Talk of being moral in the practice of therapy presupposes judgements about what constitutes the best interests of the client, the therapist, and perhaps even the greater good of society. Many consider the best ethical outcomes to be conformity with effectiveness scales, basic moral obligations, what is good or proper to do, or maybe even the development of virtue. Sceptics even argue that therapeutic practitioners endorse minimal standards of professional ethics for the pragmatic reasons of legitimising fees, obtaining prestige, and sustaining professional autonomy. Being seen to adhere to the small rules emboldens a minority to transgress the big rules.

For the most part though, the therapeutic encounter raises little in the way of what would ordinarily be considered an ethical issue for the therapist. Moral dilemmas concerning confidentiality, obligations to avoid doing harm, boundary violations and intentions to break the law are the most obvious – *and undeniably important* – red flags which, from time to time, find their way into supervision.

What is often overlooked is how therapy is a deeply value-laden activity that transcends "red flags"; the radical relationalist is aware that they are engaged in a thoroughgoing ethical endeavour. For example, a therapist who adopts a method of therapy – be it humanistic, behavioural, psychodynamic, or integrative – has already aligned themselves with a set of sometimes paradoxical values and philosophical precepts. The issue is not whether the philosophical claims of our methods can be exposed as ill founded, but rather why, since they can be so readily undermined, we continue for the most part as though this were not the case?

What goes unnoticed is how therapists see themselves as metaphorical shepherds impatiently waiting for their clients to join them in their own – unarticulated – ethical vision of the "good life". Trade magazines abound with therapists expressing their frustration towards clients who disregard invitations to engage in their theoretical models: "I had my formulation; I had my treatment plan, but I didn't have my client on board. From where I was sitting, the process of change looked obvious, but she wasn't ready to walk through the door".

There are strong grounds for rejecting the claim that therapeutic effectiveness is a morally neutral ideal. Therapeutic efficacy is entangled with a type of moral relationship which nevertheless contrives, in part, to manipulate people into compliant patterns of behaviour. It is by an appeal to their own effectiveness that therapists claim their ethical authority. When a therapist ventures into a realm beyond that which has been consensually agreed to be therapeutic (i.e., "I am interested in going back to that dream you mentioned ..."), then some moral decision has already been made. A therapist who concludes that understanding and addressing their values is a simple ("yes ... I have morals but I do not impose them), albeit "dry" matter ("I'm already bored by this subject"), then a stance on the importance of ethics has already been taken. When a therapist approves or disapproves of a goal a client selects for themselves, or when they even select a goal for therapy on behalf of the client, then too, a moral judgement has been made about what is best for the client. The therapist has responded to the other's situation *as if* from their own standpoint, rather than from the perspective of the client's actual situation.

A therapist's response to a distressed client who wants to know what to do requires that they adopt some position about the meaningfulness or truth of an ethical dilemma. Perhaps most importantly, all therapists adopt some position about the relationship of science, and the way it relates to being in the world. Even the counselling professor who believes it possible to write a textbook about psychotherapy has adopted some ethical position about their authority to objectivise and decontextualise knowledge.

Without articulating our ethical visions, therapeutic goals are likely to become implicitly guided by background relationships with childhood caregivers, social conditioning, or by a rebellion against other ethical or cultural sources. Any claim that a therapist need not take responsibility for the goals of the therapeutic enterprise because the autonomy of the client absolves them of the ethical problem is gravely mistaken. Clients are often too distressed and may not have a strong sense of their goals, at least initially. I have been with clients who simply cried throughout the first three or four hours of therapy, and it was only beyond this point that they were able to speak, let alone articulate their goals. An all too familiar refrain heard from listening to countless hours of recordings reflects this reality:

*Therapist:*   How do you think therapy will help you?
*Client:*       I do not know.

While it is important to recognise that although the goal of therapy must reflect the clients' choices, the therapist is not a taxi driver, whose purpose is to deliver a passenger – irrespective of their distress – to their destination. For the therapist to work ethically with a diverse range of people, they are compelled to make ethical decisions about client goals and whether they are *affirming*, *tolerable*, or in cases where they may be harmful, *rejected*.

The different types of relationships that therapists establish with their clients can result in different degrees of unethical influence. For example, there are the *gardeners*, who see their clients as an apple seed which can grow into the best apple tree they can be through loving care: but they are adamant that they cannot become a pear tree. The *Pygmalion* seeks to shape a client according to an ideal image based on their own experiences, histories, and value system (Tjeltveit, 1999: 173).

Seemingly benign words used to describe influential therapeutic moments, such as healing, transformative, emancipatory, actualising, and supportive, are imbued with therapist-centred values and self-perceptions. A therapist's own transformative life experiences can, irrespective of their claim to ethical neutrality, influence the client in selecting their goals and actions:

I had a real breakthrough with a client I have been seeing. I sort of suspected they were gay ... but at last ... they have realised that they are ... and I have persuaded them to come out to their parents.

An automatic *parentalism*, or sense of knowing what is good for a client, especially when they symbolise a reparative narrative of their own, risks undermining the autonomy of a client and perhaps runs the risk of disrupting their wider relational networks.

This then leads us to the philosophical and ethical assumptions of a given therapeutic method, which if homologous with liberal individualism for example, may not consider the wider impact of implicit therapist assumptions about the client's relational network. The radical relationalist understands that it is necessary to articulate not only the goals but the ethical assumptions of the goals of therapy. For this, the therapist must have the capacity to articulate their own philosophical understanding of what constitutes for them a good life.

A significant problem lies in the fact that there can be no theory of a good life which is adequately enshrined in integrative/eclectic models because of the attendant issues of ethical plurality and relativism. Professionals are thus relatively free to direct power to their own ends. People employ a diverse variety of approaches to obtain ethical knowledge and some therapists might even be able to articulate their moral sources. But it is more likely that therapists operate from a base of incoherent and variegated principles and largely unexamined ethical intuitions. Furthermore, dramatic polarities exist towards religion as a basis for ethics, with some viewing theological issues as choosing to delve into the realm of superstition, falsehood, and irrationality. Whereas others could not imagine any other approach to addressing questions of virtue, good and bad, right, and wrong, and how to live a good life.

Let us now move upstream from therapists and their clients, to consider the gatekeepers to the profession – the educators and bodies that accredit them – who function as sentinels to this value-laden enterprise. Their worthy goal is to both protect the integrity of the profession as well as safeguard future clients against the potential harm that could be done by incompetent trainees who pay to be "sheep-dipped" by their course. While trainers use carefully considered means to select candidates for their courses, the ends are nevertheless a sort of uncritical professional and economic homosocialisation, with people "just like me" judged to be the best candidates (Crago, 2003; Homrich, 2009).

It may seem ironic that when choosing potential candidates for experiential psychotherapy training, little faith is placed – by some – in the capacity of people to develop and meet the demands of the profession. Gatekeepers can adopt the value-laden position that excellent therapists – much like themselves – are "born not made". This is a phenomenon that appears to be borne out by research (Wheeler, 2000). Large-scale cross-sectional and longitudinal studies of therapists – tracked from the beginning of their training until retirement – using what are inevitably crude indicators of therapeutic success, suggests that, on average, experience does not necessarily make for better practitioners (Goldberg et al. 2016; Erekson et al. 2017).

This implies that psychotherapy training is more nuanced than simply learning a trade, or a musical instrument, as in this case, not only does practice not make perfect, but it does not even make better. Perhaps it is because trainers seek to offer a value-laden, potentially transformative, maybe even redemptive experience to novitiates who like themselves, were firstly anointed before they were appointed.

Being non-judgemental and interacting flexibly with an open mind are all worthy ethical ideals regarding the therapeutic encounter. However, the claim to ethical anonymity characterised by the term "neutrality" seems to be an unrealistic ideal. A therapist cannot achieve the impossible state of being an ethics-free zone (Tjeltveit, 1999: 177–180). When therapists can articulate their own default assumptions about what constitutes a good life, it becomes decidedly easier – though not easy – to see more clearly how a client formulates, say, what it means to be normal. When we look beyond speaking of "normal" as being free from distress and consider instead what it means to flourish, then we can admit a dazzling degree of diversity to the therapeutic encounter.

Unlike a stiff knee that can function well in only a limited number of ways, the entire human being-ness can flourish with a potentially bewildering, and occasionally delightful degree of diversity. This idea is especially important for psychotherapy because therapy has no common goals and lacks overall coherence because outcomes are often measured and articulated in terms of how the method implicitly ignores or understands what living well means. What it means to live a good life can be as unambitious as being symptom-free, complying with a method, or returning to work. If we consider therapy as a practice which enables people to live a good life, then we must consider it ethical in the most profound sense of the word.

Beneficence – which is a key virtue on which standards are set – depends on a strong ethical sense which is bound to visions shared across different communities about what it means to live a good life. Because much Western thinking considers there to be a plurality of ethics, the question of which ends are good seems both intractable and undecidable. Yet therapists face answering such questions in the routine conduct of their profession and possibly in their wider lives too. So, practitioners must attempt to offer a response to how they decide what constitutes doing good, whether it be "muddled, pragmatic, *ad hoc*, carefully thought-out or grounded in a particular ethical tradition" (Tjeltveit, 1999: 265–267, 2003, 2006).

Doing good in therapy cannot be understood in terms of reciprocity and the golden rule, which holds that we do unto others as we would have them do unto us. This forms the basis of culturally pervasive Kantian moral laws to which we turn next. The problem here is that we inadvertently impose on others a well-meaning yet distorted understanding of what living a good life looks like. The golden rule can become something of an abusive imposition of the therapists understanding of what it means to live well. To avoid such an imposition, the principle of beneficence might be better understood in terms of doing unto others *their* good – from the perspective of one who cares (Section 1.2).

Kant – The Isaac Newton of Morality. Immanuel Kant was alarmed by the relativist assertions of his contemporary David Hume, who argued that morality was a matter of emotional taste, subjectivity, or local consensus. Kant embarked on the project of creating an equally humanistic and individualistic approach to what we should *do* when faced with dilemmas. In the spirit of Isaac Newton, Kant sought to develop an action-focused guide to morality with universal injunctions, principles, and standards to guide us in choosing how to get the right answer to our moral dilemmas.

Morality, much like Newton's physics, became something narrowly concerned with actions governed by universal laws, and less to do with the greater good, or what is valuable in itself, such as what we should admire, cherish, or love. Unconditional obligations – categorical imperatives – were considered intrinsically valid regardless of our will or desires; they are a "good" in and of themselves.

Without offering insights into what gravity actually *was*, Newton was able to build a system on a phenomenon assumed to be absolute, spontaneous, acting at a distance, and obligating towards all matter with law-like certainty. Being universal, Newton's laws were assumed to extend beyond what could be seen, in the present, past, and future. The analogy of mechanical explanations was not lost on Kant, who similarly looked to address the problem of balancing morality and selfishness by invoking an absolute force of moral obligation – the *idea* of God – without necessarily acknowledging the *existence* of God.

The coherence and unity of morality were thus secured by the practical role played by the Divine. In affirming the existence of God, Kant – like Newton – was concerned with creating a coherent model of moral conduct, and not with making epistemic (theoretical) claims about the existence of God. Like gravity for Newton, it was morally necessary for Kant to affirm the universal "force" of God's existence to maintain the rationality of the absolute claims of morality over selfishness.

At the heart of Kant's system lies the powerful humanistic conviction that inward lies the source of morality which can be accessed by practical reason: it was the only route to getting the *right* answer to a dilemma. The instrumental rationality of an agent's thought was judged by *how* they thought, and not in the first instance by whether the outcome was substantively *good*. Such an intended ethical universality is not always as generous and inclusive as one would suppose.

One of the inadvertent effects of Kant's notion of procedural rationality and universality is that it dissolves particularities. It did not occur to Thomas Jefferson in the Declaration of Independence, for example, to extend universal freedom to the slaves of his neighbours. As Lenin would have it, freedom in capitalist societies is similar to that of the ancient Greek republics: it is for the slave owners. In a population of rational agents who can justify what they do,

Leslie Margolin (2020) describes how Rogers' famous "Gloria" session involved well-intentioned and benign linguistic manipulations to confer on Gloria a taken-for-granted notion of an abstracted pre-existing self, independent of social interaction. The Rogerian belief in the a priori facticity of a real or true self, both Gloria's, and his own, and indeed everybody else's, is so deeply engrained that Rogers felt no obligation to discuss the philosophical assumption behind his approach with Gloria. He repeatedly asserts its existence with such warmth and heartfelt conviction that before too long Gloria was affirming its existence too. The notion that a Rogerian client–therapist relationship can be non-directional is thus utopian. It does not imply the futility of the approach, but it does mean it should not be entered into naïvely.

The dignity of the disengaged self-responsible rational subject is founded in the attainment of happiness through the absence of pain. It is human happiness that really matters in the universe – and the only issue is how this can be maximised. The commingling of Greek philosophy – that is the dignity of self-responsible reason – with both Judaism and Christian belief transforms the power balance of Human–Divine relations into something like a patron towards their client.

The human good, the happiness which God intends for us, is purely a matter of fulfilling our natural desires and pleasures through reason. There are no final goals beyond human flourishing. Carried to its fullest limit, the Cartesian position of disengagement leads us to the injunction: as far as possible be self-fulfilled and authentic. The proud loneliness of Freud's ego is a good example of this injunction, which diminishes the importance of the spaces between human beings: the great emotions are no longer out there waiting to be discovered, they are now to be found within.

The Self-Fulfilled Authentic Individual. Many consider individualism to be the finest achievement of the Enlightenment and indeed a defining characteristic of humanism. In mainstream Western societies, we can largely choose for ourselves how we live our lives, the careers we follow, and the relationships we pursue. Although tensions exist between what we might consider to be true self-determining freedom to design our lives against the demands of external conformity, nobody seriously wants to return to the world of even our most recent ancestors. The worry is whether modern freedom has come about through the high price of discrediting all other orders. While restricting us, they also gave meaning to the world in which we live, and with their disappearance comes what has been referred to as the great "disenchantment".

As a proxy for spiritual nourishment, we feed-off the scraps of residual fascination with pop stars, celebrities, and royalty, recognising at some level that things have somehow lost their magic. The worrying thing is that the loss of purpose is linked to a kind of narrowing and flattening of individual lives. It makes us less concerned with others in our society. As if anticipating consensus becomes the pathway – amongst humans "like us" at any rate – to a good and just society.

Rational agents became defined as those people who adhere to the notion that there are universal moral laws, categorical imperatives, and unconditional obligations which are intrinsically valid regardless of our will or desire. They are good in and of themselves and must be obeyed in all situations and circumstances if our behaviour is to observe the moral law. The virtue of justice becomes nothing but the disposition to obey the rules of justice; however, they are understood at the time.

Moral law becomes something timeless, which must be obeyed in all situations and circumstances: Kant's guiding principle of universality offered little room for qualitative distinctions and indeed leads to difficulties in practice. Simply consider the categorical imperative that lying is wrong irrespective of the circumstances and consequences. A deep and intuitive sense of what is a good thing to do compels me to ignore the categorical imperative and tell a lie to the crazed knife-wielding murderer who wants to know where my loved ones are hiding (Slife & Yanchar, 2019: 11).

Rational agents understand that to live in an ethical world, all must adhere to such obligations. The only explanation for exempting oneself from such obligations is that for some reason one is irrational, and so one must pay the price. This is the source of one of our most pernicious and illusory attitudes towards morality: because we are *free* to choose the right action, doing otherwise introduces both blame and blameworthiness for those who get it wrong, use wrong reason and do otherwise.

You might conclude that being bound by inflexible obligations as opposed to virtues is the opposite of freedom: it devalues the role of mutual care and trust among people. Making obligations central to any ethical framework soon leads to coercive and unsavoury practices by a minority of enforcers over the majority of ordinary folk. The central question of who should deprive whom of what freedom soon becomes a question of whose wrath should be dreaded by whom.

Morality becomes reduced to matters of moral sanctions, the threat of public humiliation for stepping out of line, "honour amongst thieves" and oaths of silence (*omertá*). Outwardly untrustworthy manipulators agree to workable "traffic rules" to avoid getting in each other's way. Cooperation becomes something of a last resort – and even then, in a moral framework devoid of trust, it is understood that collaboration is only ever for mutual advantage (Baier, 1997: 276).

What Kant saw as the universal and necessary principles of human reason turned out to be those of a particular time, place, and stage of human development. Just as Kant saw himself to be the Newton of morality, so the principles and presuppositions of morality turned out to be the principles and presuppositions of a highly specific morality, and a secularised Protestantism which became the foundation of modern liberal individualism.

Both rational and ethical superiority exists in a similar relationship with historical contexts, where they are judged to be more or less adequate approaches for interpreting the world. This is to jump ahead, however, and a detailed discussion of interpretation – *hermeneutics* – must be delayed for now. But suffice to say there can be no universal and timeless measures of what is ethical. Ethics alter with time and context, and so there is a history of successive challenges to what prevails, by individuals who seek, not a perfect understanding, but a better understanding of living well.

*In conclusion*, Hume's view was that in a culture where moral authority seems irrational, there is little reason to choose from one of many ethical frameworks – morality becomes relative and a matter of taste. What Kant brought to our attention is the incommensurability of reason and moral authority. To avoid moral pluralism, we must submit to some higher authority, which is by definition *beyond* reason. If the ethical is to have authority over us, then we cannot derive reasons for choosing that authority. Between Kant, who sees the basis of the ethical life in reason, and Kierkegaard who sees it in radical choice, stands Hegel's *Geist*.

Radical Relationality of the Geist. Georg Hegel (1770–1831) sought to moderate the Kantian commitment to instrumental reason, which he saw as an abstract moral obligation connected to the will of the individual. Instrumental reason clashed with the ongoing practical ethical obligations to the community to which the individual was already a member (*sittlichkeit*). The doctrine of *sittlichkeit* enjoins us to bring about what already is; my ethical obligation is already established through the radical relationality towards the community to which I belong; my fulfilment of these obligations is what sustains my community and keeps it going.

The collective life of the community becomes the essence and meaning of the lives of its members. Hegel sought to resolve the problem of uniting a transcendent sense of community with the finite individual who retains the freedom to reason, with his own vision of radical relationality or *Geist*: "when we come to see ourselves not just as finite subjects, but as vehicles of thought which is more than just ours, that is in a sense, the thought of the universe as a whole" (Taylor, 2003: 46).

However, God as transcendent becomes domesticated as a cultural entity for seeing the meaning of reality in its wholeness. God becomes fully realised as *Geist*, the march of the Divine in the world. Because Hegel dispensed with a celestial transcendent entity and replaced it with a terrestrial *Geist*, he felt God Himself, was now "dead". The Kantian idea of God offered at least a basis for denying moral relativism, and for asserting the priority of morality over selfishness. Instead, Hegel marked the abandonment of moral unity, and the loss of a reliable source of ethical obligations in the landscape of human choice.

## 5.3   Existentialism and Choice

With roots in the Romantic dissatisfaction with rationalism, existentialists see themselves as offering a practical response to what they regard as the malady of modernity. Existentialism became a powerful movement particularly in Europe after the Second World War because of the widely felt need to privilege individual freedom in response to the abominations of totalitarianism. The promise of emancipation from the dominance of instrumental reason, and the ideology of humans as anonymous cogs in a profit-maximising machine led to the development of the *Frankfurt School.* The promise of a return to our original authentic selves offered a welcome alternative to the reduction of people to the mere expression of their value in the marketplace. Notable thinkers such as Max Horkheimer and Eric Fromm sought to synthesise aspects of existentialism, psychoanalysis, and early Marxism to achieve such an end.

Interest in existentialism has waned among European philosophers in the past decades, making way for postmodernism, which rejects the notion that we are individual seats of consciousness and somehow responsible for our destiny. Nevertheless, it continues to be popular among therapists, perhaps because it complements humanism and facets of the ancillary fulfilment movement, with its inevitable focus on individualism and ethical relativism.

Few dispute that existentialism is a philosophical rather than a psychological approach to therapy, claiming as it does no specific technique or method. It is characterised by an *ethereal* relationality: a disembodied consciousness which springs from an individual who exists prior to all else. It is a comforting and thus popular belief that we are personally responsible for what we do, so long as we have the insight to transcend our *nature*, that is, the socio-moral-economic-biological-temporal lottery. For the self-transcending existentialist, it can be frustrating to see others eschew the emancipating power of radical choice. An unwillingness to take personal responsibility and go beyond the *natural attitude* (see Section 9.2) seems like an intellectual, if not a moral failing. By not going beyond our nature and transcending our difficulties through *Alternate Possibilities* (Section 2.4), we somehow fail to take responsibility: it amounts to a personal deficit.

I spoke earlier about how this can lead to an implicit lack of sympathy and compassion towards those who attempt and fail, or worse, those who appear not to try and reach for a transcendent origin. It is an attitude reflected in our meritocratic society with its emphasis on effort and hard work. Those who are psychologically harmed by the world of work, or society more generally, assume they have only themselves to blame for their lack of emotional self-mastery, insight, resilience, virtue, or initiative. Without jumping too far ahead into discussions reserved for the next chapter, it is worth noting that existentialists believe there to be a place beyond false consciousness from which its falseness can be seen. It is no less a delusion than the ones that the existentialist seeks to transcend in the first place.

Existentialists invariably go beyond the bounds of investigating *being*, somehow seeing themselves as unique amongst the (humanistic) therapeutic community in terms of their commitment to Socratic questioning, truth, virtue, choice, an interest in a good life, and the complexity of relationships (van Deurzen & Arnold-Baker, 2018). Considered something of a "philosophically rudderless theory" even by its own proponents, existential therapy is nevertheless alert and open to who we are as individuals, the reality of how we relate to others, and the wonder that we exist at all.

At the core of philosophical existentialism lies the process of disclosing our way of being (*ontology*) in everyday (*quotidian*) life and examining how we relate with the other beings we encounter. It is the unavoidable stuff that takes place in days, its routines, and uneventful patterns, as captured in the poignant poem "Days" by Philip Larkin. They are, after all where we live, they come and wake us, and they are the only place we can be happy. Where else could we live but days? To answer this question Larkin warns is to bring the doctor and the priest running across the fields in their symbolic "long coats".

North American culture, stereotypically characterised by its pragmatic optimism and humanistic disposition, was suspicious of European philosophers "running across the fields" with their convoluted, turgid, and verbose existential theories. Both Rollo May and Irvin Yalom, for example, have done much to advance the popularity of existential therapy, not so much as a European-style *ontological* construct, but a powerful, philosophically informed therapeutic approach for improving how we deal with the practical *ontic* problems of existence. The latter speaks to our experience of the unexamined assumptions and beliefs we have about the nature, and the purpose of ordinary life, while the former attends to the deeper structures of existence.

By addressing our ontic concerns, we inevitably gain insight into matters which are universally and ontologically constitutive of human existence (Figure 5.1). Our everyday difficulty with **death** comes about through our *facticity*, the brute fact that we simply exist. Our difficulty with **freedom** arises because we are cast into the world with finite choices. Our concern with **isolation** comes about because we exist through relationships: *being-is-relational*. And finally, our concern with meaninglessness can only be an issue since we exist as already meaning-*full*. Humans are meaning-making story-telling creatures, and for us, **meaning** reigns in everything that is.

Our finitude and its interrelated existential concerns gather around and constitute radical relationality. Human temporality and our embodied relationship with time – our bodies become weaker and ultimately die – articulates how death relates to finitude. Freedom speaks to our limited or finite choices and these are conveyed through personal morality and systems of ethics which we discuss later. Our sense of isolation is remedied only when we reach out and create intimate relationships with others; they calm our sense of being alone in an otherwise cold and indifferent cosmos. Sovereign to our creation of meaning is language itself; it is the embodiment of how we relate, articulate, and co-create the world. It is how we understand, if not experience, time. Through narratives and discourse – temporally bound communal meaning – we may even begin to formulate the surrounding sayable of the ineffable unsayable of transcendence which completes the cycle, which began with our human frailty and the certainty of death.

Existentialism risks painting a fearful picture of solitude for the individual, a pinpoint of will, marooned on a tiny island in the centre of a vast ocean of impersonal facts. Morality only escapes from this existential isolation through what Iris Murdoch referred to as a wild leap of faith (2007: 26). For Abraham Maslow, the value of existentialism necessitates we look beyond the exclusively European habit of "harping on dread, on anguish, on despair", because "this high I.Q. whimpering on a cosmic scale occurs whenever an external source of values fails" (1999: 21). We are what we seem to be – transient mortal beings subject to necessity and chance. Movement towards the common good can appear pointless and difficult when we see life as intrinsically arbitrary and meaningless.

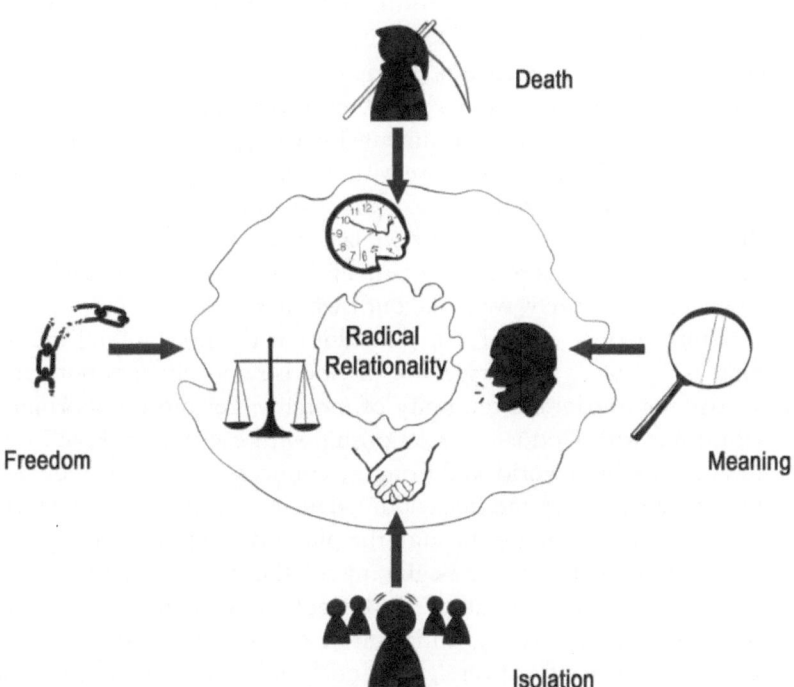

**FIGURE 5.1**　The Existential Concerns of Radical Relationality.

Ethics in a Meaningless Universe. The thinkers discussed earlier in the chapter have in common the use of reason to achieve the *ends* of realising our human potential. The *means* through which they have embarked on this quest are founded on ethical concepts which guide us beyond our untutored human selves. But how do we understand what is best when there cannot be a neutral standpoint or high watchtower from which to survey all systems of morality?

We are all, inescapably, inhabitants of advanced modernity, and as such are coloured by its social and cultural hues. The "moral high ground" implies that from among the numerous jostling systems of moral thought, there is a shared impersonal standard of virtue from which one of these systems can occupy the position of being right. Yet the poverty of arguments in support of such a belief suggests that there is no such high ground on which to stand. What seems clear is that we face a dilemma in describing what an ethical life is. Can it be understood as conformity to a set of rules, or do we allow ourselves to be guided by the naïve freedom of liberal individualism?

In the Kantian tradition, morality is based on universal imperatives, while the utilitarian ideal – which Kant implacably opposed – saw value only in subjective human wellbeing. Elizabeth Anscombe launched a famously acerbic attack on both approaches by observing that secular ethics is like the concept of the *criminal* remaining long after the structures of criminal law, the criminal courts, and indeed criminal lawyers have been "abolished and forgotten" (Anscombe, 1958).

Ethics, in the routine practice of therapy, has similarly become an idea that survives outside the framework in which it was created and made intelligible. In the absence of *God the Enforcer*, arguments for acting selfishly seem compelling when we see the underserving – those without merit – prosper through acts of immorality: it only seems irrational to politely queue for bread and go hungry while those jumping the line get to have fat bellies. Why should I act morally when being immoral leads to greater benefits for myself and those with whom I am closely related? Surely, we make our own luck?

This points to just one of the difficulties with moral pluralism. When something as unique as the perspective of God is removed from our lives, the price we pay for freedom is the unity of morality. Yet more important than our relationship with God is our relationship with each other. Free from the moorings of our ethical world, and from the connectivity and dependence that contextualise our motives and behaviours, debates about right and wrong are made interminable – in part – through the plurality of ethical perspectives.

The Enlightenment was the beginning of the move in Western culture away from a theocentric morality. As the pre-eminent modern heir to the Stoic tradition and in striking anticipation of modernity, Immanuel Kant saw morality in terms of a sovereign rational individual adhering to a set of universal rules. The profound impact of Kant can be put simply: he abolished *God* and made *humans* in *God's* stead.

The God-like status afforded to us is recognisable today in our proud, independent, lonely, powerful, rational, and heroic self-image. As reason banished transcendent reality, the once celestial ethical values collapsed into the terrestrial domain of human will. With the withdrawal of the *Divine Good* leaving an indefinable and empty void, human choice rapidly filled the space left behind. Once this transition took hold, the taken-for-granted unity of morality as an obligatory force, as well as the harmonious relationship between *being and morality* began to crumble.

Relativism in its place sees how different observers can justifiably arrive at alternative moral conclusions with their origins in different foundations and traditions. Judgements about how to live a good life are no longer a matter of ethics but determinations of approval by some or other societal standard of reference.

We are perhaps constrained to accept then that moralities are disparate and that pluralism is real: perhaps is there no common human good or ethics? There is good reason to believe that choosing definitively among competing moral viewpoints is beyond the capacity of sound rational secular argument. The problem is that all attempts to achieve an ethical perspective of good from *nowhere* turn out to require the endorsement of an ethical perspective of good from *somewhere*. Seeking endorsement from *somewhere* requires we search for what is *normal* behaviour as agreed by people affected by a particular action, assuming they can deliberate together in ideal conditions of unconstrained communication.

Contemporary approaches to ethics in counselling and psychotherapy adopt a similarly – problematic I feel – consensual approach to what constitutes doing the right thing through tests of *universality* (would you condone this action by someone else?), *publicity* (the flames of hell as it were ... Would you be willing for your course of action to be exposed to scrutiny through workshops, TV, radio....?) and *justice* (would I do the same if the client were well known or influential?) (Bond, 2016).

Context Is All. In Mesoamerica, sacrifice took many forms, though perhaps the most difficult to understand for moderns is the offering of infants. As recently as the nineteenth-century children were consigned to sacred *cenotes* or wells in the Yucatan peninsula in modern Mexico. Sacrifice was not seen as murder but the placement of a child's life in the hands of the gods. Up to the age of four, a child was considered to embody a purity that transcended the mundane world of adults. The liminality of children, and the belief of their proximity to the processes of death and rebirth, defined them as sacred and conversant with the gods. The public recognition of a parent's sacrifice accrued to them a significance and status beyond our modern understanding (Ardren, 2011).

At about the same time, schools across Germany and France would close for *justice days*, when up to a dozen or so unfortunate souls would endure public execution while serenaded by songs of death by children in attendance. In 1808, a boy described being brought to watch a public flogging while being reassured by his father that "*justice* may be severe son, but it is by no means cruel" (Spierenburg, 2008: 97–98).

Where once we gathered for the spectacle of public executions in town squares, we now come together to take café. The spectacle of public evisceration registered little alien presence within our European urban spaces and indeed were even considered both rationally and idealistically the best way to serve the judicial and penal ends of the communities to which we belonged.

Our task, therefore, is to discover what was particular to the orders of rationality and reality that informed a preceding era's own practice and experience. Imposing on the past meanings, values, and concerns of the present can never achieve such an outcome. Nor can we realise our goal by simply erasing evidence of these practices from sight because they offend contemporary sensibility.

Before we condemn historical events from the standpoint of today's understanding of what is good or just, we need to identify the important unsolved ethical *knots* of the time, and how they were ultimately resolved or loosened. What we have come to know – after centuries of scholarship – is that the certainty of being caught is the more effective deterrent than the severity of the punishment. The point I wish to make is that ethical beliefs are intelligible and justifiable only when we see them in their cultural, historical, and radically relational context.

The Myth of the Criterionless Choice. The past few decades have seen a revival of interest in Søren Kierkegaard (1813–1855), which has done much to discredit earlier interpretations of his works. A familiar caricature of the Danish theologian presents him as an advocate of the doctrine that knowledge depends on irrational faith through revelation. He was thus presented as an apostle of early existentialism who regarded belief as self-validating: *I know this to be true because it has been revealed to me.*

The revival of interest is unsurprising as Kierkegaard offers what Kant could not, which is delivering an alternative to humanistic moral relativism, and ahistorical universalism (i.e., divine command) as motivators for human beings to live virtuous lives. Kierkegaard's first book *Enten-Eller* (*Either/Or*) confronted early nineteenth-century Northern Europeans with the shocking philosophical discovery of the arbitrariness of moral culture. He was primarily and passionately opposed to Hegel's idea of Geist: the idea of a totality to which we as individuals belong as merely parts of a larger, evolving system of existence.

The idea of a *system* of existence was also unsatisfactory for Kierkegaard. Behind a system must be some individual, who by their existence, through their yearning for a system, gives the lie to the structuralist concept of a system, and any notion that there can be radical choice. Like *æthereal* relationality,

*Geist* springs from an individual who exists prior to the existence of the system. Kierkegaard's assault was not simply on Hegel's philosophy – who himself understood the problems of creating a transcendent system – but on philosophy itself.

The doctrine of "how to choose" is a recurring theme throughout Kierkegaard's reflections on ethics and the greater good, for we cannot: "constantly balance on the tip of the moment of choice ... choice is decisive ... and if we don't choose, others choose for us and then we have lost ourselves" (Kierkegaard, 2004: 486–487). What becomes important then *is not what we believe, or the object of our belief, but the way in which we believe: the focus is primarily on process, not content.* It is therefore the process of believing that defines for Kierkegaard what to believe.

Kierkegaard uses the literary genre of sub-dividing the self into parts – participant/spectator, braider/braided – in a systematic attempt to discover the rational justification for morality which he saw as defined as the process of self-becoming. In *Either/Or*, the indirectness of Kierkegaard's' approach, writing from the perspective of two pseudo anonymous authors with the added detachment of a fictitious editor coordinating the work gives the reader space to author their own selves as they explore existential radical choice. It reflects the seemingly irreconcilable struggle between sensuous aesthetic immediacy (presentation) and endless ethical reflection (re-presentation).

For Kierkegaard, there are three broad tiers of existence: aesthetic, ethical, and religious. Each tier is characterised by its own concerns and interests as well as different ways of thinking about life. As a person evolves through time – as surely, we do – there tends to be a progression from the aesthetic, to the ethical and sometimes to the religious for whom Kierkegaard chose Abraham as the paragon of faith. The aesthete is what a person immediately is and the ethical is that whereby a person becomes what they become.

Those living a hedonistic *aesthetic* life of Epicurean delight are, in fact, living in despair, alienated from themselves in an inauthentic type of existence, whether they know it or not. The aesthetic life is characterised, in a crucial sense, to be an empty one. As Kierkegaard argues, when the external validation for success in an aesthete's life disappears, it becomes clear that life is in fact built on a transient foundation. For the aesthete, boredom is the enemy. Their social world is but an arena – populated with their own attitudes and preferences – to achieve enjoyment. The aesthete does not seek coherence or intelligibility in their narratives about themselves or others, because that would require the formulation of an explicitly rational life plan (Kierkegaard, 2004: 493).

In contrast, the *ethical* life is characterised by the cultivation of complex interpersonal relationships for the inherent good they offer. It might require finding a vocation or becoming part of the community, and engaging in some challenging project whose attainment requires excellence or virtue. It involves a personal quest for radical relationality. For Kierkegaard, we only become authentic ethical selves when we are defined in terms of our cares and projects, when we are powered by a higher way of being. Moving along this path is not better insofar that I will *feel* better; it is a better way to *be*. But the ethical life does not come from nothing. It is grounded in an initial orientation or set of experiences already built into the aesthetic position of being human. Simply stated, for Kierkegaard and for those who came after, it is the absence of transcendent meaning that lies at the heart of human despair.

Carl Jung – who had little positive to say about existential thinkers and Kierkegaard, in particular – nevertheless shared significant existential perspectives with the Dane. Kierkegaard depicts human beings as having actual and ideal selves and to evolve towards the latter we must become aware of our inauthenticity, accept our shortcomings, and ask ourselves whether we find our lives meaningful, something which Jung saw as coming to terms with our *shadow*.

Both Jung and Kierkegaard considered that the matter of faith – an inexpressible transcendence beyond the sayable – was of immense therapeutic value. Such a radical participation in one's social world and personal relationships was the key to holding both rationality and faith in tension: because it is not death we fear, but the end of our relationships.

For Kierkegaard, opting for the ethical life cannot be explained in terms of agency, deliberate choice, or volition. When immersed in the aesthetic life – caring not for the past or future – then what interest can there be in choosing an alternative lifestyle unless we encounter the incentive for change? We can only resist the ethical call and refuse to ask questions of an ethical life if we have acknowledged the existence of an ethical life in the first place which could answer such questions.

Sustaining the aesthetic life requires a silent yet determined resistance to the ethical. We must be actively engaged in drowning out the voices within that tell us that this life is meaningless. In this sense, through resistance, we have already engaged in a quest for the deeper meaning of our existence. Making the ethical choice is therefore not such a groundless choice or absurd leap of faith as suggested by certain caricatures of existentialism. This is because we are never truly abstracted or detached from the call to radical relationality, with its stable dispositions, narratives, virtues, and traditions on which we can draw to act in a particular way, in each situation, to afford meaning to our lives.

Radical, criterionless choice is therefore something of an illusion because we already know what to do, or what not to do. Choices are not groundless and absurd; the criterionless choice is a myth when we see ourselves as radically related to the whole, as opposed to self-generated atoms. For existentialists such as Sartre, who see human beings becoming exactly what they choose to become, choice turns out not to be as arbitrary and groundless as he would have it: "Alone in the midst of monstrous silence, alone and free, without recourse of excuse, irrevocably condemned, condemned to be free…" (Sartre, 1945/2001).

## 5.4   Virtue and Moral Realism

When Plato sought to understand what is good, he used the Sun as a metaphor to represent the transcendent reality of virtue; its rays penetrate the veil of selfish consciousness so that we can join the world as it really is. As moral pilgrims, we seek to emerge from our dark caves and see the world in the light of the Sun. An albeit distant reality, it nevertheless gives us light and energy to know what is true. Aristotle took as his metaphor for a person who lives well, the harpist who plays well. The harp has a purpose and a function related to its context which makes it complete, perfect, and final. Similarly, to be a person who is complete, one must fulfil a set of roles which gives one a point and purpose – the more my ends are pursued for their own sake, and not for the sake of other ends, the more complete we are (Crisp & Aristotle, 2014: 1098a).

In this regard we all recognise the practices and activities of people who flourish; they cannot but help engage in the good of their communities. The arts and sciences, healthcare, schools and colleges, children's nurseries, charity shops, choirs, community gardens, food banks, those who volunteer, and those reluctantly called to arms are some of the contexts in which people become involved for the common good.

In pre-modern societies, an individual faced the world as a member of their family, household, clan, tribe, commune, or city. It is only when we see ourselves as atoms prior to and apart from our relationships that we cease to be radically relational. To consider someone good without considering their relational context is to remove our essential human purpose and understanding from what it means to flourish. Though there is no truth in relativism, this much is true: we cannot justify our beliefs to everybody, but only to those whose beliefs already overlap with ours to some appropriate degree (Rorty, 1991). To move beyond the impasse of moral relativism and begin to retrieve concepts uncontaminated by modernity, we must first challenge the persistent and corrosive dogma that morals are a matter of opinion.

<u>Against Emotivism</u>. The idea that the universe is valueless is a persistent one and gets its most celebrated articulation in David Hume's writing. Hume drew on the alleged distinction between <u>*facts*</u>, which are seen as empirical, discoverable, and interrogable by reason and science, and <u>*values*</u> which are the expression of mere emotion. This fact–value distinction is one which several philosophers – including Elizabeth Anscombe and Iris Murdoch – saw as seriously flawed. With morality considered a matter of opinion, or even a transient "whim", we are but a step away from the postmodern claim that morality is a matter of power. For if there are no rational grounds for deciding

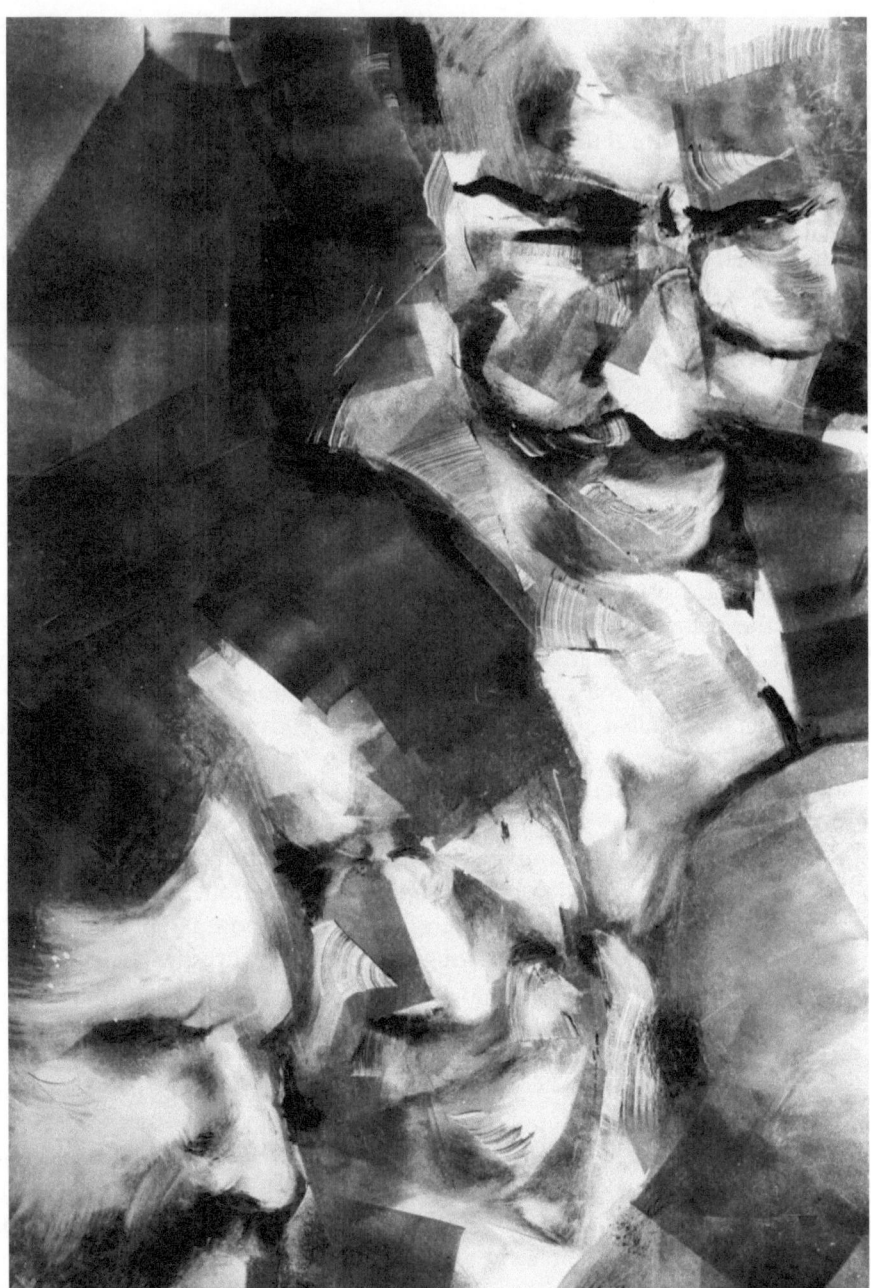

**FIGURE 5.2** Moral Pilgrims.

between moral positions, we are as Thucydides suggested, on perilous ground: "Right, as the world goes, is only in question between equals in power, while the strong do what they can and the weak suffer what they must".

The moral catastrophe of modern living is our inability to conduct rational debates about ethical disagreements. Such debates are interminable not just because they go on and on – they do – but that they lack terminus. There seems to be no way of securing moral agreement. MacIntyre's' *After Virtue* characterises a society hopelessly divided, with opposing sides of almost every argument showing little interest in engaging in authentic or reasoned debate.

MacIntyre claims that the logic of emotivism seduces us into seeing it as hopeless to expect a resolution in what would appear to be our ongoing and interminable moral debates. This is because emotivism professes that a moral judgement is nothing more than an utterance which expresses emotions or feelings. Unlike facts, feelings cannot – by any standard – be unequivocally right or wrong, and so moral judgement becomes as interminable as judgements about whether what I feel is true or false. When stripped bare of radical relationality, moral utterances become personal opinions of individual sovereign authorities which lack the guidance of the situatedness in which they were originally domesticated: "they have lost both their linguistic and practical way in the world" (MacIntyre, 2007: 60).

Emotivism is a theory socially embodied by *characters*, people in culture who are objects of regard insofar that they model an ethical ideal of being *right*. It is rare to meet a manager who genuinely believes that subordinates who disagree with them can be right. Characters, such as managers – or more broadly organisational representatives – are subject to certain kinds of moral constraint as they go about coercing and controlling subordinates, and manipulating what is thought or felt, something we refer to nowadays as *gaslighting*. We could add to this category billionaire politicians who imply that those who fail to cope with the ordinary "ups and downs" of modern life are somehow morally deficient.

To a large degree, people in modern cultures think, speak and function as if emotivism is true. The implications of believing that moral utterances are hopelessly irresolvable is a grave cultural loss because moral discourse in everyday practice loses its sense of authority. Ethics becomes reduced to relativist assertions and counter-assertions framed by the power of those in the contest because emotivism sees ethical statements – such as values – as mere preferences: "you say I have done something wrong? I am sorry – *for you* – to hear that".

The social embodiment of emotivism blurs the boundaries between manipulative and non-manipulative therapeutic relationships. When I offer – through authentic care – what I take to be good reasons for acting in one way rather than another, and then leave it to you to evaluate those reasons, then I am treating you ethically. I have appealed to criteria and resisted the temptation to imaginatively project myself into your shoes and decide *as if* I were you. To make someone an instrument of my purposes – either explicitly or implicitly – is to express my own feelings, preferences (i.e., the values implicit in a therapeutic method) as if they were obviously correct, with the aim of transforming the feelings and attitudes of others (*see* projective empathy Section 9.4). Such emotivism simulates the other and prevents me from appealing to criteria from the *actual* perspective of *your* situation. In a relationship in which emotivism is believed to be true, there can be no truly ethical relationship.

For MacIntyre emotivism risks rendering the therapist a *character* much like the manager; someone who sees others as a means to be benignly coerced to a particular end. For both professions, their sole reality is the alignment of the attitudes, values, feelings, and preferences of other people to those of the character. The moral relativism of the humanistic therapist aligns with emotivism but in the realm of someone else's life. The therapist's concern is with the technique, with effectiveness in transforming a distressed person into a numerical product – a less distressed person: "they are seen by themselves, and by those who see them through the same eyes as their own, as uncontested figures" (MacIntyre, 2007: 30–31).

MacIntyre's virtue ethics draws attention to the need to see therapy as an ethical enterprise with virtues upheld by the various theories employed. Virtue ethics invites deeper reflexivity about the myth of neutrality, what it means to live a full life, and the good that practitioners implicitly promote.

Retrieving Virtue. In conceiving of a framework which prefigures modernity and divine authority, thinkers such as Elizabeth Anscombe – who introduced the term human *flourishing* – were drawn to Aristotle's age-old notion of virtue (1958). Aristotle was radical in proposing that there was nothing worth having beyond achieving a good life through the exercise of virtue (Crisp & Aristotle, 2014). Those who promote Aristotle's ethical framework – with its roots in fourth-century Greek culture – rightly condemn the ill-founded exclusion of women, slaves, and ordinary productive working people from the possibility of achieving human goods.

Yet, after purging an Aristotelean account of virtue of its untenable elements, including unsavoury attitudes towards the "masses", the fundamental motive of human communal practice beyond the context of ancient Greece speaks to something essential about human life: radical relationality is a basic good of human existence. Central to a desire to be good is our inherent moral justification or motive (*telos*) for moving towards what is virtuous. Our *telos* is firstly to flourish and then to seek guiding frameworks to meet this desire to be good, such as creating just and ordered communities.

Is being honest or acting honestly simply a matter of refraining from cheating, lying, and stealing? Is the reason I should not lie to you because it breaks some moral law, goes against duty, violates some ethic of obligation, or impugns the wellbeing of the many. The notion of virtue then is more fundamental than the ideas at the heart of utilitarian or Kantian ethics which we discussed earlier.

*Aretē* – excellence of any kind – gives us the term *aretaic*, which describes an ethic focussed on achieving something of excellence. Virtue, in the neo-Aristotelian sense, refers to something much deeper than a desirable quality of a person. Virtue focusses on the arc of a life and not simply discrete isolated actions. An account of virtue is impossible to achieve when divorced from its relational context – virtue demands radical relationality. The virtuous therapist, for example, is not one who can act the part for 50 minutes with a client and is then dishonest in their dealings elsewhere.

Morality and social structure were one and the same in the ancient cultures which first spoke of virtue. Yet, if the idea of virtue requires for its exercise a social context that is irrevocably lost, what relevance does it have for us today? Virtues are intimately linked with culture and deeply embedded within its moral traditions. So in this sense, virtues constitute a deeply relational reality and not some abstract entity; the idea of morality as something unreal, abstract, and universal must be rejected.

The Realness of Morals. On the face of it, there seems to be something objective about the revulsion many of us feel towards sexual abuse, genocide, slavery, racism, discrimination, and terrorist atrocities. Our near universal ethical attitude to a great many actions seems to suggest that there are moral facts that constitute the bedrock or foundation of ethics, in much the same way that non-moral facts form our understanding of the natural world. Though the apparent moral facts seem only intuitively perceptible and diaphanous, they nevertheless feel real enough in the way they unite us when ethically repulsive actions are committed in the world.

Yet it seems somehow absurd to imagine that moral facts are like objects waiting to be discovered by humans. This scepticism towards moral judgements based on some independent reality says more about our metaphysical dualist compulsion to separate the world into objective and subjective, and less about ethics itself. To break out of this bind, we must employ an alternative vocabulary to understand the relationship between human self-understanding, value, and morality.

For Charles Taylor, abstract "moral beliefs" are framed in terms of the practical ways in which we are related to the world and understand how our desires, goals, and aspirations are qualitatively ranked higher than others. These strong evaluations "involve discriminations of right or wrong, better or worse, higher or lower – they are not rendered valid by our own desires, inclinations, or choices, but rather stand independent of these and offer standards by which they may be judged" (1989: 4).

The ethically "neutral", non-judgemental therapist, for example, has already decided that there is something good, something higher, perhaps even something better about being a counsellor compared to whatever else they did before. In our earlier encounter with Kierkegaard, the means through which such rankings take place about the goods we value are not the subject of criterionless choices but track some real underlying social context. There seems to be an *objective rightness* about how we experience the intrinsic value or calls to such evaluations made on us. It is clear that these hierarchical judgements transcend themselves and refer to orders of reality, which we might be either misinterpreting or getting wrong.

For example, I may be pleased with myself because I believe that my attitudes and actions are just and fair; I may even see myself as someone selflessly policing the boundaries of justice on behalf of the oppressed. In certain situations, I feel justified in my moral righteousness and my anger on behalf of others. Yet, I may be deceiving myself because my actions emanate from an unexamined sense of fear, or a desire to control others. When a therapeutic conversation clarifies what *really* concerns me – fear – it changes the shape of what matters to me because I understand my motivational force. This experience of discovery and growth is emphatically not like discovering an object, but I can come to understand something about the process of therapy – for client and therapist alike – that the interpretation of an ethical predicament can be wrong.

The change in felt intuition that comes from the field of words in an ethical conversation are brought about *within* and not through a changed understanding of how the world works in a "quasi-scientific" sense. The reality is that our moral judgements are answerable and no longer the subject of mere opinion – emotivism. Strong evaluations gesture to goods which are independent of our own desires, in that our experience of them can be faulty, wrong, and may need adjusting (i.e., wishing to appear just in my wrath when in fact I am motivated by something less worthy).

In this way, moral judgements can legitimately claim truth, reality, or objective rightness. Instead of independent moral "facts", Taylor speaks of moral "sources" that weave prescriptive ethics (How should I live my life?) with higher level *meta*-ethics (Are my moral views true?). By dissolving this dualism, the idea of the "high watchtower", or neutral perspective from which to decide our morality, becomes an illusion which distorts the transformational power of moral belief and judgement. Searching for the moral high ground becomes akin to inhabitants of a two-dimensional universe seeking a mountain. Would we recognise it even if we encountered it?

Yet regardless of our moral orientations, the important components of a good life – life *goods* – which are features of the way things really are, need referencing to some baseline moral source which explains why we believe these things to be *good*. It makes no sense to commit to life *goods*, or actions and virtues which define a good life (i.e., trying to be a good husband, an attentive father, and doing useful work), without an underlying recognition that family and work are moral sources that make – for me at least – a fulfilling life.

Affirming faith in universal human rights – a life good – cannot be separated from a deeper held belief in the "dignity and worth of the human person, in equal rights of men and women and nations large and small", which is a stated moral source of the UN Charter. Contained within the same document is an affirmation of the humanist theory of Kant and the value of living in accordance with International Law, which cannot be separated from seeing human rational agency as standing above all else in the universe, because it alone has dignity. Existentialists who confront the indifferent immensity of a meaningless universe with courage and lucidity also have a deep sense of the dignity of human life.

*Life goods then define what we find to be of moral importance and moral sources not only explain why we believe this to be so, but they also inspire and empower.*

For Taylor, ethical judgements about living well are best understood as responses to the genuine reality of our strong evaluations, moral sources, and what he calls the constitutive power of language (Section 6.4). This requires language to do much more than represent morals; language brings ethical meaning to experience. Moral sources are not merely the crucial motivators for behaving in one way rather than another; they are a deeper articulation of one's sense of value. Language then, does far more than demonstrate how our judgements reflect some external independent ethical reality.

The therapeutic encounter, therefore, must be understood in terms of a moral practice which emphasises, articulates, refines, or rejects the strong evaluations of our ethical sources. Radical relationality sees human self-understanding and ethics as inextricably linked and an expression of our ontological desire for self-interpretation, which cannot be understood without reference to the genuine reality of our underlying moral sources. To be human is to understand who we are in our ethical landscape and although moral agency is about a person articulating their values and moral goods, they do not do so in isolation: we do this dialogically through the multitude of relationships that define who and what *we* are.

We possess a tangible existential urge to engage dialogically in moral deliberation and articulate ethical horizons as indispensable aspects of being human. All these aspects are seen as radically relational; indivisibly interwoven into the plait of how a person must cultivate their ethical orientation in an existential sense. Being an ethical reasoner is not a formal intellectual process or overly abstract; it engages thought, emotion, bodies, language, and judgement in ordinary daily life. As moral judgements can legitimately claim objective rightness, it places a burden on the therapist to take themselves seriously and to "get it right" in their radical, relational, ethical, self-understanding.

*To conclude*, ethics – the way in which we participate in the world – are real and a part of our everyday lives. We are involved not only in articulating but also defending or rejecting ideas about how to live well. Ethical agency entails evaluating strong human desires, goals, and ways of life. Thoughts, words, feelings, imagination, social memory, and narrative must all be subject to active evaluation by the ethical person navigating the commonplace paradoxes of ordinary life.

## References

Anscombe, G.E.M. (1958). Modern Moral Philosophy. Reprinted in: Crisp, R. & Slote, M. (1997) *Virtue Ethics* (pp. 26–44). Oxford University Press.

Ardren, T. (2011). Empowered Children in Classic Maya Sacrificial Rites. *Childhood in the Past.* 4(1), 133–145.

Baier, A. (1997). *What do Women want in Moral Theory: in, Virtue Ethics.* Eds. R. Crisp & M. Slote. Oxford University Press.

Crago, H. (2003). Who Should Be a Family Therapist? A Personal View of Selection for Training. *Australian and New Zealand Journal of Family Therapy.* 24(3), 141–149.

Crisp, R. & Aristotle (2014). *Aristotle: Nicomachean Ethics.* Cambridge University Press.

Erekson, D.M. et al. (2017). A Longitudinal Investigation of the Impact of Psychotherapist Training: Does Training Improve Client Outcomes? *Journal of Counseling Psychology.* 64(5), 514–524.

Goldberg, S.B. et al. (2016). Do Psychotherapists Improve with Time and Experience? A Longitudinal Analysis of Outcomes in a Clinical Setting. *Journal of Counseling Psychology.* 63(1), 1–11.

Homrich, A.M. (2009). Gatekeeping for Personal and Professional Competence in Graduate Counseling Programs. *Counseling and Human Development.* 41(7), 1–23.

Kierkegaard, S. & Hannay, A. (2004). *Either/Or – A Fragment of Life.* Penguin.

MacIntyre, A.C. (2002). *A Short History of Ethics: A History of Moral Philosophy from the Homeric Age to the Twentieth Century.* 2nd edition. Routledge.

MacIntyre, A.C. (2007). *After Virtue: A Study in Moral Theory.* 3rd edition. University of Notre Dame Press.

Maslow, A.H. (1999). *Toward a Psychology of Being.* 3rd edition. Wiley.

Murdoch, I. (2007/1970). *The Sovereignty of Good.* Routledge.

Rorty, R. (1991). *Objectivity, Relativism and Truth.* Cambridge University Press.

Sartre, J-P & Sutton, E. (1945/2001). *The Age of Reason.* Penguin.

Slife, B.D. & Yanchar, S.C. (2019). *Hermeneutic Moral Realism in Psychology: Theory and Practice.* Routledge.

Spierenburg, P. (2008). *The Spectacle of Suffering: Executions and the Evolution of Repression: From a Preindustrial Metropolis to the European Experience.* Cambridge University Press.

Taylor, C. (1989). *Sources of the Self: The Making of Modern Identity.* Cambridge University Press.

Taylor, C. (2003). *Hegel and Modern Society.* Cambridge University Press.

Tjeltveit, A.C. (1999). *Ethics and Values in Psychotherapy.* Routledge.

Tjeltveit, A.C. (2003). Implicit Virtues, Divergent Goods, Multiple Communities: Explicitly Addressing Virtues in the Behavioral Sciences. *The American Behavioral Scientist.* 47(4), 395–414.

Tjeltveit, A.C. (2006). To What Ends? Psychotherapy Goals and Outcomes, the Good Life, and the Principle of Beneficence. *Psychotherapy: Theory, Research, Practice, Training.* 43(2), 186–200.

van Deurzen, E. & Arnold-Baker, C. (2018). *Existential Therapy: Distinctive Features.* Routledge.

Wheeler, S. (2000). What Makes a Good Counsellor? An Analysis of Ways in Which Counsellor Trainers Construe Good and Bad Counselling Trainees. *Counselling Psychology Quarterly.* 13(1), 65–83.

# 6

# MEANING

## A Reassuring Foundation

### 6.1 Introduction: The Play of Meaning

This part introduces the practitioner to the challenging idea that autonomy and freedom are romantic yet necessary delusions. We are more than related to the systems into which we are born – *we are their products*. Thinking, feeling, intuiting, relating, and conforming – qualities that humanistic and existential approaches in particular hold as defining features of who we are – are in fact silently defined by impersonal forces.

Structuralism is a philosophical movement that seeks to decipher, indeed dreams of deciphering the foundational truth or origin beyond the necessity of human interpretation. The structuralist presumes that the universe has a definite, discoverable set of impersonal principles, a *reassuring foundation*, an origin which resists – as Jacques Derrida put it – the play of meaning (1978).

Marx introduced the metaphor of base and superstructure, seeing economic laws as the explanatory foundational base of society. Freud also drew on the base-superstructure metaphor in his theorising about the principles of the human psyche, having been inspired by the foundational laws of physical thermodynamics. Darwin's theory of evolution can also be thought of as a base-superstructure model, as higher forms of life are necessarily based on the lower forms. Levi-Strauss too borrowed the base-superstructure perspective for the discipline of anthropology as he sought the hidden causative foundations of kinship practices.

Structuralists believe that words too are linked to reality through arbitrary linguistic conventions which derive their meanings from the structure of language itself; it is the structure that creates meaning and meaning ultimately lies in the structure. Structuralism as the apparatus for uncovering base reality

DOI: 10.4324/9781003396161-6

was introduced by the Swiss linguist Ferdinand de Saussure (1857–1913), with his posthumously published *Course in General Linguistics*. Here, de Saussure proposed that language cashiers us from control over our speech; speaking is no more than a local manifestation of the great system of language itself: *I do not speak ... I am spoken.*

Saussure argued that his insights could be applied wherever meaning was contested and this has profound implications for the practice of psychotherapy. If the fundamental structure of reality can only be ascertained by paying close attention to the structure of language, then meaning does not come from individuals but from the system that governs what any individual can do with it. It is the structures that produce meaning, not subjects: the personal pronoun "I" becomes a product of intricately webbed assumptions about language.

Structuralism sought to kick away the twin supporting ideological pillars of humanism, namely the sovereignty of rational consciousness and the authenticity of an individual's speech. Michel Foucault, in his writing about the history of ideas, avoided speaking of the sovereign subject thereby questioning the fundamental basis of liberal humanistic thought rooted in the agential individual.

By implication, structuralists see themselves resisting nostalgic humanistic notions of a literary work belonging to the genius of individual accomplishment. Structuralism calls into question the humanist ideal that an individual can deny responsibility for collective histories – including the errors of racism and colonialisation. In recognising how our lives are embedded in culture, structuralism sees the difficulty of unravelling the sovereign autonomous self from the past and its practices, because the past deforms our relationship with the present.

Structuralist hermeneutics seeks to understand texts independent of the author, or at least to understand the author's intentions better than the author understood them themselves. For example, a structuralist reading of the philosophy of Descartes undermines humanistic faith in autonomy and the inevitability of progress towards a civilised society. Descartes is seen instead as reflecting a broader structural tendency in Western European culture for self-restraint or the curbing of the more barbaric expressions of human emotion.

Sociologist Norbert Elias argued that the emotionally curbed self was a response to the development of centralised European states from preceding warrior societies. In such relatively pacified environments, people became more interconnected and dependent on civilised relationships because centralised structures intensified the obligation to be relatively pleasant to each other. In the process, human beings developed greater social self-constraint and familial cohesion, which fellow structuralist Freud would later build on through his concept of the super ego.

Elias went on to propose structural explanations for making sense of the violence that accompanies the civilising process. Western elites – extrapolating their growth in material wealth to colonial contexts – adopt an ethical and intellectual exceptionalism towards others who had yet to master their environment. Thus evolved the apparatus of colonialism; bureaucracy became the instrument which rationalised unequal status for marginalised peoples on the periphery, as well as the disenfranchised classes at the core of society (Pepperell, 2016).

The process of disseminating civilised conduct downwards through the entangling of the "colonised" into chains of interdependency was a process that also spread Western institutions and psychological attitudes. However, there lies an obvious flaw in over-relying on structuralist explanations: self-restraint in human behaviour is not a universal force.

Indeed, the twentieth century is marked by catastrophic examples of *de*-civilisation. The so-called civilising forces of colonialism secured pacification and peace within its own boundaries. Yet the trouble with colonial powers such as the British, for example, is that much of its history happened overseas, which is why so little is understood by those within its watery boundary. In deploying state-sanctioned violence outward towards vulnerable colonised populations, the colonisers deviated or regressed markedly from any principle of civilising the Other.

Paradoxically, racism, enslavement, cultural looting, destruction, exploitation, terror, and mass murder became the imperialist instruments of the civilising process. The concept of "civilisation" thus becomes an ambivalent and contradictory structuralist process whose violent nature is more often visible on the edges than within, where judicial torture, cat burning, and public execution become incompatible with domestic sensibilities.

When applied to the world, the structuralist hermeneutic process catalyses complexity and contradiction. Interpreting the world becomes a hermeneutic cyclic of prejudgment, which directs explanation, which in turn decides understanding, which defines prejudgment again. A similar circularity is suspected to attend other underlying systems presumed to shape our lives, which includes the reputed fiction of language, political systems, religion, relations of production, and our lived relationship with humanistic ideas of autonomy.

Waking from the Structuralist Dream. Almost as soon as the structuralist idiom was proposed, criticism was swift, voluminous, and specific. It was faulted for its scientific pretentions and a narcissistic relation to its own rhetoric. It seemed to allow things to mean anything to anyone, either by asserting the indeterminacy of meaning or by defining meaning as the sole experience of the powerful interpreter.

During a conference at John Hopkins University in 1966, Jacque Derrida presented a lecture entitled *Structure, Sign and Play*, which inaugurated a turn in structuralism that exposed its flawed desire to find a privileged reference point, origin, or fixed centre from which to adjudicate meaning in the systems to which it turned its gaze. In the case of language, no language can be fixed forever and this excludes the possibility that meaning can ever be anchored to reality. A significant insight of structuralism, however, is that it shows that the objective interpretation of facts neglects to reveal how those "facts" have come to have *significance* and to whom.

The experience that systems of foundational categories fail to capture the complexity of people's lives has led thinkers to become more interested in the local and particular, as opposed to universally applicable generalisations. At some point, those with interests beyond universals began to describe themselves as post-structuralists; they were characterised by seeing how useful it was to focus on contextualised meaning-making, rather than on universal truths or an all-encompassing reality. It is an approach which focusses on meaning, particularity, culture, language, and talk. All are explored here in terms of how they *relate* to the experience of people in their living present.

Proponents of poststructuralism seek specific details of a person's living present and much like the clinical case study and ethnography, insights are sought beyond the role of supporting abstract ideas. Lives are valued in terms of how they embody exceptions or uniqueness, rather than how they fit general categories. Post-structural thinkers understand that a single story cannot be told as though it were the only story to be told. A one-sided explanation or story always implies distortion. Not because it is a lie, but because a half-truth cannot be the whole truth (Hall, 2005: 36).

This more nuanced reading of structuralism proposed by Derrida no longer sought an origin but instead wanted to pass beyond the nostalgic dream of a reassuring foundation and embrace the *play* of meaning. We thus have a bifurcation in hermeneutics: one path turns away from seeking a transcendent origin while interpreting with suspicion. The other – seen more as a poetics – avoids interpretation but seeks to understand the conditions of possibilities within a lived, contextualised life.

Although those present at Derrida's lecture did not realise it, by offering two ways of proceeding within the structuralist project, they had attended what was later to be understood as the birth of *poststructuralism* – a perspective deeply coupled with postmodernism, which we explore later. Derrida's innovation was not about moving philosophy "forward", but of reading philosophy in a radically new way, which challenges the idea of eternal truths, fixed morals, the nature of being, and the illusion of a stable knowable self.

Regardless of Derrida's project, the traditional structuralist interpretation of human experience remains stubbornly entrenched in the practice of psychology, seeing people as atoms with stable internal working models amenable to classification and analysis (Slife et al., 2017). Derrida's critics see the idea of endless free play as the slippery slope to moral relativism, nihilism, and uncertainty in the meaning of everything. All that remains after any unchecked project of Derridean deconstruction is the power of deconstruction itself: *it is rightfully accused of being a sterile and impoverished philosophy which uncouples human beings from faith in anything other than the emptiness of deconstruction itself.*

## 6.2 Freedom and Autonomy – Romantic Delusions

For Marx, the economic conditions of production were the base or foundation of all other social practices: bourgeois thinking manifested itself in capitalist ideology, which acted in a classically "top-down" manner. In short, there was little room for human social agency in what became known as *vulgar* Marxism. The accompanying fatalism draws comparisons with the old philosophy of Stoicism whose aim was, similarly, to be free of suffering in a largely deterministic universe.

A radical and valuable concept within Marxist theory that helps us make sense of our social world is that of <u>ideology</u>. It is a thing that is highly consequential and "real" in that it describes the framework of meanings and values within which people exist and conduct their lives. Ideology is something we *live and do* and not something we spend too much time thinking about. Ideologies that are self-aware and self-avowed are relatively harmless – they can be necessary and good if they describe consistent ways of doing what is basically the right thing in its time.

What Marx became concerned about, however, was ideology masquerading as common sense. Indeed, "common sense" is a good example of an invisible taken-for-granted ideology that can grip us with a kind of fanatical adherence that deprives us of our freedom. The obvious, transparent, and spontaneous nature of "common sense" is characteristic of an ideology which refuses to be questioned and furthermore whose obviousness resists correction. Thus, ideology is often characterised as a false consciousness or an imagined representation of the real conditions of existence.

For Marx, autonomy is freedom from ideological capture. Yet the Marxist notion of false consciousness presumes there is a consciousness which is not false; a position of freedom from which this falseness can be apprehended and held to account. So where exactly for Marx is this high watchtower from which a critique can be made, uncontaminated by ideology? This sense of relativism did not invalidate, for example, Foucault's critical position about ideologies, because Foucault did not claim to speak from a position of scientific truth; he was aware that he too was a subject speaking within the limits imposed by the structures circulating around him (Foucault & Rabinow, 2002).

The French Marxist philosopher Louis Althusser devoted much of his career to what he saw as the problem of humanism: its tactical value, its historical beginnings, its utility, and the ultimate falsehood of universal freedom. Althusser applied structuralist methods of linguistics and anthropology to critique humanism, and the very idea that humanity is the subject, agent, and author of personal histories. In looking to dislodge tenacious humanist assumptions about autonomy and free will, Althusser sought to untangle the relationship between ideology as a *structure* (Subject), and people as *individuals* (subjects). Althusser was interested in understanding the apparatuses used to recruit incurious people into the power structures of Subjects because – he argued – rarely do they work in the interests of the individual (Althusser, 2012).

Though captured by the foundational tenet of Marxism – which holds that, in the final analysis, we are determined by economic laws – Althusser nevertheless opened the gate to a linguistic understanding of Subjects to which we turn later. Althusser revised the base and superstructure metaphor, acknowledging the important constitutive role of language for calculating, internalising, and transforming Subjects.

Althusser's most important innovation was to borrow the idea of interpellation from Freud. The term was used to describe the process wherein ideology recruits its subject (subjectivity + subjection); ideology was therefore not something produced by individual consciousness but, rather, people formulate their beliefs within positions already fixed by ideology, as if they were the true producers of ideology.

Typical apparatuses of interpellation claimed Althusser, included the church, educational institutions, the family, judiciary, political parties, trade unions, media, and culture. To this list we could also add the social practice – with its often-undeclared influences – of counselling and psychotherapy (Kearney & Proctor, 2018). The primary purpose of such apparatuses is to recruit or summon subjects so that in our thoughts, in our voluntary practices, we become willing participants in existing power operations (Althusser, 1964: Part IV):

> the rich holding forth to the poor on the most deliberate discourse ever conceived, so as to persuade them to live their slavery as their freedom …. just as a people that exploit another cannot be free, so a class that *uses* an ideology (such as humanism) is its captive too.

Althusser argued that Humanism – our lived relation with ideas of autonomy – is of practical importance and may even be essential for human society to work, but theoretically it is a romantic delusion. According to his view, even the most creative of acts – certainly discourse and writing – are less about free will than an unconscious act of subjection on the part of the speaker to innumerable complex rules of which we are necessarily unaware.

*Ignorance of the rules becomes a condition of obedience to the rules.* Politically, the implications are profound. Social revolt and opposition are seen also as illusions, whose appearance exists precisely to ensure that individuals would live their subjection as a sort of freedom.

The limitation of Althusser's philosophy was a commitment to a single unique Subject (i.e., the laws of economics), which holds the centre around which we gather. Max Weber's influential study, *The Protestant Ethic and the Spirit of Capitalism*, placed instead Protestantism as the central Subject – which is not so much a light cloak, but an "iron cage" which defines the structure of society (Weber, 2001: 123).

But this iron cage need not be our iron fate. Althusser's innovation was that he opened the gate to a more linguistic and constitutive understanding of how Subjects become internalised: there is a dynamic multiplicity of Subjects rising, falling, and decentring people's lives. The prominent cultural theorist Stuart Hall did not deny the reality of markets, but when we place the "market" at the top of the pyramid of Subjects, we continue to delude ourselves about what is really going on.

For Hall, the single explanation approach was not an adequate one because it substitutes one part to represent something about the whole – it denies the multiple disciplining factors of radical relationality. We become distracted by what manifestly announces itself, which leaves us without a plurality of Subjects to cut into our lived experience of the world at other points (Hall, 2005). No Subject can be defined by a single ideology, which for Hall had the powerful effect of expelling economics from Marxist theory once and for all; *there can be no reassuring foundation*.

A preoccupation with economic laws aside, the importance of Althusser's insights draw attention to the characteristically "obvious" nature of Subjects. Althusser uses an everyday example to communicate something of the obviousness of being *always ready* to respond to the *hail* ("Hey you!") of our Subjects. Who has not knocked on a door and announced (hailed), "it's me!" and not immediately expected to be recognised as being obviously "me"? Being interpellated is similarly to be incessantly prepared to be uncritically hailed by our Subjects.

Through interpellation, we function as we do because it seems right, natural, or obvious; we recognise ourselves as subjects of an ideological call. For Althusser, this entailed misrecognition of our participation and is central to how ideology works. In this sense there are overlaps between Althusser's Subjects, Taylor's moral sources, and Macintyre's *Traditions*, which more broadly discipline the Self (Section 1.3); they circumscribe our often-uncritical understandings, values, or ideals (orientations) about what is important for living well.

Yet plurality does not imply that Subjects are distortions. We willingly buy-into and support a multiplicity of Subjects, which function as a kind of law, be it the laws of God, economics, instrumental reason, sovereign free-will or self-determination. Human beings have a multiplicity of ethical choices or Subjects available to them, which means that we have the potential – with awareness – to adopt a radically relational stance towards interpellation; we need not be seduced by their apparent and obvious "rightness".

Perhaps it is because individualistic freedom has historically come to mean independence from something external – itself a powerful Subject – that we fail to see how the enslavement of the self *by* oneself (i.e., existentialism) is yet another ideology to which we unwittingly subscribe. The authentic human life is to be understood then as one characterised by creativity, discovery, and an openness to horizons of significance in relation to the undeniably seductive demands of our various Subjects.

While Humanism may not be the actual centre, it does offer a useful centring function, which pulls other theories into perspective, helping us consider the ethical dimensions of the therapeutic encounter. When an ideology seeks to hail, or interpellate me, I can respond from one end of the spectrum and see it as a positive proposition, or alternatively react with a bloody-minded refusal to identify with it, choosing instead to seek alternatives to what is on offer.

The implications for the therapeutic encounter are that therapist and client, when in the grip of a seemingly intractable problem framed by a shared picture of how things *must* be, have an opportunity to reach autonomy through awareness of alternative ethical possibilities. Because an unhelpful Subject is – by its nature – a collective, dialogic linguistic perspective, then autonomy equates to a liberation from the Subject towards a deeper relational effort *with* others. In short, every Subject – or therapeutic theoretical construct – has both its worthwhile benefits and readily rejected elements for the client.

But repeating an earlier point, it is only when we can achieve an equality of access that clients can actively choose to work with, say, a Humanistic therapist who is knowingly recruited into the quest for the "true self" (Section 2.3). As we see shortly, getting it right in understanding ourselves is more than a matter of aligning with the words associated with an ideology or Subject. It requires being able to grasp how multiple Subjects relate to our intuitive sense of our life as a whole and the narrative structure we look to develop.

But where do our intuitions about the correct ideological choices come from? We have already explored aspirations of the good called out in us by transcendent sources such as God, the possibility of re-enacting a nobler order of virtue from our ancestors, the felt intuitions from the pre-history of humanity, the dignity attached to our own powers, and the depths of Nature within and without. Some or all of these can be the source of our felt intuitions about how we wish to live our lives. They form the reality of what we value, and the virtues to which we aspire.

How can we be confident that we can trust our intuitions when examining our ideological assumptions? How can we be sure that we are able to refine our intuitions in the therapeutic field of words, where the meaning of talk can lead to growth, insight, and confidence in our ability to make secure judgements? To this end, we must look towards the linguistic domain of our existence.

Therapeutic Interpellations. Althusser's insights allow us to ask the question: what interpellations can we notice in the therapeutic encounter and how do we make the right choices? Earlier I described what we can now understand as Rogers' well-intentioned *interpellation* of Gloria into the notion of a pre-existing self, independent of social interaction, which calls into question the ethical ideal of a non-directional encounter.

The person-centred approach presupposes that the detached and sovereign self is the *right choice*. It reflects a ubiquitous <u>Subject</u> in contemporary psychotherapy which finds its source in the Romantic expressivist notion of an authentic inner voice, or conscience to which we must become attuned if we are to connect with our natural indwelling organismic self. Romanticism brings to our attention how we are defined by more than just the power of disengaged rational reasoning.

The power of Romantic creative imagination works in the same direction. It intensifies our sense of inner depths which are always "down there", something endless and beyond articulation which leads to even more radical subjectivism and internalisation. The modern person who recognises both these powers – objective and subjective paths to truth – is inevitably in tension with themselves because of the schism it creates.

An analysis of Aaron Beck's cognitive behavioural session with a client reveals a multiplicity of <u>Subjects</u> in play – the sovereign rational subject, a relational desire for intimate attachment, gender dynamics and heterosexual intimacy. For Beck, interpellation into the <u>Subject</u> of rationality and self-determination eclipsed the hailing power – and associated values – of alternatives including gender socialisation. Interpellation of the client into the <u>Subject</u> of the therapeutic process *becomes* the yardstick by which the success of the encounter is measured. It is the obvious, logical, right choice which reflects the therapist's preference, thereby usurping alternatives that may have been the right choice for the client (Gilfoyle, 2009).

The plurality of <u>Subjects</u> in addiction recovery and psychotherapy coincide in problematic ways with neoliberal and Humanistic notions of self-mastery and instrumental reason: they frame both the cause and the solution in terms of *recovering* the authentic self from the grip of the *self* that has been corrupted by an external substance. The idea of an authentic self, fending off the corrupted self reproduces the <u>Subject</u> of addiction as a chronic relapsing disorder with recovery understood as a never-ending personal journey towards normality.

Attributing addictive cravings to the corrupted-self calls into question the virtue and authority of the authentic-self. The authentic self has failed to exert rational control over the corrupted self: *I have got it wrong*. The authentic self fails to make the right choice when hailed by the call of virtuous self-mastery, which lies at the heart of the Humanistic ideal of the productive citizen. The burden of a failed authentic self is heavy. How does this sit with our felt intuitions and moral sources? It seems unlikely that the values of the client can be ethically accommodated by a process which conceals their participation in a preferred Subject – in this case, the modernist project of sovereign rationality and self-determination (Ekendahl et al., 2022).

*Faux* individualism dominates our society: in its various forms it presents itself as one of the most powerful, collectively constituted Subjects of our times. We uncritically put our faith in the free market, where the average of the expressed preferences of millions of consumers becomes the process – accelerated by social media – through which we come to think of ourselves as "individuals" in some way.

Allowing one Subject to eclipse all others insinuates both therapist and client into an impoverished form of relationship. The importance of recognising the pluralism of ethical Subjects available to a person is that we may be drawn to one or many of them at any given time. This has the potential to radically redefine the dynamic of the therapeutic encounter. The process of therapy becomes a mutual gateway to a field of words which helps us go deeper, through cycles of interpretation and articulation, allowing us to explore, acquire, and refine new ethical meanings and intuitions. Therapy becomes a project which helps the pursuit of new words, metaphors, and dialogues to liberate ourselves from inner-restraints, compulsions, and fears about the culture we co-create.

What place does language and ethical intuition have in the constitutive processes which are implicit in choosing between a plurality of Subjects? How do we engage in a therapeutic ethical dialogue when different therapies prize different ethical Subjects? Any Subject which sees itself impervious to critique is at risk – as Kevin Smith points out – of missing what is at stake when choosing between different visions of flourishing (2021: 75–76).

Yet it is not simply a matter of accessing an "off the shelf" Subject: our relationship with the material world, our traditions, myths, language, and relationships are entangled in the constitutive formation of Subjects. I cannot challenge my ideologies if as a therapist I do not want to give up the comfortable feeling of being the one who *knows* what truth is. In this sense, radical relationality can only hope to wake those who are genuinely asleep to the plurality of Subjects; it cannot stir those who are pretending to be asleep.

Against Relativism: Change and Therapeutic Traditions. The German term for the humanities is *Geisteswissenschaften*, which approximates to: "the organised study of the human spirit" or perhaps "the science of spirit". It understands that so long as there are practitioners of different methods, which includes the plurality of moral traditions or Subjects concerned with how to live – then there will remain competing perspectives. This creates the variety and riches of traditions which are the hallmark of studying the human spirit.

The natural sciences take it that one paradigm eventually replaces another, in much the same way that quantum mechanics and relativity replaced Newtonian concepts for understanding both the immensely small and large things in our universe. The new paradigm becomes the unquestioned ground from which normal science takes place. But this is something of a stereotype; despite the Copernican heliocentric revolution, we carry on with our technologically informed lives as if it is the sun that moves through the sky.

In the study of the humanities, which encompasses disciplines such as philosophy, history, linguistics, theology, psychology, and psychotherapy there are rarely dramatic evolutions. Moral traditions in the *science of spirit* evade crises of incoherence between belief and practice without fatal consequences for long periods of time.

The moral tradition of Buddhism, for example, can and does exist in starkly diverse forms within equally diverse cultures and contexts, that is, Japan, Sri Lanka, and Burma. There is no neutral position or centre from which to evaluate the contending claims and nuanced interpretations which such traditions embody. There can be no objective or empirical criteria for deciding whether one method – or form of Buddhism – is better than another when it comes to living a good life.

For Gadamer, all truth-claims are historical in the sense that they are framed in some "tradition" of inquiry. The "tradition" determines things like which questions seem important, which have priority at a given time, and what conceptual tools are employed to answer these questions. In short, a tradition not only decides the questions in some sense, but it also plays a role in determining what counts as the best answer to the question. For example, we might express a belief that CBT reduces the symptoms of menopause because empirical testing offers repeated and repeatable corroboration for symptom reduction. In other words, we offer a "justification" for symptom reduction inseparable from claims about the nature and reliability of empirical evidence. The particular Subject of reasoned self-mastery cannot in any empirical sense be established as being more valuable for living well compared to other competing Subjects.

Change in the therapeutic sense is usually more about a transition from one ethical perspective to another; for example as Kierkegaard would have it, from aesthete to ethicist. When a community, or client moves from one ethical perspective to another, or prioritises one Subject over another, they do so because it leads to an improvement in living, or a more convincing perspective on a matter. It is the sort of task that never finishes because it is constitutive – how we create such transitions requires the evolution of the stories we tell about our lives, which brings with it new perspectives for re-telling and refinement.

It is through the creative borrowing of concepts or vocabularies that we dissolve historically outmoded certainties between therapeutic (ethical) traditions. When, even after a period of systematic reflection issues of critical importance to a tradition remain unresolved, deeper questions arise about why progress stalls. Could it be because we lack the resources to address and solve problems and are unable to find solutions because we are slavishly committed to the presuppositions of our therapeutic methods? When we are able, through acts of imagination and questioning, to interrogate some rival perspective, it is always possible that we may conclude, indeed are compelled to conclude that it is only from the standpoint of another perspective that our difficulties can be adequately understood and overcome.

So, for long periods of time, several therapeutic traditions can and do coexist without any one of them having to take the claims of its alternatives seriously, let alone examine whether one of these alternatives works better than the others. What matters is that issues of internal incoherence can, on occasion, be decided, which makes it clear that the claims of other traditions presuppose the falsity of relativism; *the value of a tradition is real and enduring for those who live them.* The ancient idiom – which we shall return to – understands that there can be several perspectives of the same mountain, but this does not mean that there are several mountains.

*To conclude*, a more sophisticated attitude to structuralism suggests that who we are cannot be accounted for by focusing on the individual, but rather by examining the framework of a person's collective viewpoints. Our freedom comes not from within the deep structure of a person, but from recognising the fragile and contingent nature of our times, our history, and our interpellations. In short, the capillary structures of how we use language contributes to social cohesion and the plurality of Subjects. The way we engage constitutively with our Subjects, define our boundaries, and legislate the notes from which we play out our relational music, is a theme I wish to develop next.

### 6.3   Structuralism and Identity

Therapies influenced by poststructuralism suggest that language, in its broadest sense, places limits on the positions individuals can adopt, on what can be said, and on what can be thought. Language as something purely constitutive of subjectivity inadvertently undermines notions of human creativity and ethical agency.

The Russian literary critic and philosopher Mikhail Bakhtin offers a more optimistic perspective of the formative role of humans in the continual creation and recreation of meaning, while also fully acknowledging the role of language in the emergence of subjectivity. The context in which Bakhtin developed his ideas – the ideology and politics of the Soviet Union under Stalin – meant his dialogic approach evolved beyond the influence of capitalist concerns with individualism and individual freedom. For Bakhtin, there was no central "I" in charge; the self was a metaphor for a decentred, horizontalised social being suffused with the voices of others – *a society of voices within a society of voices.* Consciousness for Bakhtin was seen not as a property of the individual, somehow encased within their skin, but a communal phenomenon: the self has no internal sovereign territory but exists in a *plane* of experience (Pollard, 2018). The radical relationalist has this in mind and is aware of the subtle shifts between the self as a source of demoralising deficits and a more hopeful relational subject installed in a world of possibility, as we see next.

Noticing Shifts in Identity. Different experiences of the therapeutic encounter are possible if we can distinguish between identity as something which exists *within* a person (structuralist internal state) or alternatively as something understood to exist in the plane, in a radical relation with others. This latter non-structuralist relational self is more open to interpretation and renegotiation through a broader understanding of interpellation, Subjects, ethics, beliefs, and actions. Because we spend so much of our lives immersed in the language of structuralism, we easily miss opportunities to respond differently when a switch between structuralist and non-structuralist categories of identity occurs.

Structuralist therapeutic models incorporate humanistic attitudes which see the self as a sovereign centre of ethics, reason, and being, rather than a relational self which can be known through dialectical alternatives. The interpellated language of structuralist "internal states", so pervasive in modern psychology, describes the self as if layered, like an onion, with motives, needs, traits, and drives – all of which are indwelling. It is of little surprise then that a client – such as Kim – often sees themselves as somehow deficient in terms of structuralist characteristics, strengths, or qualities.

*Cathy:*  What would you say this means about you or what's important to you?

*Kim:*  Well, I think I'm a strong person ... but when I am with her [Kim's mother], I feel weak.

*Cathy:*  Can you tell me some more about feeling weak? Is it something you can turn-up or down, like a dial?

*Kim:*  Oh, no, somehow the dial stops working with her ... it's stuck on the lowest setting ...

The therapist's (Cathy) inquiry into Kim's structuralist concept of "weakness" will only lead to relatively superficial descriptions, as there is only so much we can say about the self as a point of existence. Yet there are opportunities here for a non-structuralist conversation, drawing on Kim's relational "horizontality" in terms of understanding her hopes, intentions (*telos*), beliefs, values, and principles (*ethics*) for living well.

For example, Cathy might ask: When you think about what you call weakness, to what use would you put your strength? Why is it important for you to use your strength in that way? What values are important for you here? When you think about these values, what hopes do they reflect? What values (or principles or ways of being) in life do they stand for? Why are these values important to you? What do they say about what you stand for? (Morgan, 2002).

Such questions invite Kim to examine how she sees herself in the world, decentred, and extending beyond the locus of her internalised states of mind. The explorative questions lead Kim away from an atomised self to a relational subject, interconnected and knotted with others, moral sources, traditions, and Subjects – even if these are not the terms she would ordinarily use.

Transactional Analysis. Eric Berne conceived of internal structures of the mind or "ego states", which he termed Adult, Parent and Child. The Subject of the technique into which practitioners interpellate their clients is the outdated goal of realising the "fully autonomous Adult" state. What defines the Adult is the structuralist ideal of a privileged reference point for ethical adjudication, hailing from mid-twentieth-century Western individualist notions that sees dependence as something shameful and embarrassing.

This sort of psychic colonialisation reflects interpellation to a Subject which eclipses cultural diversity and collectivism. For much of Asia, Central and South America, and Africa, the individualising Subject is at odds with the prioritisation of individual needs and desires over family, community, and society. As I claimed earlier, Humanistic *interpellation* fails also to reflect our environmental interdependence and the inextricable connection we have with the ecosystem – the Natural world.

Attachment Theory. Bowlby was dissatisfied with the psychoanalytic theorising of his time and the inner world of psychological representations, which were seen to spring from *within* a child, rather than emerging *through* a child's actual relationships. Yet he became drawn to the early innovators of what would become artificial intelligence, who theorised about "internal working models … carried around in our heads". Our internal pre-verbal unconscious representations served as the blueprint to live by, emerging as they did from "biologically channelled, survival-based attachment systems and the actualities of the parenting we experience" (Wallin, 2007).

Despite being among the most significant shapers of how we perceive child development and parenting across and beyond Anglophone cultures, it is widely criticised as a politically conservative research programme, "smuggling" social norms under the cover of claims of scientific objectivity. Feminist post-structural scholarship, in particular, sees attachment as oriented by a concern to police families, pathologises mothers and emphasises structural psychological notions at the expense of socio-economic realities.

To be sure, Bowlby's attachment system leans heavily on biological determinism, early twentieth-century misogyny, essentialist notions of motherhood, and anxieties about women working outside the home. Often considered a child-centred model, extrapolation to more reciprocal adult–adult relationships are fraught with ambiguity, not least of all because of attachment theory's emphasis on structuralist internal working models, which are not "internal" at all but dependent on social processes. An insistence on the importance of the mother–child dyad over and above all other childhood experience attracts further criticism from several quarters, including the exclusion of fathers, siblings, the confinement of women to the mothering role (the motherhood mandate), and a failure to acknowledge the role of the child as an agent in their social environment.

The rigid emphasis of the motherhood mandate reinforces the constraining notion that there is but one way to parent correctly, focusing attention on parenting practices as deterministic to the exclusion of broader social contexts and stressors that affect children's wellbeing. Ideas about attachment are, however, compelling, as they fit our historical moment, with its emphasis on risk-averse, intensive parenting and the professionalisation of motherhood through the consumption of expert advice (Pylypa, 2016). Nevertheless, attachment theory offers a starting point for framing the complexity of adult relationships irrespective of the "leap of faith" required to extrapolate childhood experiences to adult relationship patterns (Goodwin, 2003).

The radical relationalist seeks to understand attachment as a genuinely un-determined system, like the emergence of the biological components of puberty into the subjectivity of a young adult. Individuals are not prior to their environment but are codetermined *with* their environment. When attachment and attachment research is reduced to a child's demand for proximity with their caregiver, then it runs the risk of dovetailing with gender and political conservatism. The humanistic self-sufficient subject falls neatly within the rhetorical needs of contemporary capitalism which does not prize public investment in health, education, and social care. A non-structural approach challenges us to untangle the needs of a caregiver from the imperatives of the attachment system of the child. Softening the hierarchy which prioritises the needs of the cared-for over the relationships of caregivers requires solidarity not suspicion between those left to compete against each other rather than share in health, social and political resources (Duschinsky, 2015).

### 6.4 Language and the Emergence of Meaning

Language is perhaps our most dazzling social skill. The purpose of many conversations – particularly those in a therapeutic context – is more than an exchange of facts. The nature of talk invites joint attention, something beyond the cinematic experience of simultaneously yet independently paying attention to an object alongside another. It is an invitation to explore what we can co-create, what we can know *together*.

The embodied nature of speech only becomes apparent when say, we experience laryngitis, a heavy cold, a trip to the dentist for a filling, or an injury to the most taken-for-granted muscular organ in the body – the tongue. When we speak, we stutter, stammer, lisp, and spit; words are swallowed, stick in the throat and we become tongue-tied. We celebrate the stagecraft of ventriloquism, which denies the use of our lips when attempting to utter certain sounds (i.e., f, v, b, p, and m).

The embodied transformation I witness when my wife switches from speaking English to her native Italian is a wonder to behold. Speech is something enacted using the *entire* body, employing eye contact, gestures, facial expressions, and even posture to convey something on the way to meaning, beyond the content of an already-formed idea. Speech seems to travel in the *opposite* direction of perception in that the thought itself is formed in its externalisation – speaker and world shape and mould one another. At a fundamental level, speech embodies our desire for human contact, something many of us crave throughout our lives, from the moment we seek out our mother's nipple to our final breath.

Language is an old topic for Western philosophy. Its importance has grown since the beginning of the modern period to its zenith in the mid-twentieth century when interest reached a frenzy not least of all because Wittgenstein and Heidegger placed language at the heart of their philosophy. It is difficult to imagine how we can grasp the linguistic dimension of human experience without building on our earlier structuralist insights. Taylor adopts this perspective when he separates the theories of language into two broad categories, namely those which *enframe* experience and those which *create* experience (2016).

Language that Enframes. The family of theories referred to as *enframing* comes from a powerful tradition in Western thought that seeks to convince us that language is mainly about encoding information about the real world. Enframing theories seek to deal with descriptive coding and the transmission of information especially in scientific contexts. Here, it is at its most powerful when conveying facts and building verbal pictures for common deliberation and the coordination of actions. Language is seen as the way we represent reality from an external standpoint; it is an idea in harmony with the modern, humanistic epistemology of Descartes and the scientific revolution.

It is presumed that language precedes what it is used to explain. Language is a fixed code whose existence does not depend on the individual speaker. Language, it is believed, sits within a framework or a picture of human life which takes for granted our purpose, the way we behave, and how we think. When writing in the language of science for example, I rigidly adhere to the third person past tense format to objectify and disembody tasks and processes: "the solvent was removed *in vacuo*" and not "I stuck the flask on the evaporator and went for tea with my friends". This specialised pared-down language excludes human meaning, emotion, or understanding and is ideal for describing recipes in academic science; but this linguistic austerity is a world away from the raucous talk used by the people who conjure the recipes in the laboratory.

The parable of the fish that asks, "what the heck is water?" comes to mind again when we speak of language in the encoding frame as it is the invisible medium for fixing, communicating, and interrogating our thoughts and feelings. This verbal formulation of thoughts, feelings, and emotions allow us to adopt a disengaged stance towards them. Words give us dominion over our imagination and provides an object-like significance to our "mental contents" independent of background. The Stoic can rest assured that the mind is in control of the passions.

The ability to encode has had astonishing implications for the development of human culture and technology. Yet, language is more than an intellectual skill. We could not develop our ability to encode without creating, sustaining, and articulating meaning through our relationships. Here, I am thinking about the embodied practices that bind us to our context, such as metaphors equating time with movement (Chapter 8), expressivity (i.e., tone of voice, body language, gestures, facial expressions, hugs, kisses, and giggles – Chapter 9), and the kind of artistic portrayals (i.e., music, dance, role-play) used in ordinary conversation. This sets the stage for the second family of language theories I introduce next.

Language that Creates. The family of *constitutive* language theories are the antithesis of the enframing kind and are more difficult to retrieve because they run against the grain of how modern culture teaches us how to even think. Speech is on the way to the expression of thought; but thought is not merely language. A good deal of work in the cognitive sciences has now established that conceptual schemes are not determined by language; *concepts are prior to language*.

Studies have established that the concept of numbers and a sensitivity to statistical patterns exists for pre-verbal infants. Adults who have not acquired spoken language display sophisticated and abstract forms of thinking, the corollary being that neither vocabulary nor syntax in any way determine, force, or for that matter prevent, thought. Yet language is more than simply the face of that which exists independently. How do we create an idea or feeling for which we do not have a word? When we do have a word – say, for example, *nice* – it is undeniable that we connect this with memories, reflections, and understandings of ethical traditions and wider Subjects.

*Listen to what I mean … not what I say.* Ray Monk's biography illuminates the philosophical, spiritual, and ethical development of Ludwig Wittgenstein from a thinker who saw language as that which enframes, to one which creates (1991). The early part of Wittgenstein's career was marked by the publication of *Tractatus Logico-Philosophicus*, a book with an intimidatingly highbrow title. It explored the relationship between language and thought, and between language and the world. Such matters are intimately linked to a vision of language which, among other difficulties, tends to produce bad translations. It was essential then that the 1922 translation into English got those relationships right.

Wittgenstein's original title for the book was, in fact, quite down to earth and translates from German into something like *Essay on Logic and Philosophy* (2024). The book's early translators, however, were operating in a framework that did not address the different ways English and German work. Furthermore, Wittgenstein's supporters sought to place the text firmly in the field of technical academic philosophy. For a project aimed at examining the relationship between language and the world, this was not an auspicious start.

Devotees of the celebrated final line of his *Essay* "Whereof one cannot speak, thereof one must be silent", have to defend another clunky translation. Wittgenstein's original sentence was similar to plain English, as expressed in his 1916 notebook: "What cannot be said, *cannot* be said!". The point here is that Wittgenstein did not seek to use inaccessible or arcane language. The book nevertheless outlines a view of language that enframes and an attitude towards translation wherein every word translated corresponds to a single, consistent word in the other language. As any bilingual speaker will tell you, this is not how language works; *translation and interpretation are not the same*. While Wittgenstein does not quite admit that every English word has its German counterpart and vice versa, *Tractatus* does not account for the way language creates different images of the world.

Rueful of this early positivism which reduced language to an abstraction of logic, Wittgenstein began to turn his gaze towards language as something internally self-referential. Wittgenstein's thinking evolved to see language instead as a collective, human activity constituted through public, intersubjective use and not as he had previously believed, through its representation of some deeper structure of the world. Wittgenstein's posthumously published *Philosophical Investigations* – translated by his friend and philosophical disciple, Elizabeth Anscombe – saw how in fact, the *unsayable* could not exist without its surrounding *sayable*.

Wittgenstein was to sweep away all earlier ideas from the *Tractatus* with a single parenthetical anecdote: "A French politician once wrote that it was a peculiarity of the French language that in it words occur in the order in which one thinks them" (PI, 1974: Part 1, §336). The absurd perspective of the politician seemed to reflect the position of the younger Austrian philosopher who believed that every language in the world was German, but with the words swapped out. Wittgenstein's mature perspective was to bring to our attention how we must get the life of a speaker into view; not only their linguistic life but also their holistic way of dealing with things in the world.

In this way, *Philosophical Investigations* can be considered a work of ethics in that its central concern is our relationship with others. Only by doing so can we make it possible to articulate new purposes, experiences, and figures which shape the human experience of the world in its broadest sense. This is something Wittgenstein sought to express when he explained: "If a lion could talk, we could not understand him" (Wittgenstein, 1974: Part 2, §223e). We would first have to understand something of the concerns, cares, and relationships of a lion to understand how it uses language.

Wittgenstein insisted we see a plurality of arbitrary "language games" which work at different levels and in different contexts. The word "game" in its ordinary meaning can lead us astray here: it is not a game in the sense of an amusement, but a set of procedures which may be considered valid or invalid for producing truth. Thinking about language as a game only takes us so far. It implies fixed rules – but the games Wittgenstein had in mind are closer to the games children play. When invited to play "snuggly toys" with my daughter, there is no discernible structure to the game. It switches from playing individually with playdoh, to an invitation to smell and taste the stuff. What is clear is that the game swings between something communal to something solitary. Atomic selves cannot possibly take part in the communion of a language game. I can be a self only in relation to my interlocutors. The silent monological inner voice of which Plotinus spoke when reading to ourselves is acquired alongside the capacity for language in its openly expressed and relational form.

What characterises the game with my daughter however is that throughout it is about "our" relationship with the world "out there". It is a world we have previously co-created through trips to school, preparing food together, magical creatures, and bursts of song and dance depicting animated characters enjoyed – *together*. In fact, it can feel impossible to define a game without going beyond its object of attention. A plurality of inter-disciplinary and inter-cultural projects must be undertaken if we are to navigate our way through life. The subjective reason, rules, and ethics of the language games of a devout Christian, for example, are just as coherent as those of a particle physicist. Indeed, it is precisely how someone can be both a particle physicist and a devout Christian.

What matters is that there can be no primary language game of truth, which is something which disappoints both scientific positivists and religious fundamentalists alike. Rather than making universal claims to meaning, communities create and sustain their own language games, and by agreeing to ethical principles and values they define meaning, together: lawyers, scientists, psychologists, and physicians are good examples of this.

When one commits with awareness to speak one way rather than to speak another way, a person makes an ethical commitment: hovering over a word before alighting on a way of expressing ourselves is a process of resolving this ethical dilemma. It is important then that members of the same community see the world in a similar way prior to agreeing on the meaning of technical talk. What else is the process of training to be a therapist if not a process of homosocialisation, interpellation, and enculturation? One joins a community of belief prior to agreeing to and becoming conversant in a language which reflects those meanings. Innovation and cross-fertilisation can only begin from the point of already being established in such a language game.

Training to be a therapist mirrors the process of therapy itself; people are brought to see things differently through the practices and beliefs that help create what the theories claim to be the case. Language games are constitutive in that agreements about what it is to be a flourishing human interpellate people into <u>Subjects</u>. The same theories also shape people to accord with theory. When a client rejects interpellation into a therapeutic <u>Subject</u>, the temptation is to blame them or understand their rejection as a defence, or a pathology (alexithymia) rather than perhaps recognise their rejection to be an intuitive stand *for* an alternative that is simply not on offer.

Language games also mean there can be no such thing as context-*free* word. A word as simple as *water* can no longer correspond to a fixed reality but is connected to its context and is part of an activity which conveys the deeper relationality with which the word is imbued. For example, I have a strong memory from primary school of seeing and hearing an adult in an apron carrying jugs of water balefully crying: "water…water…water…", as they patrolled the rows of seated children.

The water carrier sought to hydrate we children and somehow encourage us to engage in the task of consuming plates of cold mashed potato and carrots. As I applied handfuls of the inedible stuff to the underside of the table, I would close my eyes and imagine that I was in a hot, dusty desert. Suddenly, the calls of "water … water … water" became transformed from an imperative into something less menacing, even comical. Unlike the food, reframing my relationship with what was being spoken transformed the experience into something more palatable.

Changing our relationship with what is spoken brings with it new meanings which re-shapes the world in ways that may make it difficult to see things in the old light ever again (Wittgenstein in Schönbaumsfeld, 2019):

> Once the new way of thinking has been established, the old problems vanish; indeed, they become hard to recapture. For they go with our way of expressing ourselves and, if we clothe ourselves in a new form of expression, the old problems are discarded along with the old garment.

The difference between "ordinary seeing" and what Wittgenstein called "aspect-perception" is to differentiate between apprehending a fact as encoded by language and instead becoming aware of a holistic configuration of the world through appreciating its relational context. For example, when looking at the famous figure of the *rabbit-duck*, I see initially the former and then later as I suddenly apprehend the aspect of latter, I do so in a way which makes it hard to unsee the duck ever again.

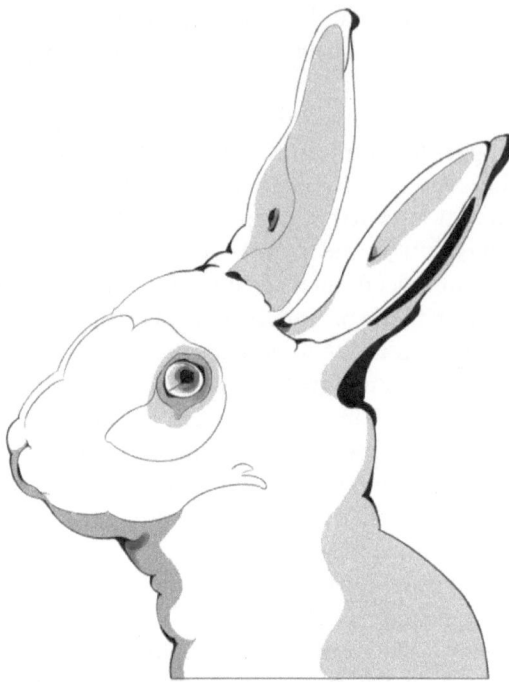

**FIGURE 6.1** Once Seen, Impossible to Unsee.

The figure conveys something of the therapeutic spirit of being able to see the world differently without altering its material facts, in this case, the lines on a page. There are no new added features to the object, but the internal relation between it and other objects in the world – a duck – are re-made. This is because we have had to go beyond the figure itself to understand this deeper relational dimension. This emergence of meaning makes the world bigger, but not in the sense of adding more items to it. Conversely, the loss of meaning reduces the limits of the world and makes it smaller. Counselling and psychotherapy have at their core this everyday task of aspect-changing, which informs our acquisition of new ethical attitudes and perspectives.

Discovery and Invention – Two Sides of the Same Emotional Coin. The idea that the way people think is shaped by the language they use is not new. Being married to a bilingual Italian for many years, I am sympathetic to the claim that language, thought, and culture are deeply interlocked, so much so that language seems to embody a distinctive way of looking at the world. I do not mean to say that the different grammatical structures of languages – Italian and English in my case – with their own unique, sometimes, roundabout way of encoding the same reality affords a wildly different sort of reality. As we see later, language, culture, time, and space are intimately entwined (Section 8.1);

but for now, we consider how constitutive theories are holistic in a way that deterministic alternatives – which bypass human motivation – are not.

Language as something which creates brings about a rotation in our understanding of the meaning of words as something embedded in a form of life. Language makes possible its own content and in this sense reminds me of organic chemistry – a practice that similarly generates its own subject. The chemist dreams of creating, of synthesising a new object (molecule), and in so doing they also discover novel performances, content, and properties, which can then alter the context in which the object was created.

The parallel with the constitutive nature of language lies in that both create alternatives, which offer gateways to new dimensions of possibility. Language is existentially constitutive: it makes the world bigger through collaboration and the uncovering of deeper meanings. We do not move *forward*; we see more *deeply*. The existential nature of being self-interpreting animals means that our search for the "right word" to articulate how I feel brings into view the experience of discovery and invention as two sides of the same emotional coin: "Everything we do consists in trying to find the liberating word" (Wittgenstein, *in* Read, 2021: 5). We devise an expression which allows what we are striving to encompass to appear. It is a crucial side of our language capability which Taylor calls "articulation" (2016: 178).

Language forms emotions through a process of articulation. Emotions can, through articulation, be re-valuated. In this sense, an incipient emotion can be refined through articulation; once articulated, the emotion is experienced differently. Emotions are, in this sense, determined both by the relational resources of the speaker and the ability of the speaker to articulate their emotions through language. Articulations are efforts to formulate what initially feels confusing or poorly formulated. But this kind of re-formulation does not leave the emotion – as *re*-presentation – unchanged. To articulate through relationships is to shape our sense of what we want or what we value in a certain way.

While people share the same neurophysiology and experiences of love, loss, childbirth, and death, we may not share the same emotional world which shapes re-presentation. The experience of emotion presents a challenge to language. The situation is not like giving a name to a physical object; emotions are less tangible and the boundaries between emotions are fuzzy. Emotional language is irreducible – there is no "thing" to which emotional language can point to beyond itself.

In essence, the reason for this – suggests Taylor – is that emotional language signifies not only a feeling, but a feeling as constituted in relation to a person's relational world. In studies with bi- and multilinguals, Aneta Pavlenko draws our attention to how emotional mismatches are one of the key sources of cross-cultural miscommunication (2014: 245–298). Language is situated not just in the mind but also in the body – something which points to a phenomenon invisible to the monolingual researcher and practitioner alike, namely, differential emotionality. With this in mind, Pavlenko asks the important question: need we be troubled by the fact that most of the world's research on human cognitive processes are conducted in English, predominantly by monolingual North Americans on other monolingual North Americans, many of whom are young students? The monolingual therapist who aspires to cross-cultural communication must recognise the limitations that their monochrome perspective may impose on their encounter with the dazzling diversity of human emotionality.

Meanings can be understood without being felt. I understand the meaning of danger when I avoid putting my fingers in a blender. This follows ordinary, designative semantic logic: we see a phenomenon and are told its name (or we give it a name). I can train a dog to respond to a signal (the name *snowy*), especially if the signal corresponds to being given a biscuit. But it does not mean that my dog recognises snow when it sees it. For a word requires more than recognition; it requires the linguistic dimension. It is rare that simply learning the name of a thing, like the name of my neighbour's cat, is going to be accompanied by a life-changing motivational force. What Taylor is getting at is that when we look to articulate something about what we are trying to understand, we have an opportunity to change the nature of our relationship with the object of our interest.

Basic distinctions – like between sadness and shame – are learnt early in our lives as the names for feelings we are beginning to have or can easily recognise in others. But there is another semantic logic that Taylor calls "constitutive". When being chased by a hippopotamus, not only do I perceive danger, but I also experience the emotion of fear. It seems plausible that all animals fear other, much larger creatures than themselves – so in this sense creatures share something universal when it comes to anger and fear. But pride, shame, jealousy, envy, indignation, or admiration seem qualitatively different from what animals feel. It seems plausible that such human sensibilities are related to their object in a form only available to beings with language. The point here is that bringing together what is "out there" with what is "in here" requires a radically relational act of linguistic communion with another human being.

The human experience is about being in touch with reality – not as some Herculean Humanistic effort on the part of an individual – but as a relational activity which requires thinking and perceiving, attention and tact, transcendent vision, and pattern recognition. Interpretation pervades our *felt* insights, making them malleable, expandable, revisable, crystalline, and questionable. It also develops from multiple ways of entering the space of reasons through emotions, metaphors, storytelling, rites, dance, symbolism, art, conversation, and the subtle play of resonance, endorsement, and recognition.

Sensibilities which go beyond an animal response presuppose an ethical sense of right or wrong. As children, our first encounter with shame might accompany being corrected for a minor misdemeanour. We want to physically hide from others: "go away … I do not want to be seen". As we develop, other behaviours such as having our bottoms wiped, or the public act of crying become things that feel somehow inapt. When we cry, shame compels us to hold our hands to our face and hide, yet again. It seems impossible to grow up without learning from those who care for us the words for these reactions and the triggers we meet through our relationships – though, of course, the triggers vary from one culture and historical context to another.

When my children learnt the word "rainbow" for example, it was not the same process through which I extended my Italian vocabulary with an extra word – *arcobaleno*. The acquisition of a novel word for a child has already been couched in hours of song ("I can sing a rainbow"), an introduction to colours, being shown rainbows and imbuing them with the kind of excitement that comes with something so fleeting and magical. The word for an object like a rainbow had already been suffused with sensations embodied in a web of other words before the bundle of social practices acquired the label "rainbow".

But let me go further into the constitutive relationship between emotions and language. Consider a child for whom there may be many triggers for the sensation that those around her call "anger". As her life experience develops, she begins to differentiate and then separate out from the anger other sensations. Frustration, indignation, irritation, and so on appear from the raw undifferentiated and unfocussed milieu of sensations that go along with her sister changing the "rules" of their game. As her relationships become more complex and the triggers diversify, an emotion labelled as anger begins to change in a way that has a greater bearing on her life. Frustration emerges as a refinement of the sensations she experiences, either when by herself struggling to make something work, or with others when things do not go her way. It is in these situations that the constitutive force of emotional development is enacted.

It is also in this sense that as therapists we should be aware that it becomes possible for emotions to be apt or inapt. While a feeling is real in the sense that it is felt, unthinking validation of a feeling by a well-meaning therapist implies that it constitutes the appropriate response to a given situation. Where then is the possibility of the emergence of new meanings, aspects being altered, or maturation? Getting it right about ourselves means more than just having the right word for a triggered sensation. The context in which the trigger occurs really matters. By context here, I mean the expectations of an ideology or Subject that has something to say about, for example, *how a girl ought to behave*.

Aligning our linguistic and emotional evolution with Subjects requires interpellation, which is invariably guided by those with whom we share *joint attention* who may already subscribe to an idea like: *angry girls are ugly*. So, a girl's understanding of anger becomes distorted or interpellated to minimise the threat to the Subject – a correctly labelled emotion can feel inapt. How we then relate to our <u>Subjects</u> becomes – in a greater sense – an articulation of the way we see our life. The kind of objectivity that engages in *interpreting* the meaning of a <u>Subject</u> is utterly different from the sort of reasoning that goes along with *aligning* with a <u>Subject</u>.

*The implications for therapy are clear.* Undifferentiated, diffuse, unrefined responses to an unusual – or persistent – relational context are open to re-valuing, re-interpretation, and re-articulation in relation to our <u>Subjects</u>. I can "tell" my four-year-old daughter about anger as if it were an independent object – perhaps something to be avoided or hidden (aligning with the <u>Subject</u>). But when it is introduced as a new constitutive expression that could alter her field of meanings, it becomes different from sticking a label on something.

The process of therapy alongside one who – from a "third-person" perspective – *cares* is similar; we learn to articulate something just out of reach, and when we have found the right word to name the feeling or sensation, we somehow know it is apt – or inapt. The point here is that there is a reality to our intuitions, to our sense of whether we have got our judgements right about how we describe ourselves. We arrive at a successful articulation that does more than begin our relationship with an emotional object: it brings about a sense of calm, or equilibrium from a state of painful confusion.

We have in the therapeutic encounter a sense that there are things we cannot properly say, something which the finite nature of a language which encodes cannot capture. We reach for metaphors or analogies to creatively extend feelings or reactions to the things around us. The rightness of an articulated emotion does more than clarify. Even when we are unable to find the right word for a feeling, experience, or virtue, the sense of being unable to articulate something would not be there if it were not for what Wittgenstein understood as the surrounding sayable.

Therapy in this way can go beyond changing behaviour, reducing symptoms, or treating disorders. When a client finds that their emotional narratives and how they are constructed are limiting and distorted, the way can be opened to a field of words which deepens self-understandings to afford new horizons of meaning. To be in therapy, to understand therapy, to do therapy without recognising its linguistically constructed ethical dimension is to overlook what is central to the social practice of living well. Making therapy more transparent requires that therapists be clear about the values, ethics, or ideologies into which they interpellate. How do they make our lives more worthwhile? What are the alternatives? How do *you* prioritise among the plurality of <u>Subjects</u>?

The next step towards being ethical and respecting the autonomy of a client requires two dimensions of introspection. The first is getting into focus and articulating what we feel. Here, it *is* possible to be apt because as we refine our sensations, we change how we see the world: discovery and invention are linked. The second dimension considers whether feeling, say, "angry" sits well or otherwise with the <u>Subject</u> that has something to tell us about how anger is acceptable more holistically? We release the tension between interpreter and interpreted – <u>Subject</u> and person – by considering alternatives: "*this beautiful girl does get angry*". And as a father of girls, that feels more *apt* to me.

<u>Metaphor and Myth</u>. The metaphor – something indispensable in life – is a beguilingly constitutive, creative form of expression that looks to take us beyond ideas of language that encodes. Metaphors are linguistic hybrids and have long stood as an invitation to recover from them something of deeper significance. The metaphor is the apparatus we use to deepen our understanding; we frame a thing *as if* it were something else. Attempting to articulate something deeper and somehow out of reach with a metaphor imbues it with embodied sensations. It can, on the one hand, offer deeper understandings, yet as Wittgenstein warned, it can also hold us captive as we shall discover in Chapter 8 (Wittgenstein, 1974: Part 1, §115).

Take, for example, the therapeutically ubiquitous yet often unnoticed metaphor of *The Journey*: we can find ourselves stuck, all at sea, losing our bearings, derailed, climbing the stairs upward, straying from the path, making progress, moving forward, going around in circles, or feeling lost. The embodiment of our senses puts us in relationship with a sort of truth in the form of a metaphor. Myths are entangled with metaphors and are similarly threads which knot together the fabric of our lives. As we grow towards adulthood and beyond, we are exposed to a multitude of fairy tales and folk allegories which communicate life lessons; perhaps to our detriment, we lose awareness of the weave of myth throughout the narratives used to make sense of the modern world. Myths belong to the apparatus of ethics; they provide a sense of continuity with ancestors and progeny orienting us towards our place in the order of things: the cosmos, the pattern of human longing, experiences, and motivations, which span histories and cultures.

Myths are pedagogical: they show us how to belong to a community of speakers and listeners by transmitting wisdom about how to negotiate life's journey. Myths point to our coexistence with all humanity, emerging as they do from accumulated insights and lessons of human experience which find their expression through semiotics – symbols and signs. Through myths, we glimpse transcendent truths that draw us towards levels of awareness shared with each other and our ancestors. Despite their tensions (truth versus fantasy and the universal versus the particular), myths nevertheless surface knowledge and interpretations about those things which transcend individuality and what it means to live a good life.

Joseph Campbell saw myths as reflecting some deeper Jungian archetypal tale whose primary purpose was to carry the human spirit forward. The *Hero*'s story centres on the prototypical sequence of a person who finds, achieves, or does something outside the bounds of the ordinary. Along the journey, the *Hero* is transformed from naïveté to deep wisdom and enlightenment. The myth is depicted as journey, a cycle, beginning with the *Hero* leaving the ordinary rhythms of their life to enter a new environment, encountering a mentor/sage, undergoing a series of trials, confronting obstacles as they go, before ultimately achieving initiation into the unknown.

The *Hero*'s Journey is a metaphor which represents personal development across individual, communal, and spiritual domains reminiscent of the journey undertaken by therapists, trainees, trainers, and clients alike. For the *Hero*, the last thing to be discovered was the beginning, arriving – as if it were possible – where we started yet knowing that place as if for the first time. The things that were not known beforehand are simply the things not searched for.

The *Hero's Journey* obviously affords a powerful framework for supporting people conceptualise their journey of transformation – it adopts an epistemic form for knowing and understanding. Yet the *Hero's Journey* also serves as a seductive <u>Subject</u>, as well as a powerful reminder to the mentor, sage, or fellow traveller (i.e., trainers and therapists alike) of their role in the process. That is, to be truly of assistance, we need to be mindful that while we a play a part in the *Hero's Journey*, the story remains that of someone else to tell (Smith, 2002).

While we do not begin our career on earth aware of the metaphoric structures, institutions, and <u>Subjects</u> into which we are born – which includes

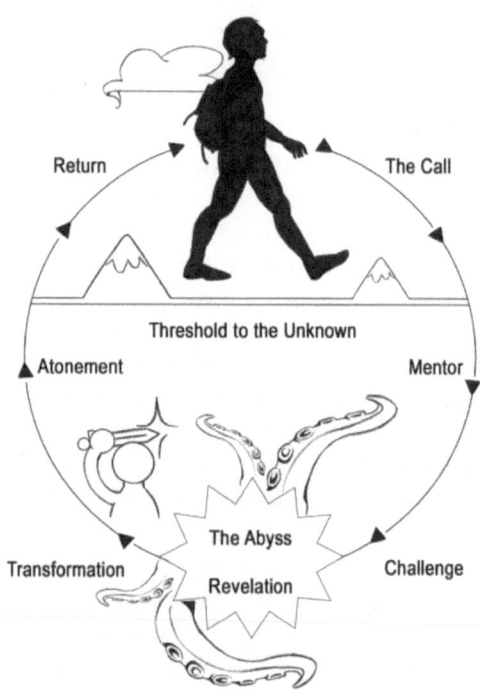

**FIGURE 6.2** The Hero's Journey.

on a larger human scale imperial rule, racism, colonialisation, and misogyny – generally speaking, seeing better and doing better tend to go hand in hand.

## References

Althusser, L. (1964). Marxism and Humanism, Cahiers de l'I.S.E.A. www.marxists. org/reference/archive/althusser/1964/marxism-humanism.htm.

Althusser, L. (1970/2012). Ideology and Ideological State Apparatuses (Notes towards an Investigation). In *Mapping Ideology*, Ed. Slavoj Žižek, Ch. 5. Verso UK.

Derrida, J. (1978). Structure, Sign and Play in the Discourse of the Human Sciences. (Trans. Alan Bass). In *Writing and Difference*. University of Chicago Press.

Duschinsky, R. et al. (2015). The Politics of Attachment: Lines of Flight with Bowlby, Deleuze and Guattari. *Theory, Culture & Society*. 32(7–8), 173–195.

Ekendahl, M. et al. (2022). Self-Interpellation in Narratives About Craving: Multiple and Unitary Selves. *Sociology of Health & Illness*. 44(9), 1391–1407.

Foucault, M. & Rabinow, P. (2002). The Ethics of the Concern for Self as a Practice of Freedom. R. Hurley et al. (Trans.). In *Michel Foucault: Ethics: Subjectivity and Truth. The Essential Works of Michel Foucault 1955–1984*, Vol. 1. Penguin.

Goodwin, I. (2003). The Relevance of Attachment Theory to the Philosophy, Organization, and Practice of Adult Mental Health Care. *Clinical Psychology Review*. 23(1), 35–56.

Guilfoyle, M. (2009). Using Althusser's Notion of Interpellation to Study the Politics of Therapeutic Practice. *Psychotherapy and Politics International*. 7(3), 159–173.

Hall, S. (2005). The problem of Ideology: Marxism without Guarantees. In *Stuart Hall: Critical Dialogues in Cultural Studies*, Eds. Morley, D. & Chen, K.-H.. Routledge.

Kearney, A. & Proctor, G. (2018). *Counselling, Class, and Politics: Undeclared Influences in Therapy*. 2nd edition. PCCS Books.

Monk, R. (1991). *Ludwig Wittgenstein: The Duty of Genius*. Vintage.

Morgan, A. (2002). Discerning between Structuralist and Non-structuralist Categories of Identity: A Training Exercise. *International Journal of Narrative Therapy and Community Work*. 4, 52–55.

Pavlenko, A. (2014). Emotional Worlds: Emotion Categorization, Affective Processing, and Ascription of Significance. In *The Bilingual Mind: And What it Tells Us about Language and Thought*. Cambridge University Press.

Pepperell, N. (2016). The Unease with Civilization: Norbert Elias and the Violence of the Civilizing Process. *Thesis Eleven*. 137(1), 3–21.

Pollard, R. (2018). *Dialogue and Desire: Mikhail Bakhtin and the Linguistic Turn in Psychotherapy*. Taylor and Francis.

Pylypa, J. (2016). The Social Construction of Attachment, Attachment Disorders and Attachment Parenting in International Adoption Discourse and Parent Education. *Children & Society*. 30(6), 434–444.

Schönbaumsfeld, G. (2019). The Aesthetic as Mirror of Faith in Kierkegaard's *Fear and Trembling*. *European Journal of Philosophy*. 27(3), 661–674.

Slife, B.D. et al. (2017). *The Hidden Worldviews of Psychology's Theory, Research, and Practice*. Routledge.

Smith, K.R. (2021). *Therapeutic Ethics in Context and in Dialogue*. Routledge.

Smith, M.C. (2002). Health, Healing, and the Myth of the Hero Journey. *Advances in Nursing Science*. 24(4), 1–13.

Taylor, C. (2016). *The Language Animal: The Full Shape of the Human Linguistic Capacity*. Harvard University Press.

Wallin, D.J. (2007). *Attachment in Psychotherapy*. Guilford Press.

Weber, M. (2001/1930). *The Protestant Ethic and the Spirit of Capitalism*. (Tr. Talcott Parsons). Routledge.

Wittgenstein, L. (1974). *Philosophical Investigations*. (Tr. G.E.M. Anscombe). 3rd edition. Blackwell.

Wittgenstein, L. (2024). *Tractatus Logico-Philosophicus*. A New Translation by Damion Searls. Liveright Corporation.

# 7

## STORIES

### Fragmented Selves

### 7.1 Introduction: Splitting the Human Atom

The self has maintained a secure, at times sacred place throughout the history of Western thought. Despite disagreements about the essential nature of the self, few have questioned that it exists. The modern sense of personal identity came to see the self as a unitary object that could be *known*. The self in this conception is not an object like a wristwatch or a fountain pen, but it seems to have the peculiar property of being able to appear to itself: the self is something inseparable from self-awareness.

Freud saw himself as the quintessential, walled-off punctuated self, insulated from non-rational intrusions, thus able to afford the reassuring foundation for scientific – psychoanalytic – objectivity. The philosophical radicalism of Freud *decentred* the self and split the psyche into unknowable parts. It mirrored the achievement of his contemporary, physicist Ernest Rutherford, who at about the same time split the atom in Manchester. Freud – unintentionally I expect – shattered the modernist dream of self-knowledge through introspection and, in so doing, presaged postmodernism and the narrative turn in therapy that we examine here.

If our inner world is unknowable, then how can we achieve consensual narratives about the world at large? For the first time, the act of introspection was de-privileged: if I cannot know myself, how can I know others? Communication becomes problematic as reality seems systematically disguised by an unconscious which recedes from view with each attempt to approach it. The tail of the uroboros will forever elude capture by the jaws of reason. The disintegration of communication thus suggests a fragmentation of the self and society, which precludes continuous discourses about culture and knowledge

DOI: 10.4324/9781003396161-7

in our contemporary world. The idea that there are no overarching meta-narratives reflects Freud's idea that we cannot know ourselves in the way that Socrates had once hoped.

Freud ensured that there could no longer be a single and correct answer to questions like: Who am I? What happened in the past? There appears to be no way out of the labyrinth: the labyrinth is all we have. If we see Freud's dictum that we are no longer sovereign in our own metaphorical kingdom as merely saying that we act in unpredictable ways, then he would have been reiterating ideas common to the time of Plato. Yet Freud's radical fragmentation of our unitary selves into metaphors of persons corresponding to internally coherent assemblies of beliefs and desires (i.e., id, ego, super ego) offered alternative stories for making sense of experience. Freud inferred a family system within, eschewing mono-mind theories, which opens the way for a compassionate acceptance of all our parts, introjects, including our inner critic.

Richard Rorty draws an important distinction between Freud's interpretation of the "unconscious" and what came before (1991). Hitherto, the unconscious stood for a seething mass of inarticulate instinctual energies, to which consistency is irrelevant: the unconscious is just another name for what Plato called the "passions" – the lower part of the soul, the unreasonable bad, false self, which must be restrained.

The radicalism of Freud's view of the unconscious was the claim that our unconscious selves is not a sullen, lurching brute, but an intellectual peer of our conscious rational selves. The unconscious becomes an intellectual mirror of our conscious selves, someone with whom we could converse. Freud untangled the link between the Platonic reason–passion and conscious–unconscious dualities. We were offered instead a more hopeful picture familiar to contemporary psychotherapists of a sophisticated transaction between two or more intellectuals, as opposed to the Platonic view of a zookeeper trying to negotiate with a pack of wild beasts. Freud gave us the freedom to create a coherent self-image, which we could then use to shape and re-engineer how we behave.

Freud's tripartite division into metaphorical selves had ample precedent. It mirrored not only the Christian idioms of Evil (id), Man (ego), and God (super ego), but Plato's earlier theory of metals. While belonging to the same unitary whole, the Greek Gods nevertheless separated the hearts of citizens in Plato's *Republic* according to their talents: gold signified the rulers, silver the auxiliaries, and bronze the farmers and artisans. Western political structures similarly adopt a tripartite division between the capricious mood swings of the masses (*id*), disengaged agents of instrumental reason in the real world (ego), and celestial wisdom (super ego): congress/parliament, Senate/Lords, and Supreme Court/Monarch, respectively. Knowledge of our internal metaphoric *persons* becomes necessary for predicting and controlling human behaviour; yet only one of them is available for introspection at any given time.

The ambiguity attending Freud's thinking was a radical epistemological breakthrough – the play of meaning was not just embraced; it was given an intense rib-cracking bear hug. The elusive nature of knowledge and its endless contestation, interpretation, and theorising ensured that truth was beyond resolution; the myriad internal contradictions of Freud's thinking have proven to be brilliantly fruitful for discovering new roads inward. Humans became something to be tinkered with through the interweaving of psychic metaphors, which would themselves become powerful strategies *for* becoming.

Freud and the Good. Irrespective of the truth value of Freud's theory one can trace its genealogy to a moment in the history of modernity. For those who want Freud to be a scientist, it would be better to see him as one of the greatest lyric poets of modernity who created a new language for thinking about emotions diffracted through the lens of nineteenth century German-Austrian positivism. Freud's metapsychology sought to formalise the axioms of psychoanalysis by knotting together the metaphor of humans as wet machines with a radical ideology of psychic energy grounded in physics.

Theories that would become the *Laws of Thermodynamics* were already familiar to nineteenth-century thinkers through the Romantic metaphysical vision of cosmic energy as something conserved (the *First Law*). The ontology of Freud's psychic energy became a metaphysics of hydraulic metaphors drawn from the age of steam to resolve the tension between the conservation of psychic energy and the universal tendency to disorder (Tran The et al. 2018, 2020; Massot, 2022). To this end, Freud produced an ingenious code for interpreting the unconscious as if definable through a set of thermodynamic laws of psychic energy, that is, displacement, condensation, sublimation, transformation, projection, parapraxis, resistance.

The talking *cure* (positivism) offered *catharsis* (Greek dramatic metaphor) or even the *remission* (medical positivism) of *symptoms* (symbolic representations) that were caused (positivism) by unconscious projections of repressed *psychic energy* (thermodynamics).

Freud's theorising about humanity was focused on making people workable, not necessarily good. His account of self-knowledge meant that what we are morally obliged to know about ourselves does not belong to some essence, or common human nature that can be identified as the source of moral responsibility. If we think of such a punctual self as neutral, then it is only reasonable to see that what it is to be human becomes an arbitrary matter.

Morality for Freud at its simplest level instructs us to tell the truth, avoid violence, sex with near relations, keep our promises, and abide by the Golden Rule. Beyond these *givens*, Freud had little to say about what it meant to be good. If we assume the demise of universally agreed values and moral frameworks, then does this not deny morality altogether? To what ends do we deploy this newfound freedom to tinker and improve with our unconscious selves?

Given the troubled times through which Freud lived and worked, which culminated in his flight from Nazi Austria in 1938, it is easy to understand why he took a pessimistic view of human nature. It is for this reason that his long friendship with the Swiss Pastor Oskar Pfister is so fascinating. Freud never hid his incredulity towards Pfister and his ability to reconcile being critical of religious tradition while also being a man of faith. Freud valued Pfister's "love of humanity, courage, candour and optimism" and was perhaps even impressed by how he himself could be loved by the Pastor despite his hostility towards religion. Conversely, Pfister struggled to accept his friend's pessimistic view of humanity, which is infamously associated with a passage Freud wrote in the autumn of 1918 – a view perhaps understandable after four years of European slaughter (Freud & Pfister, 1963: 61–62):

> I have found little that is "good" about human beings on the whole. In my experience most of them are trash, no matter whether they publicly subscribe to this or that ethical doctrine or none at all. That is something that you cannot say aloud, or even think, though your experiences of life can hardly be different from mine.

Freud concludes the note by asking: "Why was it that none of the pious ever discovered psychoanalysis? Why did it have to wait for a completely godless Jew?" Pfister responds by artfully making the distinction between piety and genius. He then goes on to conclude that if only Freud could understand his relationship within the great order of things: "... like the necessary synthesis of notes in a Beethoven symphony ...", he could then say, quite cheekily I felt of his friend: "A better Christian there never was".

Freud and Pfister ultimately came together in their critique of religion, or at least, of certain expressions of religion. In its ritualised forms, they felt religion could work on the collective level in the same way that neurotic symptoms affect individuals: both could make people unwell (Noth, & Morgenthaler, 2014). True, neither friendship nor correspondence constitute therapy, though, of course, both can be therapeutic. But the continual reflexive interpretation and re-interpretation of ideas and perspectives which characterised the dialectic relationship between the two meant that it endured, not despite their differences on religion, but because of the creative tension accompanying their differences and the way they resolved their ruptures. Difference then is not a failure, but the starting point for understanding the Other *through* the constitutive use of language.

The two agreed that although psychoanalysis may indeed have been the most fruitful part of psychology, it was nevertheless "not the whole of the science of the mind, and still less a philosophy of life and the world" (1963: 114). Shortly before his death, Freud was to confide in Pfister his hopes for the future of psychoanalysis, which seemed to reach a resolution between *Athens* and Pfister's *Jerusalem* (1963: 126):

> I should like to hand it over to a profession which does not yet exist, a profession of lay curers of souls who need not be doctors and should not be priests.

## 7.2   The Postmodern Condition

To understand *post*-modernity, we should re-direct our attention to how modernity sees itself, namely as the product of a progression of linear and inevitable phases: Greek Antiquity → Medieval Europe → Renaissance → Reformation → Enlightenment → French Revolution → Industrial Revolution. Modernity is also sociologically equated with instrumental rationality and a scientific worldview, which has been powerful in shaping our social, economic, moral, and cognitive structures.

Human reason, as exemplified by the deductive thought of mathematics and physics, came to replace the superstitious worldviews of religion and other forms of so-called irrationality (Slife et al. 2017). Philosophically, modernity also tends to be equated with the anthropocentric metaphysical emergence of Man and its ability to dominate the natural world. Together, these perspectives follow the logics of progress and development supported by two fundamental myths, namely: evolution is always forward and the ontological bifurcation of reality (dualism).

Divisions between mind–matter, human–nonhuman, and ideas–bodies becomes a concern when expressed through the social and natural sciences. But it is also more generally troublesome for framing the way moderns think of themselves as acultural, raceless, scientific beings. The height of modernity was characterised by a supreme confidence in Man's potential, and the role of – particularly white – humanity's belief that science and technology could save the world from – ironically – the errors of modernity.

Non-modern Others – as encountered by Iberians in their invasion of the Americas – became typically marked as inferior. Their cultural expressions were interpreted as a failure to domesticate nature in the way modern Europeans had. A linear perspective of history coupled with a dualist ontology of reality meant that the Other was symbolically and materially instrumentalised to both represent and justify the Occident's superiority. Non-European peoples and territories – racialised and dehumanised through colonisation – became categorised by moderns as underdeveloped, despotic, undemocratic, and traditional.

The Eurocentric vision of history and the epistemic privilege of Western Man has within it the powerful apparatus of *tunnel-vision*. It enabled historians – such as Jakob Burckhardt – to find European origins in the past while omitting the profound influences of African and Islamic civilisations which contradict the notion of European superiority.

Enrique Domingo Dussel (1934–2023) was a key figure in the philosophical movement which sought to demolish the philosophical foundations of Eurocentrism from beyond the tunnel-vision of the coloniser. Dussel was critical of the term "postmodernity", which he saw as the final moments of a peculiarly European vision of modernity. He introduces instead the theoretical proposition of <u>trans-modernity,</u> which points towards the *pluriverse*; the great unsuspected richness of non-European culture which lies beyond and prior to the colonising structures valorised by the modern Occident (Dussel, 2012). Foucault similarly saw modernity as an attitude rather than something englobed by dates "on a calendar" (Foucault & Rabinow, 1991: 39). Modernity then is seen as a mode of relating to reality, through our thinking, feeling, and the voluntary choices we make when understanding our relationship to things, to oneself, and to others. Ethics once again becomes central to what we are to do. Structuralism and modernity are therefore entangled and intimately linked.

They help integrate the study of European humanity in its various forms, yet they do so in an overly optimistic, myopic, and scientistic way. While poststructuralism shares structuralism's fundamental questioning of what it means to be human, it also challenges how structuralism's scientism became elevated to the status of a universally valid theory for understanding all aspects of what it means to be human. Western thought, as we have seen, seems habitually drawn to seeing the world as polarities, and so postmodernity slides into becoming – as Dussel saw it – the mirror of modernity. With this slide comes a blizzard of anger, despair, and pessimism as we discover that our heroes and heroic ideals may be empty and vacuous. A ripple of concern travels around a room of initiate therapists when they are asked to consider whether their *gran project* – as Satre would say – of becoming "experts" on other people is actually beyond reach.

Yet postmodernism embraces much of modernism. The epistemology of modernity becomes visible in a different context which changes its significance; rather than there being one way of knowing, there becomes many ways of knowing. It is not *what* we believe that changes, but *how* we believe: epistemology and the nature of knowledge and universal truth become more fluid and elusive, and for many this feels destabilising and relativistic. The postmodern attitude is particularly unsettling for those who see reason as a source of order and harmony. For others, it is an inspiring alternative to the disappointment of twentieth-century technical rationality – an age of fallen moral authority and the collapse of any hope of a coherent and rational account of reality.

<u>Lyotard and the Authority of Stories</u>. A decoupling of consensus (i.e., the idea of universal moral standards) between political leaders, and those they

govern, seems to have accelerated since the Nixon-Watergate crisis of the 1970s. With little regard for intellectual or ethical consistency, politicians in the pursuit of power have since become bolder in selecting whatever ideology proves useful for their goals and political ends. At about the time of the Nixon debacle, the Quebec Council of Universities set Jean-François Lyotard the task of analysing the state of knowledge in the world's most technologically developed societies. The result was *The Postmodern Condition*, which is often associated with a kind of resistance to ethical consistency and universality.

The notion of postmodernity for Lyotard stemmed from the transformational impact of scientific knowledge on contemporary societies. The way in which knowledge is produced by Indigenous cultures outside the "West" is essential to how these communities are sustained. In virtually all such cultures, every cosmic vision, every image, all systematic production of knowledge is associated with a perspective of totality.

Custom and practice were used to help people belong to and propagate communities; at the heart of such practices was the art of storytelling, or narration. To fit-in and find out what to do, a person needed to learn the tripartite practices of how to *listen*, how to *do*, and how to *tell*. It reminds me of the process of apprenticeship, be it achieving the practical mastery of a carpenter, laboratory scientist, or therapist. It applies to the practice of therapy where the client, therapist, and supervisor/trainer loop through the cycles of telling, doing, and hearing. We learn about the tradition of practice through the ancient dictum: *see one, do one, teach one*.

Members of a community find their "home" either as a speaker, audience member, or figure of the tale. The identity and desires of people belonging to the community become shaped by this structure. Narrative knowledge is thus an existential process which requires a relational understanding of how we receive and transmit knowledge. Not only do I learn a practical skill from my "ancestor", but I also learn how to listen and how to tell a story. Indigenous narrative knowledge has no need for further legitimation or validation because the authority of the narration comes from the practice of its transmission. A culture that prizes narrative does not need special procedures to authorise itself. The narrative itself holds within it, authority. Narrative statements can be neither false nor true; therefore, ideas such as agreement and disagreement are unintelligible in such storytelling cultures.

The Crisis of Legitimacy. A conflict appears when we ask the question: what happens to the idea of legitimacy when scientific knowledge expands and acquires an increasingly dominant position in society? Western science comes into conflict with Indigenous ways of creating and transmitting knowledge – the practical wisdom of *phronesis* – as scientism challenges the legitimacy of narratives which have not been exposed to "objective" argumentation or proof. With its growth, the universal appeal of science brought along with it a wider horizon of consensus. The legitimacy of claims to knowledge now required the approval of people we do not know and may never meet, that is, MacIntyre's *characters* (Section 5.5).

Their role was to formulate agreements about what it meant to follow the new standards of knowledge. With the rising tide of modernity also came the need for it to provide its own stories to legitimise statements about how the world worked. While few can dispute that science gets things done and makes things happen, it cannot use itself to legitimise its methods – there can be no experiment to show that science is the path to truth. Scientific knowledge cannot know and make known that it is true knowledge, without resorting to external narratives from which point of view it can validate itself.

When scientific knowledge is turned towards "talk", a birds-eye view of a pendulum swinging between the binary categories of *materialistic* and *discursive* is uncritically assumed. In the former category sits the idea that there is a material reality that exists beyond words. This reality exists prior to – if not separate from – language. It exists, and we use language to enframe, make sense of, and give meaning to the world. The other extremity of the pendulum is <u>discursive</u>, where language, or more properly – discourse – is seen to create rather than discover meaning. The discursive turn holds that the things we assume to be given in the world – for example, emotions – are created solely through language (Section 6.4).

The twentieth-century preoccupation of philosophy with language has oriented the pendulum firmly towards the <u>discursive</u>. The result amounts to a naïve social constructionism which distances the world from the observer to the extent that reality becomes inaccessible, and inquiry is limited to the territory of discourse alone. To reduce all human experience to something linguistically constructed and purely metaphorical takes things too far. Suggesting that language is unmoored from external references and the material world makes much of human experience unintelligible.

There is clearly a world beyond words, but it is not a blank slate for human metaphorical projections – culture and traditions have stability. The scientific method has proven powerful in the context of the material world. Technologies for extending life and transporting millions of people safely at great heights above the surface of the planet via the implausible means of combustible pressurised winged tubes are not social constructions but material facts. The problem, however, comes with metaphors of a disembodied, objective bird's-eye view of the binaries over which the pendulum hovers. We will address this more specifically in the context of Barad's radical post-humanism (Section 7.4) and Merleau-Ponty's phenomenology later. But any philosophy that strays too far towards the discursive potentially undermines physical realities such as climate destruction and the consequences of exploiting finite resources.

Equally, little good comes from scientism and its empirical justifications for therapeutic techniques or matters of human experience. There is no empirical justification for empiricism and no scientific validation for science: "empiricism and the philosophies underlying science are just that – philosophies" (Slife, 2004: 50). The formulation of any scientific method must assume – even before the investigation begins – that a certain type of world exists in which the method is effective. In fact, each time the scientific method is turned towards a new group, place, or time, it must make assumptions about the group, place, and time.

Practitioners are interpellated by the ideology of science even before the investigation begins. It is no coincidence that CBT has almost identical epistemological values as traditional science, that is, empiricism and rationalism. If I feel anxious about flying in an airplane, for example, my emotions are not reliable evidence that something bad will happen. When I put my *faith* in science (i.e., statistics), I can – allegedly – deny my feelings about the risks of flying because the probability of an accident is so small. Statistics are powerful, but they do not make emotions evaporate; what really matters is the practical consequences we place on dismissing our intuition about a situation. The scientific validation of CBT is the result of systematic bias rather than bias-free efficacy. The method, in this sense, is not a value-free, transparent tool of investigation, but a narrative for naming itself among other narratives, thus therapeutic models. There can be no intellectual position and no scientific method or therapeutic technique that does not have values embedded within, at least implicitly.

Lyotard contrasts Indigenous forms of narrative knowledge which connect people in the present to traditions of the past, and the grand narratives of modernity which point towards a future where the problems we face will be resolved, and progress is inevitable. Lyotard was not the first to be sceptical of such assumptions about knowledge and the meta-narratives that shape our stories. Nietzsche before him implored: "*Mankind* does not advance; it does not even exist" (1968: 55). The most level-headed are led astray by the illusion of Hegel's notion of the absolute human spirit or *Geist*, which ensures society progresses through the ongoing, smooth accumulation of knowledge.

Postmodern thinkers assert that we can only see clearly and comprehend the world if we abandon our commitment to historical continuity and the uncritical assumption that all changes are necessarily progress. When we imagine that we live through a seamless parade of events towards an improved future, it disallows the material fact that things deteriorate and that all change is not necessarily progress. To accept that we live through discontinuities requires we disregard our commitment to grand narratives. The idea that each *episteme* – or historically related way of structuring understanding and knowledge – is necessarily an improvement on an earlier one, must be rejected.

The postmodern turn means we must abandon our commitment to the inevitable civilising processes imagined by the likes of Norbert Elias. We do not necessarily become more *civilised*, but lurch from one system of barbarity to another. Though we profess higher standards and possess greater ethical insights, we do not – on the whole – act more morally than our forebears. Lyotard saw post-industrialisation as the tipping point where Western culture lost faith in the credibility of grand narratives. Knowledge was no longer organised towards the fulfilment of universal goals which drew consensus. Thinking lacked a fixed resting point from which legitimate judgements about what may be right or wrong could be made. Instead, neoliberal values such as efficiency and profitability became what mattered in a global market-driven economy. Society – as Margaret Thatcher notoriously argued – was nothing more than the individual or traditional family unit motivated by self-interest.

It is hardly necessary to emphasise that the political and economic promotion of individual self-interest is unlikely to advance radical relationality, social cohesion, or indeed enhance the economic and social prospects of the typical household. Yet Thatcher generated and then capitalised on a grand narrative of economic improvement founded on the disposal of finite resources (North Sea petrochemicals and accumulated public assets) to fuel the myth of progress.

The aim of promoting the wellbeing of the traditional family was paradoxically undermined by the impact of her neoliberal policies. Calamitous social fragmentation followed the stripping of assets previously held in common. At least I can agree on one thing that Thatcher said: "Those who think they know, but are mistaken, and act upon their mistakes, are the most dangerous people to have in charge" (Albertson & Stepney, 2020: 337).

<u>Universality without Consensus</u>. Unlike Indigenous narratives, science makes robust claims to universality. If true knowledge consists of generalities and universals, then understanding people requires a focus on the stable things that do not change rather than particularities and one-time happenings: *universalism leads therapists to be incurious about what does not fit diagnostic categories and theoretical constructs.* So long as universality is equated with consensus, its opposite must be explained away as stemming from prejudice, backwardness, or some other kind of fault.

Radical relationality aligns with the postmodern vision in that both see formal monolithic theories and systems of therapy as limiting the project of an authentic openness to others. The solution to the limitations of universalism is to multiply the number of totalising – and often philosophically incompatible – theories on which a therapist draws, that is, theoretical integration (Slife & Reber, 2001: 213–234). Beyond this lies the tossed salad of techniques and therapeutic categories more aligned with technical eclecticism.

I am again reminded of the "Manchester" screwdriver: when the sharp end encounters a slotted screw, then all was well; but for all other cases, use the blunt end as a hammer. In spurning single theories and single sets of practices, both the integrator and the eclectic reflect the muddled thinking of those who seek to particularise with the universal.

Lyotard's radical claim was that consensus is an outmoded idea, as it cannot reflect the plurality of language games characteristic of contemporary cultures and society (Section 6.4). It is a misreading of Lyotard, however, to equate his rejection of consensus with a rejection of universality. So, can universality have a stable relationship with what is particular and unique about the human experience? To address this, Lyotard introduced us to the situation produced by the heterogeneity of language games: the *differend*. It happens when a problem or injustice that we want to be put into words cannot yet occur.

To convey the idea of the *differend*, I wish to draw a parallel with survivorship bias, and the contributions of Abraham Wald, a statistician working on the problem of aircraft vulnerability during the Second World War. A statistical analysis of the damage that an aircraft could – or more importantly could not – sustain for the purpose of reinforcing the structure was hindered by the fact that the fatally damaged aircraft were missing. The aircraft that *did* return from hazardous missions endured sustainable damage throughout their entire structure, with the exception of the engine. This led to the common practice – up to that point – of reinforcing all the damaged areas of the aircraft *except* the engines.

In short, the aircraft that had been "wronged" – that is destroyed – and did not return were invisible to the analytical paradigm. A universal truth – that an aircraft is vulnerable to engine damage – was therefore invisible because of an unrepresentative "consensus", that is, the population of aircraft that *had* successfully returned to tell their stories of survival. The *differend* then is the condition where a harm, wrong, injustice or exclusion is invisible to the standard of judgement inherent to the paradigm with which we view the world. *Consensus then, is not necessarily equated with universality;* clearly a new paradigm or framework is required to make visible what was hitherto invisible.

The example of *differend* that Lyotard offers is one drawn from the injustices of colonial imperialism. An inhabitant of Martinique – currently an Overseas Department of France – was peopled by those who, under French law, were considered French citizens. In being considered a French citizen and not a Martinican, a wrong is suffered by those who do not consider themselves to be French. Yet resistance to the fact that Martinicans do not consider themselves French could only happen using French law, which only recognises French citizens. The *wrong* therefore lacks an Indigenous language game to express itself, because what it is to be wronged is always understood as a discourse external to itself.

Foucault took the language of psychiatry as yet another example of the *differend*. Psychiatry is a monologue of reason about unreason, which ignores and silences those voices made absent by the conversation. The sense of wrong suffered by one of the parties in a *differend* produces both a silence and a sense that something cannot be uttered, yet this something is sensed as a call to create new phrases with which it can be expressed. It seems paradoxical that the creation of new ways of communicating would stem from feeling there is no communication, or that there exist incommunicable sensations. Yet this is precisely why communication depends – as discussed earlier – on a process of creation entangled with discovery (Section 6.4).

Discourse in this sense is not an abstract set of textual practices performed by academics in universities. As I proposed at the outset, life is not lived as if we are reading a book; we do not live lives which unfold sequentially in print, but in the reality of relationships. Discourse infers that our daily activities, the way we speak, and act are shaped by structures of power which go beyond texts and the grammar of a sentence. The question that follows is: if an omission or an injustice lacks an idiom through which it can be expressed, can it be communicated at all? Can we even know it is there?

For Lyotard, the sense that we must search for new ways of expressing ourselves summons us to idioms which do not yet exist. It has nothing to do with the discovery of common ground or establishing a compromise between two standpoints, which depend on the practices of argumentation, justification, and reason-giving. The idea to which we continually return is that resistance relies on the situation against which it struggles.

Therapists who integrate a multitude of universal theories to fix particularity offer no guarantee of escaping the *differend*. The civil rights advocate and scholar Kimberlé Crenshaw emphasises this point when using the term *intersectionality* to voice the problems of how the law responds to violence against Black women, naming injustices so that they may be addressed (1991). Sensing the abyss between separate discourses or language games requires the creation of passages and pathways that allow communication rather than subordinating the *Other* (i.e., Black women) to a particular universalising procedure (Law).

There is, however, a link between communication and disagreement – as modelled by Freud and Pfister – which introduces the possibility of discovering universal judgements independent of consensus. The plurality of moral sources contained in multiple language games or discourses – which can often seem incompatible – produces a new ethic of responsibility that compels us to create alternative discourses. *Difference – yet again – is not a failure but a starting point for understanding Others through the constitutive use of language.*

*To conclude*, the postmodern turn seeks to undermine hierarchies of meaning, what is good or bad, higher, or lower. It seeks to move us towards a world in which all interpretations can be taken seriously if not necessarily believed. We have previously rejected relativism as the only alternative to modern dogmatism (Sections 5.4 and and 6.2). This is because we can never be truly abstracted from the stable dispositions, narratives, virtues, and traditions on which we can draw to act. The demand for universality is a complex feeling that nevertheless calls on us to create new ways of communicating with each other. It is an open-ended, inherently unfinished understanding of universalism that for Lyotard and Foucault is characterised by the narrative approach to therapy to which we turn next.

## 7.3   The Narrative Turn in Therapy

Therapeutic interest in narrative emerged from the ground of family therapy and the broader linguistic turn in philosophy, the humanities, and the social sciences (White & Epston, 1990). As I shall argue, only when we abandon the naïve relativism of narrative approaches can we accept its radically relationality. Released from its sterile deconstructionism, it becomes more than a tool in the bag of tricks for a therapist. The strength of the narrative turn is that it truly sees the interlocking nature of philosophy, ethics, and practice as transcending method; it is an attitude to living, a political project, and an alternative to prevailing, pragmatic, empiricist, instrumental approaches to therapy. It forces a re-evaluation of the unquestioned or unquestionable truths of traditional psychological discourses.

The importance of language and meaning, especially as articulated by Foucault has had a profound effect on the development of narrative therapy. Foucault sought to read history without the "subject", or the liberal humanist notion of a stable cohesive ego. Rather than focusing on the self as a fragmented and unstable amalgam of conscious/unconscious – as perceived by Freud – the self was for Foucault the effect of discursive structures which align with the disciplining factors I spoke of earlier: 'I' am not the foundation of my world.

The key features of Foucault's philosophy are characterised by its radical relationality; *we are our relationships*. Who we are as individuals is deeply connected with who *we* are as a group or collective. Who we are is embedded in *our* historical legacy. But the matter of determination is not simple – it is deeply complex. I argue instead that rather than a singular self who vanishes without trace in the movement of historical life, who we are emerges through an intricate weaving together of historical themes that split, transform, and reform. Self-relatedness is thus inseparable from knowing oneself as part of a greater whole. When we look at ourselves, it must be through the lens of the things *we* do, which is not just about how we act, but how we go about knowing ourselves.

For Foucault, power was important (Foucault & Faubion, 2002). It is not a thing to treat as a possession, defined in individual terms like a physical characteristic such as having large biceps. Empowerment in this sense becomes easily equated with liberal humanistic ideals of self-assertion, upward mobility, sports utility vehicles (SUVs), and the psychological experience of feeling powerful. Foucault saw power as something which circulates rather than something owned by a person or group of people. It is not inherently bad, repressive, or negative, but it is constitutive, actively shaping people's lives and outlooks.

But it is naïve to believe that in the real world power is not abused and misused; it can be difficult to recognise and corruption is not easy to challenge and uproot. The web-like structure of power relations is one that feminist theorists find invaluable since it enables people to resist oppressive practices. Resistance is a political act leading to concrete change which improves the real, material conditions of people living in a fiercely unjust reality. It includes redressing the problems of sex discrimination, rape law reform, the criminalisation of abortion, domestic violence, sexual harassment, and sex trafficking.

Focusing on narrative has both hopeful and benevolent political implications. In a social world which is both discovered and constructed by people, there is the possibility that it can be revalued and reconstructed to make things better. Action can be brought about by making visible, challenging, and reforming the way we use language to tell stories about power.

Unlike the stereotype of the modernist therapist who assumes they know best about what is good for you, the narrative turn considers whether there is something suspicious about a profession which proposes a specific vision of what constitutes health, the common good or reality for that matter. At most, the narrative therapist is an expert at conversations of change, focusing on the need to be sceptical towards prevailing theories of what it means to be a person, and whose interests they represent.

While resisting being drawn into the destructive nihilistic vortex of unintelligible deconstruction, it is necessary that scepticism extends to the narrative approach itself. Deconstruction in this sense has emancipatory possibilities to glimpse a world that is yet to be. Narrative therapists see – as did the Stoics – that we inadvertently contribute to problems in the way we interpret experience. The linguistic turn, however, takes us a step further in seeing that meaning is not static, but embodied by language and the contexts which shape thoughts, emotions, and ultimately, narratives.

Radicalising the Client–Therapist Relationship. Perhaps the most significant contribution of the narrative approach is to radically decentre the practices of the therapist and question the nature of the relationship between the therapist and the client. Despite the many differences between Rogerian, cognitive, and psychodynamic therapies, they have in common a tendency to position the problem squarely "in" the person of the client. Although Rogers rejected an expert role for the counsellor, the person-centred tradition nevertheless risks idealising the role of therapist as "liberator". The unrelenting focus on the counsellor–client relationship "puts the therapy room at the centre of the process of therapy, with the relationship between the person and the therapist comprising the crucial agent of change" (Payne, 2006: 170).

In doing so, a person's relationships and life beyond the therapy room are excluded and marginalising when it comes to understanding how they contribute to overcoming problems. Not only is the therapist in a powerful position in terms of relations emanating from their power knowledge, but the therapeutic relationship develops its own mystique. It becomes elevated to a position above all other relationships in the client's life, so that the oft repeated mantra: "this is *your space*" comes to promote the absurd notion of a context-free therapeutic relationship.

Anchoring focus on the client and their problems – abstracted from their relational context – results in therapy as a one-way street, deepening ideas of personal deficits. A person's identity becomes defined as the *other* whose life requires change. While the life of the client is seen as dynamic and open to reform, the therapist on the other hand is seen as static; the reassuring "congruent" foundation to which the client's progress is indexed. Narrative therapy, instead, resists interpellation into the humanistic ideology of an essential self by seeing how *we* – client and therapist – are constituted through the braiding of radical relationality; it is an attitude which seeks to dissociate itself from the ideology of therapy itself. Foucault explains the project of emancipation which so often characterises the intentions of the well-meaning humanistic therapist (Foucault & Rabinow, 2002: 281–301):

I have always been somewhat suspicious of the notion of liberation, because if it is not treated with precaution and within certain limits, one runs the risk of falling back on the idea that there exists a human nature or base that, as a consequence of certain historical, economic, and social processes, has been concealed, alienated, or imprisoned in and by mechanisms of repression. According to this hypothesis, all that is required is to break these repressive deadlocks and Man will be reconciled with himself, rediscover his nature or regain contact with his origin, and re-establish a full and positive relationship with himself. I think this idea should not be accepted without scrutiny.

Psychotherapy, which promises to liberate the "true self" at some time in the (far) future, prevents clients from inquiring about alternative possibilities for living *now*. The ideology of personal development does not disturb, worry, or challenge the socio-cultural political forces that shape how the problem experienced by a person came about. Indeed, the well-intentioned therapist becomes an unwitting accomplice, reproducing the dominant, culturally sanctioned ideologies of popular and revered forms of personhood. In its poststructuralist critique of humanism, the narrative therapist does not look to exhume some pre-existing dormant knowledge, be it of the mind, heart, nor any true, real, authentic, or essential self.

Foucault was fascinated by the practices used to produce and promote truth which he saw in terms of two broad yet contrasting forms of discourse, namely *polemics* and *problematisation*. The former proceeds with privileges possessed in advance which are rarely questioned. Those who the polemicist encounters are not partners in the search for truth, but an adversary who is wrong, yet to self-transcend, mistaken, incongruent, potentially harmful, or whose existence is a threat. Their final goal is not to come as close as possible to a difficult truth, but to bring about the triumph of the cause they have manifestly upheld from the start. For the polemicist, difference signals a failure of the Other.

This is because the polemicist understands themselves as already knowing the truth, and any challengers to their authority are assessed as being wrong, morally failed, or plain guilty. Consider the practices of politics, religious dogma, and the judiciary, respectively. The practice of polemics was, for Foucault something sterile, of which he asked: "has anyone ever seen a new idea come out of a polemic?" (Foucault & Rabinow, 2002: 111–119).

*Problematisation* is founded on reciprocal, interrogative approaches which privilege curiosity about the things we silently believe or take for granted. It is the ethical practice of going some way towards disentangling ourselves from the disciplining circumstances that make us what we are. It resembles a therapeutic encounter in which people who are serious about "disturbing" habits look to uncover the limitations of their thinking and attitudes. Difference does not signal some catastrophe, but the fertile ground from which language can build understanding.

Narrative therapists look to suspend judgement and remain mindful of the obligations afforded to them by the client within the language game of therapy: they remain unconvinced, can perceive contradictions, and draw attention to faulty reasoning. They are aware of how the practice of therapy is linked to power structures, in the way it is taught, and the way in which consensus – such as it is – is organised within the closed circuit of those who regularly troop off to the same conferences. As for the client, they too exercise obligations delimited by the nature of the encounter, such as a slow and arduous commitment to transformation through constant care for the truth.

Against Relativism. Having already sketched out arguments against relativism (Sections 5.4 and 6.2), the great disturbance posed by postmodernism must be settled in relation to questions of ethics and values: if we value the autonomy of clients, then what is the moral ground – knowingly or otherwise – for the interpellation of clients into a particular therapeutic method?

The antidote is a radical questioning of contemporary and historical understandings of benign ideologies and practices that silence, confine, or dominate people; freedom for Foucault meant making visible the *differend* through the endless practice of de-familiarising conventional beliefs which discipline the Self. The falsity of relativism is thus uncovered when considering the facticity of our relational entanglement, attitudes to authority, delusions of neutrality, and the more general realities of life beyond the bubble of therapy.

The potential for interpretative circularity cannot be avoided by any approach which claims that there is *no* truth; a claim to truth in itself. Though truth and authority are unavoidable, they are not inherently oppressive – what matters is how they are interpreted and deployed. In this sense, all theories have the potential to be abused through circular means as truth and authority become monopolised in ways which silence and oppress those who seek the services of a therapist.

By way of illustration, let me suppose I no longer love my partner and wish to end the relationship (categorically not true!). When I discuss this with my narrative therapist, they take the view that romantic love is just one of several stories (constructs) about relationships that I have (uncritically) chosen to tell myself to make life more intelligible. In principle, there is no way within the relativism of the narrative paradigm that I can convince my therapist that my predicament is <u>not</u> a metaphor. In telling my story, I only confirm the therapist's worldview that to resolve my problem I must choose another – equally arbitrary – story.

Next, I consult my psychodynamic therapist. I reject their stance that the problem stems from the past, most likely the early relationship with my mother. My belligerence in response to this suggestion is interpreted as a defence. My lack of emotional availability is obviously projected towards the therapist, which only reinforces their view that the problem rests ultimately with my attachment style, or my mother. The therapist gets to be right either way.

During the next session with my cognitive therapist, I claim not to suffer from automatic thoughts regarding my partner; this too is interpreted as an automatic thought. My humanistic therapist validates *all* my feelings yet seems preoccupied by what seems to be absent from my emotional repertoire. Problems with my congruence most likely? Why else would I have problems relating to my partner? My Gestalt therapist has gone fishing! When I complain to my existential therapist that nobody is taking me seriously, I am told that the problem lies in allowing others (presumably therapists) to take responsibility for my choices. As we are born without reason, live out of weakness, and die by chance, what difference does it make anyway?

Postmodern – and humanistic – approaches to therapy suggest that the possibilities of living are limitless for the self-aware, empowered, authentic person: we can fashion whatever kind of life we please. This can leave postmodern therapy vulnerable to accusations of ethical, theoretical, and methodological nihilism. In practice, therapists do not adopt a relativistic position towards indisputable facts, including those about the physical world, or past traumatic events.

What happens in practice is that how we respond to facts can be refashioned and re-evaluated. The ethical and historical constraints in which we live indisputably create the conditions for our freedoms and responsibilities. But to imagine that our possibilities are boundless assumes we are isolated atoms living in static communities, rather than relationally dynamic entangled beings. We simply cannot reinvent at will practices and understandings, individually or collectively. Thus, our ethical context too, is a condition of our creative selves, not just an arbitrary limitation placed on it.

Relativism in psychotherapy is often aligned with the long tradition of resisting both authority and its power to stigmatise and is most notably characterised by the activism of Thomas Szasz (2010). Szasz highlighted the danger of stigmatising and alienating people through medical categorisation and in this sense his anti-authoritarian stance seems justifiable. Indeed, Szasz was among the first to resist the idea that same-sex relationships were a form of mental illness. Again, as Foucault reminds us: "Resistance really always relies upon the situation against which it struggles" (Foucault & Rabinow, 2002: 168).

While an unquestioning trust in diagnostic categories can stigmatise, so too does rejection of all authority which includes therapists, social workers, teachers, psychologists, families, and local communities – cynically termed the carceral archipelago by Foucault. All that can be claimed is that authority is unavoidable. If we assume that authority and power are neither inherently good nor bad, then we can decouple the automatic insinuation between authority and stigma. Another reason for opting for a relativist position is thus eliminated (Skovlund, 2011).

Stories Are Real. A Pastor sought therapy because of their debilitating, decades-long struggle with low mood. Over time, they had come to accept that it was a cross given to them by God. Scores of therapists had failed to "cure" the Pastor, which only seemed to prove that not only was God real, but that the Pastor had been equal to this terrible burden. A carefully curated résumé showed how few of the therapists got beyond a couple of consultations. The symbolic evidence for the transcendent reality of God remained intact and secure from the objectifying practices of the terrestrially bound agents of reason.

Therapy for the Pastor adopted a symbolic – idiographic – identity which would seem alien to the therapist, their profession, and indeed the project of modernity itself. All were required to flunk the test for the Pastor's faith to survive. What was to be done depended on how helpful the prevailing narrative was for the Pastor: Did it offer succour? Was yet another therapeutic failure necessary to avoid a crisis of faith? Did the Pastor's family support the narrative and to what extent did it help them live with distress in terms of their own relational context?

Rather than taking the Pastors stance to be erroneous, reducing their logical alterity – or difference – to being plain wrong and irrational, a more creative approach is to investigate the world of the Other, and the relations and practices made possible by this person's unique manner of engaging with therapy. To understand that the role of the therapist was to fail transforms nomothetic – empirical – truth to a more pragmatic idiographic truth. Truth acquires a quality aligned to the wisdom of Frank Sinatra: "I'm for anything that gets you through the night". In rejecting what is nomothetic we are not appealing to relativism but acknowledging instead that what matters is interpretation and how it makes people's social and cultural environments function.

Though not universal or scientific in nature, <u>reality</u> for the Pastor was nevertheless non-negotiable and resistant to change. Acknowledging alternative realities need not be understood as a commitment to relativism, but a more compassionate attitude to realities which cannot be wished away or exchanged at will – even if they *are* built on idiographic understanding. Within such realities, personal authority, resistance, and most importantly, the lived experience of a person privileges the interpretation of certain truths over others.

As the history of anti-racism within feminist struggles has shown, the "Master's tools" – in this case theoretical abstraction – can never dismantle the "Master's" house. Instead, what is required is a sober acknowledgement of the epistemological, metaphysical, ethical, and political value of the lived experiences of human beings on the planet, who are not white, male, heterosexual, able-bodied, or relatively wealthy. It is necessary to understand what real people say about the varied and complex ways in which they act on, and are acted on by, each other and the world. This is especially the case with race and gender, mired as they are in the messy realities of our material world. Such an interpretation of human identity lies at the core of the concept of *intersectionality*, calling us to take sober account of the wide array of factors affecting the lived experience of people (Crenshaw, 1991).

Our encounter with alterity – or what makes people different from ourselves – is an ethical call to acknowledge the complexity of human experience. The Enlightenment's focus on identity, sameness, and the individual subject reflects an extreme neglect for the Other that is indicative of a deeper neglect of the ethical. Focusing on the ethical needs of others means understanding the experiences of others. When Foucault observed that while not everything is bad, everything was nevertheless dangerous, he was reminding us that there can be no absolute answers or definitive theories. As Tina Botts remarks (2017: 348).

> The retelling of the real details of a real story about a real experience of a real woman who underwent a ludicrously racist and sexist experience reminds us that these sorts of things actually occur, not just in theory but in life … simplistic, theoretical solutions to the lived experience of oppression cannot and do not exist.

As relational therapists, we must be alert to the ways in which our attempts to ameliorate distress can inadvertently oppress the people we want to help. Telling and re-telling stories rests at the heart therapy and indeed autoethnography. It implies the discipline of observing ourselves observing, interrogating what we believe, feel, and think in a way that challenges our assumptions. It requires asking repeatedly whether we have penetrated as many layers as possible of our defences, anxieties, and insecurities. It asks that we undergo a revolution and rethink and revise our lives. The joy of such a revolution is not just a reaction against former oppression. It lies in the delight that comes with a rich, intense, eventful life. One in which humans no longer feel lonely, but experience unity, connectedness, and collective strength.

If a newly generated narrative is to be regarded as a source of change at all and not something arbitrary, the therapist presupposes that something understood in therapy can be exported – like an object owned – to other parts of a person's life. Theoretical paradoxes abound in the use of narrative therapy unless we distinguish between transferring a *process* as opposed to *content* beyond the bubble of therapy. A perspective created in the bubble of therapy for export beyond its context risks elevating itself to the status of yet another meta-narrative.

The problem has always been that unless the context of a person changes, then no amount of re-storying will alter the behaviour of an abusive partner, the socioeconomic conditions of a client, or a toxic organisational culture for example. The shortcomings of therapeutically generated narratives become clear: they cannot be implemented in contexts that continually and persistently reject them.

The problem of ethical neutrality and the frailty of exported narratives cannot be resolved while at the same time insisting on relativism: therapeutically generated narratives all too often evaporate on contact with reality. The social and cultural circumstances of people in the real-world force restrictions on new narratives that make them resistant to change, since they are dependent on the actions of others, as in the case of abusive relational dynamics.

Changing people's minds was less important for Foucault than changing political, economic, and institutional regimes that produce truth. A commitment to the greater good understands that what is needed is not the means for making all people the same, but of creating new relationships, language games, and social forms: "we should fight against the impoverishment of the relational fabric" (Foucault & Rabinow, 2002: 158).

The risk of domination arises precisely because one has not cared for the self, become a slave to one's desires, and so cannot conceive of the greater good. Such *care* for self is not a form of first-person selfishness or self-interest which clashes with the interests of others (Section 1.2). It reflects the neo-Aristotelian attitudes of understanding one's place in the order of things. Foucault's *ēthos* then was not to dissolve games of power to create some utopia of transparent communication, but to play these games of power between liberties with as little domination as possible.

## 7.4   The *Other*

In the second decade of the twenty-first century, two pandemics converged to highlight the legacies of global racialised oppression and injustice. When the World Health Organization declared coronavirus disease (COVID-19) a global pandemic, it soon became apparent that racialised persons experienced heightened disease contraction and mortality rates, as well as worsened social and economic inequality. To do anti-racism we must first bring to the surface the inescapable Eurocentric contexts of living which are grounded in modernity and its projects of colonialism.

In much of postmodern thought, and especially in the practice of counselling and psychotherapy – the epistemological and hermeneutical role of the Other takes on a critical importance. Experiences that are not within a dominant Eurocentric power–knowledge paradigm can offer critical perspectives on reality – amplifying alterities entails making alternative knowledges, worlds, and practices more visible. The postmodern reading of difference and Otherness often presents itself as having an ethical and emancipatory function, in that it looks to make visible subjugated knowledges within a dominant power–knowledge relationship. Foucault employed this ethical method to highlight how modern totalising forces – particularly in prisons and mental hospitals – oppressed, marginalised, racialised, and dehumanised Others.

The aim of decolonising institutions by teaching the dark side of colonialism, which includes the role of Nations such as Britain in the transatlantic slave trade, is to promote anti-racism and anti-colonialism. However, revealing atrocities is inadequate for restoring and revitalising lives affected by colonial rule, and therefore, it is not decolonising – it perpetuates the myth that imperial history is separate from its context, from regular history. Decolonising requires more than telling the stories of how we got here. It involves incorporating the imperial dimensions of our history, so that we can deepen and widen our understanding of the past and access alternative viewpoints.

Decolonial theory works against the grain of modernity with its ceaseless domination, exploitation, and ecological destruction, which eliminates alternative methods of understanding (epistemological), relating (ethical), and being (ontological). It is a theory that attempts to disrupt the notion that colonialism is separate from ordinary history, and something situated in the past "on a calendar", rather than a persistent structure that creates discourses about who belongs and who does not. We must also acknowledge that the process of expanding our horizons is unsettling for colonisers and colonised alike: "I am myself a settler, like many of my ancestors before me, and I have nowhere else to go" (Macoun & Strakosch, 2013).

The time has long since passed when Europeans could consider their experience and culture to be the goal towards which the rest of humanity should travel; from this perspective, the Other was but an earlier step on a path already trodden by the Occident. There too, was the presumption that Europeans already understood something of other cultures and their histories. But to truly understand Others requires that I am prepared to give ground on what I seek to achieve through that understanding.

The end of the process of understanding then is not to control or manipulate the person with whom I seek to understand, but to learn to live alongside them; this means listening as well as speaking. To understand the Other comes not from negotiating how you sit within my identity, but about experiencing your challenge to my identity. Understanding requires different and sometimes disconcerting ways of being another way, while also being able to live my way too.

Frantz Fanon was an early exponent of the idea that psychotherapy needed to cure its institutions before it could cure others. Fanon left his home in Martinique after the Second World War to study medicine in Lyon. Like Germany and Japan, France was beginning to understand the implications of colonialisation through the lens of its own occupation. As fortune would have it, Fanon attended lectures by Maurice Merleau-Ponty and was introduced to the ideas of Lévi-Strauss, Marx, Lenin, Heidegger, Sartre, Freud, and the philosophy of Gestalt through Kurt Goldstein. Fanon would come to appreciate the decisive effects of wider political and social structures on the human condition.

Having become the medical director of a psychiatric hospital in Algeria, Fanon quickly resigned. In a fiery letter to the Governor General, he stated that he had quit despite years of toil in the service of the Indigenous people, due to the reality of colonialism and its: "tissue of lies, cowardice, [and] contempt for man". He was expelled from the country and moved to recently independent Tunisia where he continued his work on "deterritorialising" the universal practices and totalising theories that he had been taught in the metropole (Robcis, 2020).

What was the significance of these totalising metropolitan theories? The concept of reality in Eurocentric culture perpetuates the assumed ontic division – especially in psychology – between inner and outer. Individualism in psychotherapy becomes something expressed through an inward turn, which isolates experiences, thoughts, and feelings so that the essence of a thing can be examined before concluding what is to be done. This leads to the erroneous assumption – not necessarily explicitly – that injustices are a social phenomenon "out there" and therefore of little relevance to the subject of therapy.

Psychodynamic explanations of how racism operates tend to draw on the dynamics of projection, introjection, and splitting. It helps to illuminate how an individual relates to the system of racism that exists in society, but it does not explain the system itself. Racism and the creation of the races is a social, political, and economic phenomenon. It is the structure of power relations within which we live that renders a statement like: "I am not a racist" meaningless. While the individual may use the sentiment, the radical relationalist understands that this is not where the cause, nor the remedy lies.

Therapists embarking on training do so with a sincere desire to help other people. The relationalist understands that innocent, benevolent, helping professionals armed with individualising psychological interventions risk perpetuating civilising colonial attitudes towards trainees, supervisees, and clients. Believing that I have the capacity to help, "hold" or other such euphemism for rescuing and civilising the Other, relies on the notion that I have the competence, right and permission to do so. At the same time, the capacity to help depends on the presence of a marginalised and subjugated Other. The apparent need for "interventions" or "treatments" for distress creates for client's the colonial relations of dependency which sustain logics of imperial practices as enlightened, competent, independent, able-bodied, benevolent helpers of those who need help/civilising.

Though critical of pedagogical institutions, Foucault saw little that was inherently problematic about the practice of people familiar with specific "truth games" sharing their knowledge and techniques. The risk for Foucault was the effects of power relations and domination, where a person inadvertently attempts to control the Other. This he felt, only comes about when one fails to care for the Other, for their sake, rather than becoming subordinate to their own desires, fears, and anxieties. The well-meaning psychotherapy trainer who projects their anxiety onto their students falls into this category: "Yes ... I know that *my* students are in therapy, and supervised practice ... I know all that ... but *my* role is to hold *their* process".

The Jungian archetype of the "Hero's Journey" risks entangling the mentor, trainer, facilitator, or therapist in a journey that is not their own. The language of the coloniser of Other's psyche is invisible – like water. The inherent rightness of tutoring the untutored, civilising the uncivilised, rendering the irrational intelligible, and turning the child towards the ways of adulthood, is already presumed. Given mental health's legacy of colonialism, notions of helping "should not be accepted without scrutiny".

A short-cut to colour blindness would have me insist that all people are the same irrespective of their outward appearance. Yet such an assertion is not only untrue, but it denies the experience of our social world. By focusing on the universality of humans, the message I risk conveying is that seeing difference is the cause of racism; it denies the fact that we are born into a social system inspired by white heterosexual disembodied males which flattens difference and conflates histories. Unless this is acknowledged, how can we begin to understand and think through reorganising our social world? We risk convincing ourselves that if there is a problem then only small adjustments are required – we collude with the loud silence.

Frequently, the majority community remains silent because of a fear of making mistakes, saying the wrong thing, and experiencing social shame. For therapists, inscrutability becomes the mask to wear when we cannot trust our spontaneous selves; what becomes "difficult" about difficult conversations is avoiding missteps. Studies find that once in possession of a greater awareness of unconscious biases, we withdraw from encounters which might reveal ourselves and our biases for fear of offending (Noon, 2018). Yet by avoiding these conversations, the status quo persists because people lean into their power and privilege, disavowing the salience of structural and interpersonal prejudices.

Colour-blind therapies following this way of thinking overlook crucial relations to context. In Māoridom, for example, interdependence indicates healthy functioning, whereas independence is considered immature or irrational. Support is something done by the *whole* and so limiting therapy to the individual or indeed a single-family unit, segments clients from their relational, meaning-making systems. To many Māori clients, a spiritual encounter with a therapist can be more enlightening than any scientific explanation about chemical imbalances and rational self-control. Similarly, in Samoan cultures, the self is considered a deeply relational subject. The relational space between an individual and their kin suggests that therapy neglectful of a client's relationship to others denies the most important source of healing (Durie, 2011).

The radically relational therapist recognises that people and the practice of therapy do not exist in an ahistorical vacuum: we are culturally, politically, structurally, and systemically located. Anti-oppressive therapeutic practice explicitly recognises structural inequalities and the mechanisms through which powerful or privileged social groups engage in relational oppression. Indeed, there appears to be some mechanism of oppression – be it ideological, institutional, interpersonal, or internalised – for nearly all characteristics of being in the world, that is, age, gender, racialised identity, ethnicity, ability/disability, faith, sexuality, and class.

Diversity is not an additional concept to remember, or something that the therapist "adds on" or "works with". Diversity transcends the therapeutic relationship. To see it otherwise is to risk a relational dynamic where the client is *Othered* while the therapist inhabits the normative position from which the practice is conducted: it remains oppressive as it is something "done to" the Other.

To focus on the client and their "diversity" or its impact on the therapeutic relationship is to ignore the impact of the therapist's identity. This denial of the therapist's identity, or who they represent to the client, transfers responsibility and understanding to the client. It does not acknowledge that the therapeutic relationship is constituted by two identities, two histories, two worldviews. To be "inclusive" is equally problematic because it is to enjoin the outsider – the

Other – to come alongside the invisible, normative, centred, and dominant identity: to put my arm around your minoritised shoulder and "take you in".

Supporting engagement by minoritised communities requires building a relationship which simultaneously invites while also raises awareness about the co-created nature of the exercise. It requires the Rawlsian concept I spoke of earlier, where the client and therapist take the opportunity to be explicit about their values, and whether they are near or far regarding culture, faith, and traditions (Section 2.3). The idea of "working within" diversity means holding two, simultaneous, embodied and potentially conflictual claims to meaning without dismissing or denying their validity.

For example, playfulness and attention to what emerges, on one hand, or directiveness and structure, on the other, encapsulate the polarities of Eurocentric talking therapies which may be unfamiliar beyond its own "territory". Explaining cultural assumptions in therapy can avoid people feeling anxious about getting it right or wrong. A further illustration of this relates to Honour codes, which are prevalent in collectivist cultures and are connected to a group's social and relational systems of dependence. In ways which may seem alien to a Eurocentric humanistic ideal, power rests with the group – and in particular with women – and not with individual autonomy (Khan, 2023).

Barad's Post-Humanism. Because it was originally intended to challenge the idea of biology-is-destiny, the distinction between gender and sex served the argument that the former is culturally constructed whatever the material facts of sex appear to be. In which case it was not biology but culture that became destiny. The uncritical reproduction of such a mind–body distinction inadvertently established an ontological binary, which reflected systems of compulsory heterosexuality (Butler, 1999: 8–26). To uphold then, the emancipatory goals of feminism, scholars have emphasised how philosophy and psychology must work to define the ground that lies between the dualities of the material (i.e., bodies, spaces, objects, and practices/traditions) and social worlds (discourse).

Agential realism is a radical post-humanistic movement that responds to philosophy's twentieth-century preoccupation with language, and dualist narratives which reflect the idea of a pendulum that swings between either material or discourse. It seeks to avoid the primacy of human agency in social life, and if not dissolve, then transcend the binary distinction between knowing and being. To move beyond the distinction between mind and matter, agential realism emphasises how discourse is knotted and entangled with materiality. Particle physicist and philosopher Karen Barad sought to reconceptualise the pendulum that swings between the material–discursive realms into a non-dualistic radically relational ontology.

By extending the insights of poststructuralist thinkers – particularly Judith Butler and Michel Foucault – Barad leads us away from discourse as something that constructs reality, to seeing both discourse and materiality as mutually constitutive – again, reminiscent of the uroboros I introduced at the outset. From Barad's perspective, the world is not made of separate human and nonhuman entities. The world comes about through entangled phenomena that engage in and become determinate through intra-actions – a term of art which avoids the presumption of pre-existing, separable entities to be synthesised as entailed by the alternative inter-action (Hollin et al. 2017).

As a physicist, Barad draws inspiration from the interpretive framework of Niels Bohr, Werner Heisenberg, and the quantum experiments of the early twentieth century. In the quantum context, matter was shown to display both wave-like and particle-like behaviour, depending on the apparatus used to do the observing. Wave–particle duality remains a revolutionary and counterintuitive observation, suggesting that quantum systems can remain entangled and superposed in theory, while in practice they appear "classically" – as wave or particle – but not simultaneously both to the observer.

Another example familiar to the practice of spectroscopy is the Heisenberg uncertainty principle which acknowledges the impossibility of simultaneously measuring nuclear position *and* momentum. This is because the experiment for identifying the position of a particle necessarily alters its velocity, and vice versa. Barad extends the quantum idiom to the either/or situation of a pendulum which hovers between the material–discursive domains, to persuade us that it is the methods that produce rather than describe the world, and the things we do in it. The swinging pendulum is no longer an object to be witnessed from some aerial vantage point from above which aspires to the notion of objectivity. The embodied self and physical, meaningful, and symbolic world are so thoroughly entwined that we cannot fully untangle the body as *intelligible* zero point from the body as *sensible* zero-point.

Anticipating Lyotard's *differend* by almost 50 years, Bohr saw how concepts are embodied within, and defined by, the technologies used for their measurement. Bohr was thus able to make sense of wave–particle duality by suggesting not just that matter exhibits mutually exclusive characteristics (particle or wave) under different experimental conditions, but that matter really is *either* a wave *or* a particle under different arrangements. In agential realism, subject and object are mutually exclusive positions, enacted differentially by different practices.

Barad – and before them phenomenologist Maurice Merleau-Ponty – draws on the thought experiment known as the Heisenberg cut to emphasise how human agency is at work in the process of shifting between exterior and interior moments. Consider holding a stick in a dark room. If the stick is held tightly, then it can become an instrument for exploring and navigating the room; through poking and prodding it becomes entangled with the subject (me) in the practice of investigating the room. If, however, the stick is held in a different way and is felt and touched to explore its texture, it becomes an object to be investigated as part of the room; a separation or cut has taken place which excludes the stick (object) from the measuring apparatus (me).

Similar phenomena accompany the mundane everyday activities of say, using a pencil, fountain pen, or paint brush. The object becomes entangled in the flow of human expression, and when the lead snaps, the ink runs dry, or the brush needs re-loading, then there is a withdrawal of entanglement – or cut – and the *object* appears once more. Instead of an unnoticed aspect of my engagement with the world, I now hold in my hand a useless wooden stick or piece of metal and plastic. It follows that the boundaries of how a person goes about understanding the world do not coincide with the boundaries of what we assume being human is about. Indeed, being human becomes a category which emerges within our intra-actions; that is by either sensing with a stick or sensing the stick itself. Objects and subjects do not pre-exist in their interrelating; different intra-actions, through different apparatuses, enact ontologically different subjects and objects.

Barad argues that the entanglement of mind and matter is not simply an overlap between separate independent, self-contained entities. To get a sense of what this means we must go beyond Wittgenstein's Rabbit-Duck (Section 6.4). Here, we have already noticed that we cannot – simultaneously – recognise a duck and rabbit in the optical illusion. An agential cut must be made between the two images which renders a sense of separation or dualism by withdrawing one of the images from the other. The entanglement peculiar to Heisenberg's electron, Barad's stick, my fountain pen, and Wittgenstein's' Rabbit-Duck have in common two apparently distinct systems that are more than the mere combination of their respective individual states.

A zebra, for example, is not brought into existence through an overlap between the separate entities of a black horse with white stripes and a white horse with black stripes. Yet, my experience of a zebra – constituted through the lens of white Eurocentrism – sees a white horse with black markings. Conversely, a black horse with white markings is a zebra constituted through the lens of Black African Heritage.

Materiality and discourse are constitutive – it makes no sense to separate the material facts of a zebra (arguments about whether a zebra is a black horse or a white horse) from the context of the subject or observer be they of European or African heritage. What matters is that the Heisenberg "cut" excludes other realities from my being. A Eurocentric "cut" for example *excludes* other ways of experiencing the material reality of a zebra.

Agential realism emphasises the value of understanding the discursive effects of an encounter along with the material, and the material effects of the discursive. While there is clearly a world beyond words, discourse shapes what we notice and exclude about the material world. Though matter itself has stability I still need to be accountable for the ethical consequences of agential cuts and the exclusions that underpin them.

An everyday example may help to show how agential realism offers a more nuanced approach for reckoning with human and nonhuman interactions. Before the emergence of social media, visitors to a hotel would provide feedback using comment cards or even a visitor's book, for example, lovely stay, home from home. Hoteliers might also frame feedback through the material boundaries of a card with text boxes that conditioned what could be said, that is, length and style. The feedback was further conditioned as it was available to only a few staff who would read, discuss, discard or perhaps even act in the feedback (Orlikowski & Scott, 2015).

Technology – social media – gradually altered the material facts about how visitor and hotelier related. Instead of a card being sheepishly passed across the desk when paying, technology meant comments became relatively unconstrained as the audience for the reviews became focused on other travellers and not necessarily hoteliers. Where once materiality confined discourse to the boundaries of the business, social media made it visible to a wider audience. A shift in material–discursive practices from captive-private to public-consequential meant that where once hoteliers saw a *guest* standing across the counter, now they saw a *reviewer*. Over time, changes in how human communication became materialised – from comment cards to online reviews – produced different discourses, different guests, different hoteliers, and different hotels.

Barad brings to our attention how we are responsible for the changes we enact. This is not because we <u>do</u> the choosing; equally, we do not escape responsibility because we are <u>hailed</u> by our <u>Subjects</u>. We are an agential part of the material becoming of the world. The agentive – yet superficially passive – role of technology and how it changes the balance of power between visitor and hotelier becomes acknowledged. Though entangled, the capacity for intentional action keeps humans at the top of the agential ethical pyramid – for now at least.

Why should this be of interest to psychotherapists? By apparatus, we can mean a set of materials and practices that, by being used in a specific situation for a specific purpose, afford the boundaries of what can happen in that situation. The experience of transference, for example, can be understood as something simultaneously produced by the apparatus of therapy (i.e., the beige or highly personalised consulting room, regular meeting times, the scent of the therapist which reminds the client of their father, the methods used, and style of interaction), as well as being constitutive of the therapeutic relationship.

Psychotherapy practitioners who used technology during the COVID-19 pandemic will be familiar with the distinct and disembodying effects brought about through using technology for therapy (Section 9.1). Agential realism offers a powerful tool for anticipating the ethical problems arising from the burgeoning augmentation of technologies which seek to offer artificial empathy, for example. Specifically, the concern lies with the unchallenged biases inherent in STEM practices, where AI technologists tend to be unrepresentative of the humanity that consumes their inventions.

*In conclusion*, the material world and discourse are knotted together and unfold over time. Time then, is not like an inert, yawning chasm between separate events that wait to be bridged. It is textured by embodied customs and practices – material shapes communication and communication becomes materialised – as we have seen above. Time is the supportive ground of events, and where the present has its roots, which is why as therapists, it is imperative that we turn our attention to time itself.

## References

Albertson, K. & Stepney, P. (2020). 1979 and All That: A 40-year Reassessment of Margaret Thatcher's Legacy on Her Own Terms. *Cambridge Journal of Economics.* 44(2), 319–342.

Botts, T.F. (2017). The Genealogy and Viability of the Concept of Intersectionality (Chapter 28). In Garry, A., Khader, S.J., & Stone, A. (Eds.). *The Routledge Companion to Feminist Philosophy.* 1st edition. Routledge.

Butler, J.P. (1999). *Gender Trouble: Feminism and the Subversion of Identity.* Routledge.

Crenshaw, K. (1991). Mapping the Margins: Intersectionality, Identity Politics, and Violence against Women of Color. *Stanford Law Review.* 43(6), 1241–1299.

Durie, M. (2011). Indigenizing Mental Health Services: New Zealand Experience. *Transcultural Psychiatry.* 48(1–2), 24–36.

Dussel, E. D. (2012). Transmodernity and Interculturality: An Interpretation from the Perspective of Philosophy of Liberation. *Transmodernity.* 1(3), 28–59.

Foucault, M. & Faubion, J.D. (2002). Power. *Essential Works of Foucault 1954–1984.* Vol. 3. Penguin.

Foucault, M. & Rabinow, P. (1991). *The Foucault Reader.* Penguin.

Foucault, M. & Rabinow, P. (2002). The Ethics of the Concern for Self as a Practice of Freedom. R. Hurley et al. (Trans.). In *Michel Foucault: Ethics: Subjectivity and Truth. Essential Works of Foucault 1955–1984*, Vol. 1. Penguin.

Freud, S. & Pfister, O. (1963). *Psychoanalysis and Faith: The Letters of Sigmund Freud and Oskar Pfister.* Eds. Heinrich Meng & Ernst L. Freud. Trans. Eric Mosbacher. Hogarth Press.

Hollin, G. et al. (2017). (Dis)entangling Barad: Materialisms and Ethics. *Social Studies of Science.* 47(6), 918–941.

Khan, M. (2023). *Working Within Diversity: A Reflective Guide to Anti-oppressive Practice in Counselling and Therapy.* 1st edition. Jessica Kingsley Publishers.

Macoun, A. & Strakosch, E. (2013). The Ethical Demands of Settler Colonial Theory. *Settler Colonial Studies.* 3(3–4), 426–443.

Massot, A. (2022). Psychoanalysis, Thermodynamics, and the Matter of Scarcity: A Genealogy of Freud's Death Drive Hypothesis. *Theory & Psychology.* 32(4), 571–589.

Nietzsche, F. (1968). *The Will to Power.* W. Kaufmann and R.J. Hollingdale (Eds). Vintage Books.

Noon, M. (2018). Pointless Diversity Training: Unconscious Bias, New Racism and Agency. *Work, Employment and Society.* 32(1) 198–209.

Noth, I. & Morgenthaler, C. (2014). The Friendship Between Sigmund Freud and Oskar Pfister as Seen in the Correspondence between the Jewish Atheist Founder of Psychoanalysis and the Swiss Pastor Who Pioneered Pastoral Psychology. *Pastoral Psychology*. 63(1), 81–90.

Orlikowski, W.J. & Scott, S.V. (2015). Exploring Material-Discursive Practices. *Journal of Management Studies*. 52(5), 697–705.

Payne, M. (2006). *Narrative Therapy: An Introduction for Counsellors*. 2nd edition. Sage.

Robcis, C. (2020). Frantz Fanon, Institutional Psychotherapy, and the Decolonization of Psychiatry. *Journal of the History of Ideas*. 81(2), 303–325.

Rorty, R. (1991). *Freud and Moral Reflection*. In, *Habermas and Lyotard on Postmodernity*. Cambridge University Press.

Skovlund, H. (2011). Overcoming Problems of Relativism in Postmodern Psychotherapy. *Journal of Contemporary Psychotherapy*. 41(3), 187–198.

Slife, B.D. (2004). Theoretical Challenges to Therapy Practice and Research: The Constraint of Naturalism. In M. Lambert (Ed.), *Handbook of Psychotherapy and Behavior Change* (p. 50). 5the edition. Wiley.

Slife, B.D. et al. (2017). *The Hidden Worldviews of Psychology's Theory, Research, and Practice*. Routledge.

Slife, B.D. & Reber, J. (2001). Eclecticism in Psychotherapy: Is It Really the Best Substitute for Traditional Theories? In B. Slife, R. Williams, & S. Barlow (Eds.), *Critical Issues in Psychotherapy: Translating New Ideas into Practice* (pp. 213–234). Sage Publications.

Szasz, T. (2010). *The Myth of Mental Illness – Foundations of a Theory of Personal Conduct*. Harper Perennial.

Tran The, J. et al. (2018). The Epistemological Foundations of Freud's Energetics Model. *Frontiers in Psychology*. 9, 1861–1871.

Tran The, J. et al. (2020). From the Principle of Inertia to the Death Drive: The Influence of the Second Law of Thermodynamics on the Freudian Theory of the Psychical Apparatus. *Frontiers in Psychology*. 11, 325–333.

White, M. & Epston, D. (1990). *Narrative Means to Therapeutic Ends*. W.W. Norton.

# 8

# TIME

## 8.1   Introduction: Fidelity to Experience

The foremost of human concerns is time. Our inescapable awareness of time and the ever-dwindling amount of time that remains to us: "Time is the means offered to all that is destined to be, to come into existence in order for it to no longer be" (Merleau-Ponty, 1962: 419). Time is at once familiar, banal, elusive, and strange. We never have enough of it.

Doomed King Richard reflected on how profligate he was with this most valuable of commodities: "I wasted time, and now doth time waste me". Wasting time – for some – is immoral; especially wasting *my* time, because it is tantamount to depriving me of something I can never get back. Every experience I have had, my thoughts, what I do, and my achievements, happen in time. It is the movements of a clock, the burning of a candle, another sunrise, the changing seasons, and schedules of one kind or another. A future event is ascribed a moment in time – a date – as if it already exists, with time being the void for me to traverse before I can arrive, on time.

Time is rarely consistent. It rushes, drags, or simply passes; it can change us too. As well as being arranged in time, my experiences come with a distinct sensation of living presentness in what Husserl called the "extended now". I am aware of writing this now, while also feeling time pressing as I must leave to join my family. This time I know will "fly". I have heard it said, often by those nearing the end of their lives: "time goes so quickly". Watching children grow – as parents often report – is an oddly distorted temporal experience of long days and short weeks.

These are a few of the things which point to something curiously elusive about time. It informs how we think about free will, the influence of the past

DOI: 10.4324/9781003396161-8

on the present, and in connection to space, it leads us to the foundations of the natural sciences and our cosmic origins. Psychological distress disrupts the continuity of our lives and in doing so it also radically distorts the subjective experience of time.

Boredom, impatience, agitation, and, at worst, mania are associated with subjective time seeming to accelerate. Conversely, when we fall ill, experience grief and loss, or suffer depression, time seems to slow down or even stop. How I experience time cannot be grasped without some appreciation of the basic structures of subjective temporality, and our implicit and explicit experiences of living alongside others and their time.

When my mind goes blank, I slide into timelessness – I am uninvolved and no longer present or available to you. I have decoupled from the march of time. My field of perception right now as I write this, is filled with colours, noises, and fleeting tactile sensations: my bare elbow feels the pressure of the desk at which I sit; my awareness drifts dreamlike – accompanied by the background noise of children playing in the next room – out through the window. I am in a trance-like state, *participating* in a timeless flow of absorption and assimilation. I am lost among the rain-lashed trees of the November gale outside, which seems to represent to me something of this reverie: I recall people and fragments of conversations from the past, whose presence drifts in and out of my temporal flow.

This is the ground from which these words and thoughts emerge. I return to the room, a *spectator* of my own existence. Time stops flowing and once again becomes the object of my interest. What do I make of this ordinary mundane *hovering* between my experiencing and observing selves? I unloosed myself as a viewer of myself, to an experiencing self, to become lost in a sensation, drawn to what emerged from my field of experience beyond the window of my room.

As I watch my children play with their toys, it seems clear to me that they are oblivious to the world and do not notice the passing of time. This lived time, where I am absorbed in the flow of life, is *implicit* in children's experience of being engaged in play and directed towards some immediate goal. Neither the past, the future, or even calls to eat stand out from this pre-reflective existence, which constitutes the undercurrent of experience. To use Husserl's terminology again, implicit time is a passive or involuntary synthesis of anticipation, momentary impressions, and the retention of what sinks away. We do not actively perform this process, yet this original impression signals the birth of subjectivity.

Augustine drew on a deeply personal knowledge for his investigations, arguing that no mortal could readily express the nature of time (2021: 230): "For what is time. Who can readily and briefly explain this? If no one asks me, I know … if I wish to explain it, then I know not". The remark was made in anticipation of the reader's patience as his explorations unfolded, pausing from time to time to pray for God's assistance as he was driven close to despair. Through prayer, Augustine was modelling the "contemplative now" an elongated field of attention incorporating a *past-now*, the *here-now* and a *future-now* (2021):

> I know, that if nothing passed away, time past were not; and if nothing were coming, a time to come were not; and if nothing were, time present were not.

The Augustinian fidelity to experience was to influence Edmund Husserl 1,500 years later as he too reflected on how we synthesise sensations of inner time consciousness. The mere succession of atomised conscious moments cannot hope to establish our experience of flow and continuity. It is only when moments are mutually related to each other in a forward and backward direction, flowing in and sinking away, that the sequence of sensations are integrated into a unified and experienced whole.

Time consciousness for Husserl integrates the experience of single moments into an integrated intentional arc, helping me move towards goals which have meaning. This intentionality can be illustrated by what is going on right now. As you read these letters, you perceive and understand them as a meaningful sequence of words; automatic, multiple syntheses of *gestalts* combine into sentences, which hopefully direct you towards the totality of their meaning. Unless a typographical error interrupts your sense of flow, the letters are only *implicitly* present in your perception. The arc of intentionality relates to the temporal dimension of your experience: to form a meaningful sentence, succeeding words (or moments) have to be integrated into a coherent sequence. Similarly, my experience of consciousness which flows is more than a succession of now's.

Retentions and protentions are deep temporal structures that make anticipations and recollections possible. They are necessary for you to understand my sentences as well as being necessary for me, the speaker, to guide my sentence to its conclusion. If my retentions evaporate, I am lost mid-sentence. If my protention deserts me, I will not know how to go on. This prophetic process does more than merely catch what is coming: "it has already caught it" (Husserl, 1991: 54).

Retention and protention are not to be thought of as separate components of temporal experience. The former shapes the latter; *what* we anticipate and *how* we anticipate are shaped by what has just passed. Protentions are fulfilled and we are conscious of this in recollections. In this way, each moment retains its predecessors and anticipates the future. Succeeding events refer to and bleed into one another.

Thus, awareness is not momentary but is made possible and run through by its dual facets of retention and protention. Through this retention–protention structure, every conscious act and process suggest an awareness of itself: it is what constitutes the unity of consciousness over time. It suggests an intentional arc which joins the start and the end. The process seems more illusory when I speak because I am often only aware of my intention once the talk has got hold of me and I am already launched into what I hope to say. What I have to say seems to emerge while I am already in the flow of saying it to you, the listener, who also seeks to anticipate where this is all going. While Husserl articulates something profound about the experience of time as it is presented to my consciousness, Merleau-Ponty saw that something was missing from this picture, which radicalises and perhaps even undermines our understanding of time.

## 8.2 Thinking about Time

A deep philosophical tension exists between the contrasting tendencies we have for thinking about time. The first tendency privileges our subjective or common-sense experience of time, and it argues that the structure of temporality is identical with the structure of subjectivity; the subject – that is you, me, and we – *are* time. This family of views which stresses the role played by the activity of the human mind in building knowledge out of and beyond sensible experience is termed **idealism**. Objectivity itself is the greatest creative accomplishment of our subjective and intersubjective experience of the world. While there are unique forms of idealism, they all agree that deep down, time is not real.

Beyond philosophy, it was becoming commonplace in the eighteenth century to represent time using space. Joseph Priestley created the first timeline, depicting lives with lines. Today, we unthinkingly accept the use of timelines for training and with clients when figuring our lives like trains calling at various events along the fixed tracks of time. By the beginning of the twentieth century, the spatialisation of time seemed complete. Modernity and the techniques of science – Einstein's relativity and Maxwell's electromagnetism – led some to question whether the human experience of time was a figment, an illusion which gets in the way of how time really is. For Bertrand Russell, **realism** meant that past, present, and future were just so: they have a reality which exists beyond human experience. There was nothing special about any one part of space or any one part of time and our belief in a present moment was just that – a figment, the product of human psychology.

Many railed against idealism, but it refused to perish because it is rooted in human subjective experience. The British logician John McTaggart sought to reconcile the tensions that existed between our experience of time and what we learn about time from science. The analytical arguments proposed in *The Unreality of Time* (1908) examined the implications of how we order events in time. The common sense, or folk theory of time seeks to do justice to our perspective of a durationless boundary – the present – that separates the past and future.

But as we know, time is not experienced as a static distribution of moments or events like beads on a string. We experience time as moments which come to be and then pass away – it flows from one temporal moment to the next. We take it that time has a direction, and I experience a dynamic future flowing, whooshing towards me as I occupy what feels like a privileged static present. The sentiment captured by the idiom: "there is no time like the present", speaks to the view that lacking a future or past reality, we must inhabit the sovereign viewpoint of *now*.

Yet without the idea of before and after, our understanding of the passing of time could not exist and any sense of "now" becomes meaningless. When we think about the ordering of events in common-sense time, we recognise that every event is in the past or future. But we also recognise that the ordering in the future is fluid, and that the future will become the present before receding into the past. McTaggart called this ordering of events the A-series, where the future seems to push its way into a durationless present before becoming ordered and immutable in the past. Like a zipper, the present moment is where the strands of the future are gathered together and bound into an immutable past that extends beyond.

A second, unchanging series of successive events becomes apparent. McTaggart called this the B-series, a perspective that appeals to the Stoic view which sees time as a succession of events already standing in some temporal relation to all other events. This ordering is not so fluid and adopts a more "objective" mind-independent perspective of time, which speaks well to the *realism* of science. Time in this framework refers to earlier, later than, and concomitant with – there is no objective distinction between past, present, and future.

The dynamic flow of time is a figment, something which says more about what it is to be human than of the reality of time itself. Most importantly for our purposes, the B-series is understood as grounded in relationships between events and facts which are fixed, unchanging and without tense. Time becomes a landscape of successively related temporal events; the passage of time is the unremarkable presentation to our awareness of the successive moments of the world. Temporal realists claim that all times are the same, equally real, and capable of containing events.

When analysed in this way, time for McTaggart becomes paradoxical and thus *unreal*: if change is real, then the A- and B-series are simply incompatible. Granted, it is unusual for philosophers to take McTaggart's arguments to this conclusion. But it does bring to our attention how **analysing** time draws attention away from the **experience** of time. It is a tendency shared by psychology and psychodynamic theories in particular, which side with a B-series ordering of events which presumes that the past pushes – deterministically – into the present, thereby shaping the future. It undermines lived experience and our faith in therapy which claims that changing the present in turn changes the past and the future. But a closer examination exposes the flaws of McTaggart's analysis, which presumes that the future contains the whole of the past which proceeds through a point-like *durationless present*.

Against the Durationless Present. An irresistible component of our common-sense attitude to time is that the moment we occupy – the present – is privileged. The only reality we can speak of manifests itself in the absolute now. From the progression of instants comes the impression of duration. The imponderable question of the stationary present has puzzled thinkers since Zeno of Elea who introduced a variety of paradoxes to challenge the so-called common-sense ideas about reality. Perhaps the most celebrated example is the absurd conclusion reached in the flight of an arrow.

At any given instant, a moving arrow must occupy a space equal to itself; it cannot extend into another instant, which is to say that at any given moment it is at the place where it is, and nowhere else. Yet places do not move. So, if in each instant the arrow occupies a space equal to itself, then the arrow is not moving in that instant because it has no time in which to move; it is simply there at that place. The same holds for any other instant we take to be the flight of the arrow. Thus, the arrow is never moving, and by extension neither is the present.

There are no transitions, merely the occupation of different places at different times. An objective distinction between past, present, and future can only be drawn at the moment Zeno's arrow appears stationary. And yet if the present moment is stationary – accurate for just a moment – how does time pass? If, through right reason we arrive at an absurd conclusion then the initial premise of the argument must be wrong, that is, there is something fishy about the durationless now. The paradox of Zeno can only be formulated if we equate time with movement and take it that now is devoid of duration. This is the false paradox at the heart of McTaggart's argument against time's reality.

One of the difficulties which friends of the "durationless moment" must face is that it is incompatible with Einstein's theory of relativity. Relativistic space–time is inhospitable to the idea that time flows through joined-together atomised moments, as its structure does not admit temporal partitioning. The movement of the present is a process that takes time to happen, and for that to be the case, there needs to be a second-time dimension (hypertime) relative to the movement of the present along the ordinary temporal dimension. To accommodate innumerable present moments, we need to invent an infinite number of temporal dimensions to permit the sensation of time passing.

By contrast, the present is a radically intersubjective feature of the B-series. Every moment is present relative to itself. This is far more consistent with our experience of occupying different times and having different temporal perspectives at those times, and referring to each of those times as being present. From each temporal perspective, we can designate a different moment as being *present* and a different distribution of the past, present, and future. The experience of observing light from a distant galaxy, for example, is not something which lies behind us at our remote beginnings but is, in fact, before us in our cultural milieu (Merleau-Ponty, 1962: 432).

*The only way to envision free will or agency is to reject the idea of the durationless present.* Psychologists who objectify time fail to see that a privileged present is an assumption; the present is not an object in any conventional sense and cannot be objectively observed. The paradoxes within the A-series alert us to its idealist constructs that have been discarded by many of the natural sciences. If we view past and present as synchronous, then theorists must view the present as a mere extension of the immutable past; clients <u>and</u> therapists are thus rendered utterly determined in their thoughts and actions.

Conversely, denying the influence of the past eliminates its role in the present – where therapy takes place – rendering therapy less meaningful at best and incomprehensible at worst. Modernists traditionally assume that a person's will must take place exclusively in the present. The presumption of a linear arrangement of past and future centred on a privileged now mandates that it take place exclusively in one of these dimensions, as each exists independently. Common-sense attitudes to time would consider it ludicrous to assert that free will occurs in the future, and we can only be free if we are free of the past. The ethical problem lies with the privileged present, something which psychotherapists often place at the heart of their practice.

The present makes little sense without the past, whether that past be our cultural or personal histories. This is one of the reasons why psychotherapists have difficulty adopting a purely existential free will perspective. It is impossible to understand a client's – or therapist's – will without their history in context. The A-series perspective makes no provision for the experiential commingling of the past, present, and future. Yet the A-series captures something of our intuition that the past is different from the future. If the past were in the present, the two dimensions would not be sequential. The past would be synchronous with the present and this contradicts the idea of a privileged now. As nothing can be both past and present – with the past fixed and done, and the future in principle open – the A-series nevertheless imparts a sense of radical freedom to human action.

But this frozen picture of time, accurate for a just moment, soon to be succeeded in the A-series by a different temporal perspective suggests that we see reality from no perspective – or *nowhen*. Relational time, on the other hand, extends beyond the experience of the "instant" to consider the trace which an event leaves in the immediate memory (Section 8.4). For Augustine, to whom meditative scriptural chant was a way of life, this meant recognising the reality of the contemplative "now" which possesses duration beyond the moment itself. Though not a physical quantity, this contemplative "now" is nevertheless a true quantity.

This suprahistorical "sacred time" where the present is not the fleeting moment of the A-series but the *fullness* of time, can be seen from an existential perspective as solemn, with the character of epiphany about it (Gadamer, 2013: 124–125). Our lived experience is aware of its milieu and need not be trapped by the myth of a durationless present moment interfacing past and future. Consciousness is a synthesis or intentional weave – a communion as Merleau-Ponty puts it – of future and past perspectives. It changes as it advances, processing relationships between events in a way we are not ordinarily aware of but may become so as soon as our attention is drawn to some prominent figure among a field of activities (1962: 320).

The future is different from the past. It consists of possibilities which might or might not occur in the present. The present is not a passive gateway through which events must proceed from the future to the past. Indeed, McTaggart's obligation to the categories of past/future and a durationless present lead us astray. It is a modernist illusion to project the acquired temporal order of the past into the possible order of the future; both are subject to change in the present. Rather than reduce human consciousness to a passive observer which exists in an immobile present, intersubjective time invokes an active subjective communication with its field (Section 8.4). The past and future are shaped by this field of presence, which for Augustine meant prophecies and revelations, but for atheist Merleau-Ponty, referred to a network of intentionalities, expectations, and anticipations (1962: 416–417):

> It is in my "field of presence" in the broadest sense – this moment spent working, with the horizon of the day behind it, and the horizon of the evening and night ahead, that I make contact with time ... I do not think of the evening to come and its consequences, and yet it "is there", like the back of a house of which I can only see the façade, or like the background beneath a figure ... Our future is not made up exclusively of guesswork and daydreams ... but carried forward by lines of intentionality which trace out in advance the style of what is to come.

McTaggart's thesis matters because it offers a way of understanding how moderns think about time. The B-series does not include an objective present or temporal passage – moments do not flow into one another. This only happens when our self abstains from separating lived moments from past moments. So is our temporal experience illusory, mistaken, or irrelevant in the face of cosmic time? Is lived time simply what we should expect of who we are: creatures embedded within temporal reality, who encounter it subjectively, and interact with it, from our uniquely human perspective? Radical relationality appreciates the inescapable, culturally bound, and often contradictory linguistic expressions that characterise the experience of slipping in and out of lived time. But however important it may seem, separating the world into idealist and realist perspectives is just one of the things we do; it is the product of one (modernist) stance to the world, among others.

Hazardous Metaphors. What shall we make of this apparent conflict between idealist and realist perspectives? Is physics wrong to exclude features of time as experienced by human beings? Can we explain away our anthropocentric experience of time as an illusion? The confusion stems from subjectivity becoming the object of examination by an objective attitude – itself, the creation of subjectivity. If you could imagine the fictional scientist Victor Frankenstein stepping out of Mary Shelley's novel and regarding the author, then we are close to seeing what happens when we assume a place of absolute contemplation from which to explain the world: the creator becomes the object of what seems to be detached conscious reflection.

The impartial spectator – the so called third person perspective – imagines it can observe its subject from a distance and thereby objectify its own subjectivity. Husserl was adamant that objectivity was an achievement of our subjective experience. The *implicit* timeless "now" I spoke of earlier unfurls itself into the *explicit* dimensions of an observed and remembered past and a chasm-like future in waiting. Science – Husserl argued – seems dishonest in its blindness to the embodied experience of the eating, drinking, jealous, angry, dancing, loving, frightened people doing the observing. No wonder we feel remorseful about our finite lives, thrown as we are into what we are led to believe is the flow of an inexorable and independent river of time.

Merleau-Ponty rejects this persistent and distracting metaphor often used to think about time, pointing out that time is not a river: it is not a fluid-like substance at all. The metaphor based on this comparison has persisted for millennia, beguiling us into the surreptitious placing of ourselves in the scene as witnesses looking on from a God-like perspective. The metaphorical observer folds in on themselves and becomes an ontological blind-spot, exempt from reflection (Section 3.1).

This unnoticed and disembodied witness – hovering in a continuous aerial vantage point above – aspires to the notion of objectivity, seeing consciousness as something washed along by the river of time, transported through a stationary landscape. Alternatively, consciousness is positioned as a stationary observer watching the moving torrent of time from the bank. Depending on whether the observer is in the flow of the river, or whether they observe its passage from the riverbank, temporal relations are readily inverted by this two-dimensional abstraction of consciousness (Merleau-Ponty, 1962: 411–412). They are figure-ground reversals of one another: for the former, *time is ground* – a fixed location – and it is the observer who is moving; for the latter, *observer is ground*, and it is times that are moving.

Such figure-ground structures of perception are the invisible, dynamic ways we have for sorting the wildness of the world into intelligible, manipulable structures for creating meaning. Neither metaphor captures reality because time cannot be stopped, but then neither does time go on without me. What is more, the age of steam brought forth new technologically inspired versions of the "time as river" metaphor involving – as we shall see – figure-ground reversals of perspectives employing trains, carriages, and observers facing this way or that.

Merleau-Ponty avoids this impasse by arguing that the embodied self and the physical, meaningful, and symbolic world are so thoroughly entwined that we cannot distinguish between the body as intelligible zero-point and the body as sensible zero-point of orientation. Our relationship with time is not one of consciousness projected into the metaphor of flow, but a spatialising-temporalising vortex where time is not confined to the objective two-dimensional future-past flood plain of a river but possesses some vertical quality or temporal "depth". It is the past that adheres to the present and not the *consciousness* of the past which adheres to the *consciousness* of the present (1968, 244).

To this end, we are not to think of combining substances, such as body and spirit, future and past, because then we would be seeking a union of contradictories. We are badly placed to see this "depth" because we are already caught within space and time. There are no two leaves or two layers of the sensible and the intelligible. Fundamentally, it is neither thing seen nor seer but a reciprocal and reversible insertion and intertwining of one in the other, in what Merleau-Ponty termed the *chiasma* of time (Merleau-Ponty, 1968: 244).

The semantic force of Merleau-Ponty's imagery seeks to displace the Cartesian view of experience – a mind taking in and analysing information – as the foundational way of knowing the world. I perceive and take in the world, but I am also part of the world I come to grasp. Within the momentary sense of any one moment and place, there is a host of other times and incidents packed within such moments. Each aspect of the world about us belongs to that depth of time which "piles up", stretching back and forth indefinitely, shaped and given meaning by our personal history, cultural legacy, desires, and embodied involvements.

The Ecstasies of Embodied Time. The smell of freshly cut grass has a powerful effect on me. Perhaps you too? I am called to long, hot summer days of my childhood, making hay on the family farm in the West of Ireland, or playing football in the local park with brothers and friends. The mere whiff brings about temporal ecstasies in the emotional unfolding now of time. It is this temporal depth – stimulated by what is sensible – which opens up space in a way I can readily pass over. I can never be a point of existence, because even though I am here and now, I am not here and now.

As an indifferent teenager visiting a research laboratory for the first time on a school trip, I caught a whiff of benzaldehyde; it smells like freshly cut grass. Time unfolded for me, meaning that at that moment I became layered in the depth of the span of my existence, both in its history and relationships. In that present I became absent from myself and was pulled within the vortices of embodied time to ecstasies I will always associate with the freedom and play of the laboratory. As embodied creatures, we are in a continuous relation with the world, adapting to and synchronising with the cosmic rhythms of days, months, seasons, and years.

Such synchronisation also involves a person's relationship with their social environment; my time aligns with the time of the world around me. Connected with this is the tacit sensation of feeling temporally connected with others, of living with them contemporaneously, in the same intersubjective time. We are aware of this through daily and weekly routines, schedules, punctuality, and in a broader sense mutual commitments to share time. Then there is the basic contemporising of people sharing cultures, traditions, values, ethics, and forms of behaviour. All of this synchronisation of time requires language.

Whether we like it or not we persist with the habit of linking time with metaphors of movement through space. Merleau-Ponty recognised that our lived experience of time appears to us as a mobile setting which escapes from us, like a landscape seen through the window of a railway carriage: it is compelling even though we do not believe the landscape is moving at all (1962: 419–420). For English speakers, time is depicted like a train travelling

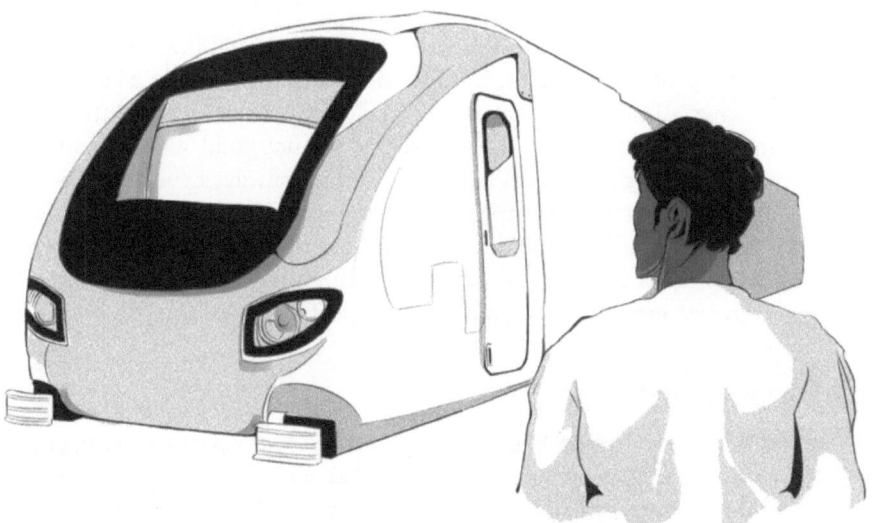

**FIGURE 8.1** Time and the English Speaker.

from the future to the past, with the static ego facing the oncoming future with "now" being the carriage which is parallel to our position in space. From the static ego's reference point of now, earlier events (or carriages of the train which have passed) are before later events (carriages yet to pass), and it is reality that zooms towards us, before receding into the past to be replaced by yet another present moment.

Events appear ordered in time to pass through this privileged "A-moment" of the ego-reference-point, with earlier events behind the ego, in the past. Despite its problems, there seems to be a compulsive privileging of the durationless present moment. We can accept the experiential perspective which has it that multiple temporal perspectives need not be considered discrete at all; each moment has its horizons of past and future which allow an unbroken chain of moments. To separate one from another requires the *deliberate* act of intellectual abstraction and Merleau-Ponty reminds us that it need not be this way (1962: 432).

Unfortunately, this does not halt discussions about the powerful influence of the past on the present, a notion embraced by some of our therapeutic methods. How do theorists bridge the gap between the immediate (or distant) objective past and the present? The answer lies in the linear view of time, of causality, and the much-favoured role of scientism, which serves a bridging function between past and present. It is a synchronous past and present that gives causality its apparent sequence, where the cause is thought to <u>necessarily</u> precede the effect. It enables modernist theorists to talk about the past in the present when the nature of the A-series alone would prohibit this. The present becomes – problematically – the leading edge of the past (Slife & Fisher, 2000).

For Merleau-Ponty, this was the hazard of such metaphors – which have language at their core: they seduce us into believing that there is a certain void that has its own dimensions that must be filled by a defined quantity called the present (1968: 195–197). The present does not fulfil what is somehow absent but impending in time. What has passed has always been there as itself, indeterminable like some haunting of what might emerge for us. What is present is not necessarily in the dept of time; it is not captured by its promises or ensnared by its grasp, but gives the past as a lining to itself, allowing what has passed to become itself revealed in its intensification of the present.

## 8.3 Language and Time

There has been a prevailing belief throughout the latter part of the twentieth century that we can apprehend the fundamental nature of reality by inspecting the structure of the language we use to describe it. This implies that we can argue *from* the nature of language *to* the foundation of reality, and this is no different when it comes to explaining time. Language contains within its structure distinctions between past, present, and future; some argue that language accurately reflects reality whereas others point out that tensed language simply reveals facts about our representational faculties.

To see these assumptions at work, we need to look no further than the abstract "hieroglyphs" of mathematics and physics, which serve as good examples of how theories about reality can be couched in terms which sit uneasily with our common-sense habits of comprehension. How we represent and articulate our ideas about the world through language reflects something important about our cultural contexts, perceptions, and perspectives of a reality that we seek to convey. Different languages have different means of locating events within their structure, and to this extent, all languages are culturally "tensed".

Are we thinking differently when we talk differently about time? A series of papers published in the 1930s by Benjamin Whorf and Edward Sapir made spectacular claims about how the structure of language shapes the way we perceive, understand, and think about the world. In the intervening years, there have been impassioned debates amongst psychologists, anthropologists, and linguists about the confusion created by conflating two distinct questions about the relationship between language and thought, namely, do we think in language? and does language shape thinking? Objections against the former have become misrepresented as arguments against the latter (Casasanto, 2008).

A *deterministic* interpretation of the Sapir-Whorf perspective has it that the language we speak locks us into a worldview such that we cannot see the world as speakers of other languages do. A *relativistic* stance on the other hand sees it that because languages differ in their grammatical structures, so the worldviews encoded by one language need not necessarily carry over into the worldviews encoded by other languages. This matters since different languages employ different spatial metaphors to represent time, meaning speakers talk differently about time in their native languages.

The idea that people think in the medium of language – in which case language is equated with thought – is inconsistent with empirical studies: a great deal of thinking happens without human language. Non-humans can use tools, navigate, reason, communicate, build shelters, cooperate, deceive one another, and create complex social hierarchies. The cognitive sciences too have established that concepts are not determined by language; concepts are prior to language. Studies with pre-verbal human infants have shown that they possess the concept of numbers and can reason with statistical patterns. Aural isolates lacking any form of language display a plethora of abstract forms of thinking, and others argue that neither vocabulary nor syntax determines or indeed hinders thought.

Spatial metaphors seem irresistible when we speak about time. English speakers talk of going a *long* way for a *short* break; I drive my car *back* but move my meeting *forward*. Therapy is a journey which nevertheless happens in the same place each week. Though the tendency to conflate may be universal, the way we index *from* space *to* time varies across languages. When we talk differently about time, we also think and feel differently about time. We do this in ways that are linked not only to the preferred metaphors of our native language but also to cultural attitudes towards past and future. In English, the ego faces a future which is *before* us, and time that has passed is *behind* (Section 8.2). This seems to be consistent with the embodied experience of walking in a certain direction; the route travelled represents the past and the direction into which we are heading is the future.

These space–time mappings are influenced by culture, language, embodiment religion, and individual attention to time. The trend in English is not reflected for speakers of other languages such as the Indigenous peoples of the Andes, where the ego faces the past and so the future lies *behind*. This is not so strange, given that what we can see and know – visually – lies before us (the past), and what is unknown (the future) lies out of view, behind.

The case of Mandarin Chinese represents an interesting combination in that the words *front* (*qián*) and *back* (*hóu*) are used as temporal conceptions of before/past and after/future, respectively. Chinese culture also employs a stationary "ego" in relation to the temporal axis. If time resembled a moving train, then a stationary Chinese speaker facing the past experiences a future rushing from behind, which is the inverse (figure-ground) of the English speaker's experience (Gu et al., 2019).

So not only does language reflect the structure of our temporal representations, but it can also shape those representations. But the fact that language influences thought does not mean we *think* in languagé. Mapping from space to time correlates with our universal physical experiences which are then conditioned by the languages we speak. Language itself has no influence – causal or otherwise – on the nature of non-linguistic entities such as tables, chairs, space, and time. Language does not determine what reality is like. The point here is that there are potentially profound yet unappreciated linguistic figure-ground reversals – ordinarily unappreciated by mono-linguists – that thwarts transcultural understanding.

Research with bilingual and trilingual people goes a long way to support the view that language acts like a temporal lens which distorts and diffracts information as we go about making sense of emotions and reality (Montemayor, 2019: 149). Thus, a tentative interpretation of Whorf's determinism seems about right; it entails that speakers of different languages are not, in principle, denied access to each other's worldviews. The issues raised by Sapir and Whorf are highly relevant to the way in which human relationships are founded. People have linguistically nuanced experiences of the same reality, of a common world. This is a far more optimistic perspective than that offered by Wittgenstein (1963. I: Section 521):

> One human being can be a complete enigma to another … we can fail to understand people and not surely because of not knowing what they are saying … but because we cannot find our feet with them.

The mental representations of things we cannot see, or touch – like time and emotions – may be built out of representations of universal physical experiences of perception and action. To view the bilingual or trilingual speaker as a person who speaks the monolinguist's language but with an odd accent is to misunderstand a life informed by different footings, ethics, virtues, and ideals, which requires patient mutual consideration.

*To conclude*, language shapes thought, but it is not the foundation of thinking. All languages have some way of locating events in time by mapping the speaker's temporal location as an embodied "point-like" observer in an A-series, which flows – either rushing towards or away from the "body". The A-series does some justice to *implicit* time – it is involuntary and embodied, but it does not segment time into future and past. *To get things done and to synchronise with others in the modern world, we actively invert figure and ground – lived time and observed time.*

This means using language from the B-series perspective too. Time as a resource – the piece time of the assembly line comes to mind – needs to be managed and organised. This is so we may synchronise – but importantly for therapists, desynchronise – narratives and events in *explicit* time, to shape and structure non-linguistic reality, retrospectively living forward. Yet the modern era over privileges time as something to control. This leaves us disconnected from lived time, which is why we need the ardent connection offered by Maurice Merleau-Ponty's concept of relational entwinement: being both an object of experience and also that through which we experience objects. How else are we to connect with the rhythms of reality?

## 8.4 Intersubjective Time

Storytelling is more than a cognitive instrument for imposing order on an otherwise meaningless series of isolated episodes in our lives. It is an ontological category which constitutes human existence – we cannot do without the idea of our lives as narrative. When an intentional act seems baffling, it is because it has lost its place – become desynchronised – in a broader intelligible narrative which describes our relationship with others.

Passing someone on the street engaged in a boisterous, animated conversation with an invisible interlocutor raises little interest nowadays because their actions are made intelligible by technology. Yet not so long ago, when mobile telecommunication meant queuing by a kiosk with a handful of coins, such self-talk was a sign of losing touch with reality. The unity of human life and the role of narrative speaks of our ability to tell coherent stories about ourselves, which is crucial for ethical self-understanding. In the absence of meaningful temporal continuity or synchronisation with others, life dissolves into uncoupled, atomised, point-like experiences unrelated to the past or future, and thus any sense of responsibility for our actions. To isolate a moment from the flow of time is to denature it. Like eviscerating a vital organ from the being to which it belongs, it is a process which renders the tissue different, and the vitality of the being from which it came no more.

Edmund Husserl had a strong intuitive sense that our past pervades the present, which in turn opens out into our future. How I interpret events depends on memories and happenings from the past which cohabit now. This is why memory can be changed by present moods and situations. The radical relationalist has an intuitive sense of the presentness of the future because actions in the present are oriented towards the future in terms of our dreams, expectations, anticipations, and goals of a future yet to unfurl.

Hope, often identified as a critical feature of the therapeutic encounter and something valued by therapists, is the expectation of a future which exists in order to affect our actions in the present by drawing on memories of the past (Bartholomew et al. 2019). Temporal intersubjectivity or relationality allows for the past to be a meaningful influence in the present without the present being a mere effect of the past. It does not assume that the dimensions of time are separate from each other. As Heidegger put it: "The unity of time's three dimensions consists in the interplay of each toward each" (Slife & Fisher, 2000).

The "present" of the B-series is not the durationless instant of the A-series "now". The present is always coming-from and going-to somewhere in Heidegger's view (1926/1962). This *becoming* and *going-to* does not require objective dimensions of time – past and future – independent of one another. The intersubjective now encompasses all three dimensions of our relationships, memories of others, traditions, and culture, as well as future-oriented anticipations and expectations.

Understanding life as a narrative requires *knowing* in the present what has happened *before* in the past, while anticipating what is *about* to happen in the future. Similarly, any moment of time requires a commingling between the past and co-occurring future. In this sense, the synchrony of past, present, and future is not counterintuitive; it is deeply intuitive, culturally enmeshed, and furthermore experiential.

The maxim "the past is gone, the future is unknown, and so we only have today" conveys something of the radical freedom of Sartre. Yet Sartre saw reality as lacking an organising narrative structure. There was no rationale, no overall plan, no intrinsic meaning to events. The view that narratives are the retrospective order we impose on disconnected units of meaningless existence independent of the humans who impose meaning, presupposes a chaotic universe that presents itself for inspection.

Hermeneutics rejects the idea of life as unmediated point-like atomised experiences. When existence is seen as a process of interpretation, of a constant commingling of the past, present, and future, it is impossible to envisage a raw, undistorted level of immediate experience that has not traversed the lens of self-interpretation and the horizons of past and future. Our existence cannot be separated from the stories we tell of ourselves, but as we shall see, our existence means more than stories because we are forever having new experiences which challenge and renew our interpretations of what is an ethical life.

When making sense of how we exist in the course of time, Strawson draws a useful distinction between narrative forms which reflect McTaggart's analysis of time (Strawson, 2004). A _psychological_ narrative is the banal, straightforward way we have of describing, sequencing, and ordering things in our lives from birth to death. Indeed, this "tombstone" telling of life as a series of events lacking any structure seems too banal to dignify with the term narrative. It correlates with the dimensionless now of the A-series where we do not figure to any interesting degree in the past or future – our existence lacks narrative and indeed the absence of a framework renders the task of acknowledging, engaging with, or even bracketing the paradoxical and inconsistent aspects of our lives redundant. Why be troubled by the fact that nothing adds up when nobody – least of all me – figures in the calculus?

When we eschew an overarching narrative structure to index our actions and values, paradoxes fade into the background. For Strawson, living in the episodic A-series is, as it was for Sartre, the only true expression of freedom. It represents individualisation, the Humanists picture of the atomised self, bracketed from future and past, ethically quarantined from the things we have done in the past, and the things we may do in the future.

_Ethical_ narrative, on the other hand, is the task undertaken when we want to conceive of our life as synchronised with others, inherently good, something essential to the task of living well. Ethical narratives situate a person in a wider temporal context which reflects the diachronous B-series: the self is pictured as being present in _both_ the future _and_ the past. Time exists _tenselessly_ not simultaneously with other times. Time as a succession of temporal moments does not entail that the future is fixed, in the sense that it cannot be affected by our actions. The reality of the future does not mean that what happens is causally determined. Things could turn out the way we anticipate precisely because of our chosen actions.

From the fact that there are truths about the future, it does not follow that future events are inevitable. If we see the future as something that exists _now_, just like each frame of this summer's blockbuster movie, it need not infer that my response to those events must be fixed _now_. To think that the reality of a future event determines my present choice is to get the cause and effect the wrong way round. It is choices made in the lived *now* that influences the way future events turn out the way they do (Slife & Fisher, 2000).

The aliveness and possibility inherent in relational temporality do not equate to traditional free will in the sense we are independent of the past; there remains latitude for change even though the present can never be divorced from the past. Though entanglement with the past is not traditional determinism, there is always some historic grounding to any change. Unlike the humanist who advocates naïve free will, we can never be independent of our history and traditions. History and tradition are the font of possibility and change. Possibilities, choices, options, and opportunities must always be understood in the context of our past and future. Far from being determinant of our behaviour, history and tradition are a rich source of options and opportunities (Gadamer, 1993).

The radical relationalist contends that the unifying bridge of causality is unnecessary, as past, and future cannot be understood without the other. This diachrony does not imply that the present is the leading edge of the past, however. Unlike the A-series where the past is considered static and immutable, an experiential understanding of the B-series sees the past as alive and dynamic. Research showing the fragility and changeableness of memory in response to present circumstances and mood only supports this perspective.

Although traditional psychotherapy typically concerns our personal pasts, the impersonal or "objective" past must also be interpreted by human beings, so it is inevitable that it too is subject to the same vagaries. Modernist thinkers argue that the past itself does not change, only the <u>meaning</u> we make of the past changes. This distinction is, again, a result of the modernist's separation of time dimensions by privileging the present moment. Meaning is in the <u>present</u>, whereas past events are viewed as in the past. Relationalists, however, do not separate meaning and memory, present and past. Recollection without meaning, and a meaning without recollection is experientially irrelevant, if not ontologically impossible.

<u>Relational Time in Practice</u>. Thinking and theorising about time speaks to something already understood in the practice of psychotherapy, its attitudes to the living present, and the approach taken to the histories of our clients and their communities. Our existence cannot be anything unless it is seen in its entirety; an attitude embodied in the view that relational depth transcends any method with which a therapist might identify. Dave Mearns sees the fundamental unit of therapy – the punctuating 50-minute session – as something which *narrows* the therapeutic context to suite the practitioner (Mearns & Cooper, 2017:162). When services are sculpted to the needs of our clients, for example when we offer therapy in the home space, then the context of a person becomes more visible (Costello, 2007). A seemingly mild-mannered client who – inexplicably it appeared – could not forge amicable

relationships with their children leapt explosively from their chair and hurled expletive-laden abuse at the postal worker crossing their lawn.

A person and their environment are not separate, isolated entities. Rather, a person is embedded in a surrounding field which affords their relationship with the environment. By extension, no single function of a person can be considered separate from the relations and interactions of their whole being. It is in the realm of sleep that this becomes most readily apparent. By falling asleep, I productively retire from myself in the world, and in so doing, come to understand my timeless simultaneity with it. My sleeping self is an undifferentiated unity; a self which cannot distinguish between what is me and what is not me, what is my mind, and what is my body. This is why dreams are so vivid because I am no longer able to differentiate between what is me, and what is not me. And when I emerge from sleep, I come back to setting myself apart from the world again – I return to a self which differentiates between me and not me (Nancy, 2009).

An important focus of Gestalt therapy is describing – not necessarily explaining – the processes that occur at the boundary of where the self and world emerge. Here, the self is not seen as a fixed point-like being, but a regulating process at the boundary of contact. As if to emphasise the risks of assuming homogeneity within a given therapeutic modality, Fritz Perls infamously claimed that there is no other reality than the present. Of course, Perls worked on past and future issues with his clients, but he insisted on a break with traditional psychoanalytical processes in that therapy ought not limit itself to "talking about" the past or future. Therapy for Perls was a process of engaging with the *present* for change and growth to take place in the future and the past. Laura Perls, wife of Fritz, student of Martin Buber and an influential psychologist in her own right, sought to set the record straight about Gestalt's commitment to intersubjective time (Sabar, 2013: 23):

> [The] emphasis on the *Here and Now* does not imply, as is often assumed, that past and future are unimportant or non-existent for Gestalt therapy. On the contrary, the past is ever present in our total life experience, our memories, nostalgia, or resentments, and particularly in our habits and hang-ups, in all the unfinished business. The future is present in our preparations and beginnings, in expectation and hope, or dread and despair.

Gestalt psychology presumes that we cannot encounter the world objectively. Rather, the phenomena we perceive are not the sum of sensations but an interpretation of a meaningful and organised whole. Even if we knew nothing of rods and cones and other details of our retinal structure, when my gaze falls on an object of interest it becomes the figure against a now blurred ground. Because we think of time and space in similar ways, our experience of a phenomenon which comes to the fore renders its context opaque.

Merleau-Ponty understood this dance between implicit and explicit time, my experiencing self and my observing self who strives to re-integrate experience into an intelligible whole (1962: 408):

> I understand the world because there are for me things near and far, foregrounds and horizons, and because in this way it forms a picture and acquires significance before me, and this finally is because I am situated in it [the world] and it [the world] understands me.

*Synchronising with Others.* It is common to feel as if we dance between first- and third-person experiences of time. *Implicit* time describes a living present when I am absorbed by an activity, such as listening to my client: time seems to fly because time is not the object of my experience. *Explicit* time on the other hand, is when I feel detached from my projects and temporal properties become the object of my experience. I fall out of involvement with my client as they speak, and I glance at the clock. For this brief moment, there is a transition from one relational state of affairs to another. It is a transition in temporal direction from being absorbed in the intersubjective flow of time with you and falling out of contact. Perception of time loses its onward momentum as I emerge from this shared temporal flow.

Attachment theory is predicated on the belief that children have a sense of moving towards an inviting future when they feel synchronised with caring adults who present the world as a promising place to be. More generally, when I synchronise with the world of others, I experience an explicit awareness, an intersubjective "now" through our simultaneous or joint attention to some task or activity. Intersubjective time is this relational arrangement characterised by synchronisation and inevitable desynchronisation. While implicit time and our sense of flow is fundamentally correlated with synchrony, explicit time comes about through desynchronisation. To build back to coherent structures, we must be active in our relationships and our engagement with our environment. We must be curious about when our involvement drifts, our attention wanes, or when our mind goes blank.

The ebb and flow of such brief transitions belong to everyday experience, but a state of profound desynchronisation is thought commonplace in complex and heterogeneous experiences such as "depression" – Matthew Ratcliffe reminds us that we need not be preoccupied with classifying experiences to engage with them. Decoupling from a sense of temporal flow – or the living present – in the experience of depression means an absence of certain sorts of possibility: the anticipated future and, in extreme cases, any imaginable hopeful future or recollected past. The conviction that one cannot recover is similarly bound up with what the future offers, which includes the experiences of hopelessness and diminished agency (Ratcliffe, 2015: Chapter 7).

A common sensation associated with depression is *remanence*, which means feeling "left behind" in our social relationships. Our inability to grieve is similarly linked to a desynchronisation of our lived experience with expectations about how we *ought* to adjust to life's sometimes unavoidable losses (i.e., a significant bereavement, becoming a parent, divorce, children leaving home, retirement, or moving house). When it seems too frightening to abandon familiar patterns because we fear being overwhelmed by loss, it can feel safer to remain frozen in the past. Such grief is complex and physically raw and has nothing whatsoever to do with thinking sad thoughts or with mourning. It is the blurring of past and future which contributes to the experience of time as somehow static. The future looks like more of the past, and the future therefore cannot offer the possibility of significant change (Ratcliffe, 2015: 194):

When you are depressed, the past and future are absorbed entirely by the present moment, as in the world of a three-year-old. You cannot remember a time when you felt better, at least not clearly; and you certainly cannot imagine a time when you will feel better.

As we can often find when we talk of the past, disputes about the reality of events as experienced by those who were there can be unproductive, descending into the downward cycle of accusations, denials and ultimately disengagement. Several parties to the same historical event may, for manifold reasons, admit different perceptions, figures, interpretations, and experiences of that event.

If an event did not occur in the way that a client claims, or recalls, then how does a therapist who sees the present as the leading edge of the past help someone with what could be an imagined, or at least a different perception of the past? To think in this way means that a person's feelings and relationships may have no factual or causal legitimacy – they are simply *wrong*. The client would presumably have no right to their feelings, and their actions would have no meaning in relation to their past. How do we know what we know about situations, life histories, challenges, and strengths?

A happily married – yet restless – couple who migrated for work decided that having raised their three daughters, it was time to return to their country of birth and re-integrate with their extended family, culture, and community. The youngest daughter returned with her parents to what was for her a foreign land. The middle child was given the choice to return with her parents but chose to remain and run the family business, and the eldest left for college. Twenty years later, the three siblings found that the same family event had been experienced quite differently. The youngest and eldest children saw the unfolding of the family as a difficult yet rewarding transformation. They had forged successful careers and created happy, stable families.

Yet the middle child never really got over their sense of feeling abandoned; she had become stuck in the past and felt emotionally and physically desynchronised from her family and those around her. She blamed the others for the pain she experienced in feeling left behind, for not "seeing the world", finding the right partner, or creating a family. How realistic was it for the "abandoned" child to simply let go of the meaning they had attached to a past event experienced differently by her siblings? For the "abandoned" child, their direction of attention, or figure against the ground of the dispersing family unit was desynchronising and became the foundation of her existence. The only relationships she could tolerate were with those who she could control. In therapy, it made sense for her to forgive and forget the past, but this meant that she must somehow deny what was "figure"; that is, her lived experience of being abandoned.

The past is integral to the present and cannot be avoided. But how do we acknowledge the futility of contesting what will be the figure and what will be the ground? The things we have chosen to be our figures, our tastes, relationships, and attitudes require we reject other possibilities, other figures. Indeed, what we choose to see as prominent in our lives depends on our projects, our ontological choices or as Sartre put it, our *projet fondamental* (Nilsen, 2008).

Remaining frozen in the past means we are unable to process our difficult emotions. The active synthesis of past and future in explicit time – which affords a self who has experienced loss – does not occur. Without closure, which is an idea central to Gestalt therapy, the pain of loss from the past continues to intrude on the present. Our attunement to others becomes frozen, and the ability to connect, empathise and be affected by others leads to a painful sense of lifelessness relative to those around us (Fuchs, 2013). Desynchronisation from the social world, loss of a meaningful future, and the absence of "temporal flow" are what binds the person who no longer feels they belong to the world.

In focussing on what Gestalt therapy refers to as "the present moment", we can acknowledge that our perceptions and feelings about a phenomenon which foregrounds need not be determined by past events. The difficulty is that as therapists, we rarely, if ever, have direct access to the past through the confusing hurly-burly of a life recounted. If speech is not the translation of our thoughts, but rather the accomplishment of them, then what is often taken to be the objective past may be the client's rendition of a desynchronised history; it being established that people can remember traumatic events that did not happen, such as being sexually abused in a previous life, or being abducted by aliens (Bookbinder & Brainerd, 2016).

Further from the objective truth of an event is the therapist's speculations based on reasoning backward from what a client says. Even if the past is somehow known with certainty, the deterministic foundation of modern therapeutic methods presume that the client is unable to be free from their past; freedom from the past, autonomy and any hope of change that can be generated by the client, become mere illusions.

Of interest to the relational therapist are interruptions in the temporal synthesis of what has *just-passed* (retention) and what is *to-come* (protention), which can mean disturbing thoughts or physical movements that can intrude into the crevices of our intentional arc (Section 8.1). Such "intruders" appear to consciousness as a *surprise*. Not in the ordinary sense, but in a way that consciousness appears to *startle* even itself. I no longer have an eye on the temporal horizon but am distracted by what just turned-up on the doorstep of my consciousness, so to speak. Fuchs proposes that such profound desynchronisation may be regarded as the essence of schizophrenic auditory hallucinations, and the feeling of physical disconnection from my own body, and time itself (2007).

It is the intrusive thoughts which break into the fragmented intentional arc which undermine any sense of agency; the voices no longer belong to me but appear against my intention. It seems to explain what helps those experiencing the distressing process of interrupted or disrupted Gestalts. Compensatory behaviours which minimise change, create order, and avoid overstimulation – including social withdrawal – can slow down or even freeze the apparent passage of time. Hoarding, counting, handwashing, self-stimulation (stimming) and social isolation are behaviours which help us sustain our narratives and prevent the world from fragmenting. Yet particularly in the case of the latter, it is the separation from others which entrenches desynchronisation. Separation is what impedes our attempts to re-build sentences from single words.

There are ways of addressing our expectations of the future in the present which can liberate us from wrangling over events from an elusive past. We free ourselves from being ensnared by the past in the present, if we focus on the past like a lining to the present, where each presently lived moment will become situated, thereby "deepening" the lining once it too has passed. That is to say, there is no retrievable truth to be articulated since time does not allow us to "step outside" of its unfolding. The work of interpretation is thus not one of extracting meaning from the past, but rather allowing for the fullness of sense to come forth in the encounter with the Other.

We need not search for explanations that presume that the past – through its deterministic mechanisms – is the only way to understand the present and the future. It is possible to legitimise the stories of others, asking ourselves as therapists: "what do we overlook or disregard when listening to your story", without the need to establish the elusive, true account of an event – as in the case of the Pastor who needs mortals to fail (Section 7.3). After all, understanding is not an understanding better, but an understanding differently. The final chapter takes forward Merleau-Ponty's concept of enmeshment, focussing more forcefully on being involved with Others in the therapeutic encounter.

## References

Bartholomew, T.T. et al. (2019). The Meaning of Therapists' Hope for Their Clients: A Phenomenological Study. *Journal of Counseling Psychology*. 66(4), 496–507.

Casasanto, D. (2008). Who's Afraid of the Big Bad Whorf? Crosslinguistic Differences in Temporal Language and Thought. *Language Learning*. 58, 63–79.

Costello, J. (2007). Nightmare or Needed Strategy? *Therapy Today*. 18(1), 32–34.

Fuchs, T. (2007). The Temporal Structure of Intentionality and Its Disturbance in Schizophrenia. *Psychopathology*. 40(4), 229–235.

Fuchs, T. (2013). Temporality and Psychopathology. *Phenomenology and the Cognitive Sciences*. 12(1), 75–104.

Gadamer, H.-G. (2013). *Truth and Method*. Trans. and Revised J. Weinsheimer & D.G. Marshall. Bloomsbury.

Gu, Y. et al. (2019). Which is in Front of Chinese People, Past or Future? The Effect of Language and Culture on Temporal Gestures and Spatial Conceptions of Time. *Cognitive Science*. 43(12), e12804.

Heidegger, M. (1962). *Being and Time*. Trans. J. Macquarrie & E. Robinson. Harper Collins. (Original work published 1926.)

Husserl, E. (1991). *On the Phenomenology of the Consciousness of Internal Time (1893–1917)*. Trans. J.B. Brough. Kluwer Academic.

Mearns, D. & Cooper, M. (2017). *Working at Relational Depth in Counselling and Psychotherapy*. Sage Publications.

Merleau-Ponty, M. (1962). *The Phenomenology of Perception*. Trans. C. Smith. Routledge & Kegan Paul Ltd. (Original work published 1945.)

Merleau-Ponty, M. (1968). *The Visible and the Invisible: Followed by Working Notes*. Trans. Lingis, A. Northwestern University Press.

Montemayor, C. (2019). Early and Late Time Perception: On the Narrow Scope of the Whorfian Hypothesis. *Review of Philosophy and Psychology*. 10(1), 133–154.

Nancy, J-L. (2009). *The Fall of Sleep*. Trans. C. Mandell. Fordham University Press.

Nilsen, H. (2008). Gestalt and Totality. The Case of Merleau-Ponty and Gestalt Psychology. *Nordicum-Mediterraneum*. 3(2), 1–17.

Ratcliffe, M. (2015). *Experiences of Depression: A Study in Phenomenology*. Oxford University Press.

Sabar, S. (2013). What's a Gestalt? *Gestalt Review*. 17(1), 6–34.

Saint Augustine (397, 2021). *Confessions*. Harper Collins.

Slife, B.D. & Fisher, A.M. (2000). Modern and Postmodern Approaches to the Free Will/Determinism Dilemma in Psychotherapy. *The Journal of Humanistic Psychology*. 40(1), 80–107.

Strawson, G. (2004). Against Narrativity. *Ratio (Oxford)*. 17(4), 428–452.

Wittgenstein, L. (1963). *Philosophical Investigations*. Trans. Anscombe, G.E.M.. Blackwell.

# 9
# BEING *WITH* OTHERS

## 9.1  Introduction: Vital Beings

Classical Humanism is portrayed as something of a beleaguered philosophical perspective. We are more than wet machines controlled by genetic programmes. Consciousness is not attributable to neuronal processing of input to output in a way that can be simulated by artificial systems. The related and widespread attitude of constructivism, which argues that perception is an illusory assemblage of subjective realities, undermines our primordial trust in a shared relational world. Humans are not dualistically separated entities of mind and body but beings of flesh and blood, embodied and simultaneously aware of themselves.

I argue here for an alternative to this naturalistic-reductive Humanism, which recognises that we are embodied vital beings. It is a position that requires no abstract indwelling spirit or disembodied consciousness. I am present in my body. In fact, I *am* my body. I feel, perceive, act, and express myself with my whole body in a manner which is coextensive with it. In acknowledging this, I become liberated from the inaccessible inner space of conscious life, from where only words can escape like signals indistinguishable from the algorithms of artificial intelligence. You are real to me, and I am real to you *because* we are embodied.

There is no communication or empathy *between* brains, even if scientists – and therapists – like to believe this. Intersubjectivity is co-created through intra-corporeality. I come to understand you not through a "theory of mind", but intuitively through your bodily expressions, gestures, and behaviour. I also come to understand that theory – while a useful abstraction is wholly dependent on my embodied being in the world. When transferred online,

DOI: 10.4324/9781003396161-9

ordinarily intimate encounters such as psychotherapy become a meeting with someone who is nowhere because they have lost their physical presence.

The cognitive and "figuring-out" aspects of disembodied communication come to dominate because what it lacks is inter-affectivity. Feedback from embodied contact – emotional cues, expressive gestures, the crossing or uncrossing of legs, flexing of the hands, and changes in posture – are missing. Illusions insert themselves between seeing and what is seen, saying and what is said, communicating and what is communicated, feelings and their expression.

The term phenomenology is commonplace in the field of human behaviour. But its meaning when used in disciplines allied to therapy has drifted from its original sense and come to mean something as banal as appreciating first-person experiences. Yet, Merleau-Ponty expressed sympathy for the reader "pressed for time" who considered giving up on a phenomenology – a philosophy of everything – which struggled to define itself (1962: vii).

It seems obvious why phenomenology is misunderstood in therapeutic circles; it has become equated with a method that reflects on aggregate first-person descriptions of experience. Phenomenology has become oversimplified, meandering from its origins in the analysis of the structures of conscious life and the intersubjective achievements of objectivity. In becoming associated with first-person subjective experience, it is regarded by hard-shell empiricists as an unreliable "science". Once phenomenology becomes synonymous with subjectivity, it is confined to a meaning, which its pioneers sought to escape. The extent of this simplification is that therapists see little value in studying the philosophy of phenomenology.

Untangling the influence of phenomenology on therapy is not easy because its founders – often seeking a new home following the horrors of European wars – sought to emulate a North American pragmatism unconcerned by Old World habits. In his first book *Ego, Hunger and Aggression*, Fritz Perls – who disliked theorising – declared an antipathy towards questions of philosophy. In his autobiography, Perls states he had little knowledge of Gestalt psychology, emphasising instead a greater intuitive interest in phenomenality (i.e., figure-ground), unfinished situations, and body-awareness (Sabar, 2013).

Phenomenology constitutes an attitude to experience as the source of all knowing and the basis of our actions, like "an underground stream enriching the ground" (Moran, 2000:18). For Maurice Merleau-Ponty, and those who call themselves phenomenologists, the world of reason and abstract generalisation are but secondary expressions of the spectacle and plane of experience.

Trying to understand the world of the other is not sufficient in and of itself to warrant the label phenomenological. In this context, the term throws a wide – and arguably undisciplined – net over subjective experiences. *Phenomenality* is a better term to describe what we get up to when we amass examples of awareness, be it therapeutic, contemplative, meditative, or mystical (Stone &

Zahavi, 2021). The radical claim of Husserlian phenomenology was to uncover how our concern with objectivity – the simultaneous back and forth between participant/spectator, braided/braider – comes about in the first place. How we encounter the world really does matter.

To properly recognise the philosophical nature of phenomenology, more is required than simply describing what I feel "here and now". It demands going beyond amassing descriptions which neglect deeper questions about meaning. Phenomenology is at heart a philosophical endeavour concerned with the theoretical implications of the mind–world correlation. There is much to be learnt from hovering between self as observer, and self as sensual experiencer adrift among the storm-tossed trees. Can I deepen my awareness of a client, while simultaneously being an internal supervisor? How far can I go in achieving pure awareness? How can I use this in understanding compassion, projections, empathy and intersubjectivity? What can I understand about the experience of depression, anxiety, trauma, menopause, dementia, and healing beyond words? If this practice can be learnt, then can it be taught?

As to what perception is, Merleau-Ponty had little to say; it is neither this, nor that, nor something else. The *Phenomenology of Perception* is a four-hundred-page assault on the notion of perception as conceived by modern philosophy; it simply does not exist: "perception independent of background is inconceivable" (1962: 281). Merleau-Ponty denies the notion of perception as the way an individual, aware only of their inner sensations, somehow manages to represent to themselves an "external" world. We do not have such *perceptions* but exist in the flow of experiences which imply and explain each other.

Rejecting modernist visions of reproductive, mirroring processes whereby what is "outside" is duplicated "inside", Merleau-Ponty and others make a broader, richer case for language as a linguistic expression not reducible to words inserting themselves into silence. My body speaks and my words are on the way to expression. Living speech thus not only requires but embodies its performance. In other words, perception is a process of semiotic or symbolic relationality where the perceiver and the perceived are, or become, what *is* in terms of the other. His radical enterprise amounts to questioning what modern philosophy had hitherto termed the "mind", because for Merleau-Ponty, there is no such thing as the *mind*.

For Martin Heidegger, the world of objects was predicated on a much more primordial layer of pre-reflective existential engagement with and understanding of the world, seeing the purpose of phenomenology as twofold. Existence is our entwinement with the world, or better, our existence is constitutively worldly. Here he saw German as the most apt language for philosophising (along with Greek … at a push), as it offered access to terms such as *Dasein*. It commingles *both* the entity that is the human being, *and* the act of being human which understands our own humanity and what it means when we say something *is*. Phenomenology then is not about investigating either the subject or the object, the mind, or the world, but their fused interrelation as a whole *gestalt*.

The world of *Dasein* is not one where we are on our own, but one in which we share the world with others as part of our constitution. This being-with-others – *Mitsein* as Heidegger termed it – acknowledges that we are always in relation and the world is a shared world. My being a person is not simply my own achievement but the result of my communicative entwinement with others.

Even our aloneness or capacity for solitude must be understood in relation to the existence of others, without which it would not be possible. In the breathless delirium of our final moments, uncoupled from protension and those physically in attendance, we continue to reach out and seek to touch those retained in embodied memory. Though I was unrecognised while standing by my father's bedside, it gave me comfort to believe that it may have been my head, as a young boy, that he seemed to reach for and caress.

The long-established influence of Augustinian thought on phenomenology, and its attention to human restlessness, sees religious belief, intimacy, friendship, love, faith, and hope as legitimate concerns, and not just supernatural illusions. Phenomenology then requires more than describing things such as time, motion, colour, or indeed any property dependent on the human observer as it appears to consciousness. As argued earlier, the world is encountered perspectivally, within a temporal flow. So, irrespective of how paradoxical, the human perspective has to be assumed whenever we consider experience. This innovative way of interpreting the world sees our relationship with the world as less about what I take from it and more about understanding my experience as primordially relational, and therefore ethically *mitsein* in the world.

As one would hope with a branch of knowledge dealing with interpretation (hermeneutics), the story of phenomenology is one of re-telling and re-interpretation, even if its method is one of descriptive analysis aiming to become a grounding science of appearances. We might see the story beginning with Franz Brentano's lectures on descriptive psychology, which were attended by both Edmund Husserl and Sigmund Freud.

Brentano emphasised the rationalist continental tradition of internality, which begins by theorising what goes on inside (i.e., the soul, psyche, cogito, mind, consciousness), before attempting to work our way out into the external realm of the material or real world. Husserl's thinking influenced Martin Heidegger, Hannah Arendt, Hans-Georg Gadamer, and Emanuel Levinas. The latter took phenomenology to France from where it continued to influence generations of philosophers: Simone de Beauvoir, Jean-Paul Sartre, and Maurice Merleau-Ponty, and then Jean-Francois Lyotard and Jacques Derrida.

Phenomenology then is not some add-on perspective; it is a fundamental modification of attitude and attention critical to the practice of good therapeutic practice. It is about accessing a position, witnessing the grand act of creation, and meaning-making where thoughts are clarified, emotions understood, memories reconsidered, time and memory become shifted, and lives reimagined.

## 9.2   The Verity of Intuition

Husserl rejected the naturalistic view that all phenomena are ultimately encompassed and explicable using the laws of nature. The science of psychology, with concepts modelled on the mechanical laws of physics, creates the absurdity of denying the consciousness which gave rise to the naturalistic picture in the first place. All rationality depends on conscious acts which cannot be properly understood from the natural perspective of ordinary appearances. The distance from something gives one a perspective on that from which one takes distance. Since consciousness is something presupposed in all scientific endeavours, the only appropriate approach to the study of consciousness itself must be transcendental. By which I mean adopting an attitude which brings the world into view from a position distinct from the world being viewed.

Husserl then took the radical path of exploring experience in its purest form, unsullied by the distortions of assumption and prejudice. His paradigm was to see perceptually embodied experiences as something dependable and available to inspection and description. The experience of anger, for example, is something distorted through introspection, linguistic processing, and assumptions about an event; the purity of the phenomena evaporates, its contents modified by reflection and time. Yet the buzzing in my chest, and the sensation of the trigger is something steady and repeatable, a source of insight not just about the world – like a factual discovery – but as a way to reveal meaning of a phenomenological kind.

Husserl made the ambitious claim that phenomenology was the means to uncover the foundational essences of human consciousness, the invariable structures, or the necessary qualities that cannot be doubted or called into question but rather brought into view or made manifest. Because, when we know ourselves, we can overcome our concerns about bridging the gap between the internal world of my experience and the external world of my environment. In this regard, Husserl's task was to adopt a different starting point, taking a step back to apprehend the pre-givenness of nature as the basis of knowledge itself, returning to the "things in themselves" as always and already given to intentional consciousness.

For Husserl, it was not inherently preposterous to trust intuitive knowledge drawn from my internal world. I can rely on the subjective experience of feeling bored say, without having to provide evidence that the object of my attention is in essence *boring*. This idea has taken an interesting turn in contemporary life as it suggests that I need not challenge, inspect, or be suspicious of my intuitions. Indeed, should you challenge my subjective experience of being bored by saying something like: "only boring people feel bored", then we enter the realm of gaslighting. Yet the sensation of "feeling bored" constitutes meaningful subjective information: "there is not a human word, not a gesture, even one which is the outcome of habit or absent-mindedness, which has not some meaning" (Merleau-Ponty, 1962: xviii).

Such mundane lapses are familiar to the therapist, yet they signal vital experience. When I presume that I withdraw and fall silent because I am tired, or feel bored by my client, or utter a lazy platitude: "I'm sorry to hear that", or "how does that make you feel?", then something is going on. Disengaging, falling out of contact, falling back on ready-made formulas are not accidents, for they express a lack of interest, presence, or involvement, and hence a definite position in relation to the situation or the client.

There are no pure accidents in existence or indeed co-existence; both integrate chance events and transform them into the rational and the meaningful. The term "lived experience", for example, has come to communicate something problematical beyond a report of my "experience" of a thing; the term seeks to extend the power of my claim to experience as foundational, utterly certain, and what is more, *infallible*. Perception in this context does more than presume to be true; it becomes defined as access to truth.

Merleau-Ponty points to the flaw with such idealistic principles. The real has to be described, achieved and re-achieved, not constructed, or formed. In basing my framework of the world on such infallible thoughts, we prove ourselves unfaithful to our experience of the world; instead of looking for what the world is, we should be looking for what makes the experience of the world even possible.

> The self-evidence of perception is not adequate thought or apodeictic self-evidence. The world is not what I think, but what I live through ... Perception is not a science ... not even an act; it is the background from which all acts stand out and is presupposed by them.
>
> *(1962: xvi–xvii)*

A mathematician by training, Husserl – like many scientists and I include myself here – rejected classical structuralism, which prioritises impersonal systems of relations that downplay the centrality of rational subjectivity. He was knowingly committed to the profound purpose of his project, which was no less than arriving at the universal common ground of human experience. For Husserl, phenomenology seemed to be an extension of his mathematical pursuit of tautology, or the expression of relationships in more intelligible ways. The ubiquitous "=" sign even finds its way into

Husserl's writing as a means for re-*presenting* experience in a different way (Husserl, 1991: 45).

The concern then was to transform the universal obviousness of the being of the world, as the correlate of the being of consciousness, into something I can understand and find meaning in. I do this by penetrating the curtain of the ordinary and taken-for-granted world of appearances, known as the *natural attitude*, to widen my access to things as they are in themselves and yet given to me. The process of *reduction* was Husserl's attempt to achieve a clearer, deeper, and unbiased perception of phenomena and their emergence of meaning.

The reduction is often talked about as a series of steps: epoché, eidetic, and transcendental. Like the rationalist Descartes before him, Husserl felt that before we can know others and the world, we must make known to ourselves how we see and understand the world, as well as how we are affected and in turn constituted by the givenness of the world.

Husserl was not so different from his contemporary Freud, who also believed that what lies within is not an undifferentiated pack of wild beasts, but something we can approach with rational subjectivity. But for Husserl, the disembodied third-person perspective is the domain of contemporary experimental psychologists. Phenomenology is interested in the general structures of consciousness. How it is directed to the world and not *what* it is, starting from my consciousness and then achieving an understanding of consciousness per se, and not just in a third-person empirical objective sense.

Recovering the Socratic Ideal – Husserl's Reduction. Husserl first used the term *reduction* to describe a radical self-reflective process for withholding, disregarding, or bracketing the natural world and the business of interpretation in pursuit of phenomena in their essential form. It seems to me that Husserl sought to retrieve the Socratic ideal of returning to things in themselves through: "being wiser to a small extent … in that I do not think that I know what I do not know" (*Apology:21d*, 2003).

While calling for a systematic theory of phenomenological reduction, in practice, Husserl was relaxed – for good reason I believe – about its organising principles and how such a transcendent view from "nowhere and nowhen" could be achieved. Nevertheless, his three-tiered process sought to deliver us from prejudice and prior understanding, to afford a level of detachment that would allow us – in principle – to encounter the world as it appears to consciousness. In his mind, the epoché and reduction mark a radical methodical shift towards a more complex phenomenological attitude that forbids the practitioner from asking questions which rest on taken-for-granted assumptions about the world at hand.

Questions about being or not-being, about valuable or not valuable, useful, beautiful, or good and bad are put out of play or made no use of. The world does not disappear and its validities continue to obtain, yet it becomes for the phenomenological practitioner, in quite a peculiar sense, a *phenomenon*, allied to the achievement of consciousness.

The practice of reduction was the means through which we could "bracket", or as the Greek *sceptics* saw it, achieve a state of suspended judgement – *epoché* – towards the ordinary psycho-mundane way of understanding the world. Bracketing is a term Husserl borrows from mathematics to describe a function which "suspends" an operation until later, rather than ignore or dismiss it. Bracketing does not support unregulated or unexamined assertions, nor the rejection of science or what is real. But it does recognise that subjectivity is inextricably involved in the process of constituting objectivity and vice versa. Indeed, Husserl held that objectivity was the greatest achievement of our subjective experience of the world.

Through a process of evaporating what seems superfluous or naïve, reduction returns consciousness to its essential subjectivity by stepping back from – without invalidating – cultural, familial, and educational preconceptions (Subjects) which go to make up the natural attitude. It is an attempt to allow all that appears to perception, including what is meant or thought, to be seen in the way in which it seeks to reveal itself. Nothing must be assumed or taken for granted external to the experiences themselves. The phenomenologist must begin their study, therefore in absolute poverty, with an absolute lack of knowledge, free of *interpellation* as Althusser might say (Section 6.2).

You will recall how Gadamer argued that if we seek *Truth*, then we cannot have *Method* (2013). What I have been exploring throughout is what do our therapeutic methods reveal about the truth of our encounters, and whether such truths are of service to our clients? The epoché gestures to such a method, but this idea must be held lightly. Awareness can only ever be relative. There can be no experience that we can – with confidence – consider to be wholly in our awareness; that would require an unimaginable wholeness and perfection beyond what it means to be human – something understood in Husserl's transcendental reduction.

Rather than be absorbed in the intentions of our therapeutic *methods*, a radically relational attitude has it that we step back and become more aware of the structures shaping our intentions when theorising. I have argued throughout for a "wariness" towards the paradoxical stories, signs, metaphors, virtues, ethics, moral sources, and transcendent symbols from which we draw to create this practice of "healing souls". I have sought to "bridle" what I can and question the psycho-mundane: as far as possible, I seek to overcome the more obvious Subjects of my world.

Yet I do so for the sake of the world and the suspension is conducted with the world in mind. But can we come to know the overarching communal spirit of this many-headed subjectivity and intersubjectivity which shapes our dreams, intentions, and theories? Though psychology thinks of itself as a science, its ground is one inherited from traditions, passed down over generations which regulates, orients, and organises our experiences and actions and guides us in how we ought to act and behave as practitioners.

Radical relationality is not a method, theory, or psychoeducational "tool" to add to the toolbox. It is a process of stepping back from the natural attitude, and realising, as did Husserl, that we do not encounter an individual in therapy, but the temporal nexus of histories, including my own. What are the realistic limitations of what we can bracket as therapists? Bracketing is an open-ended striving for more wholeness in the knowledge that each and every attempt is going to fall short. It signals a perpetual beginning that conceives and re-conceives the reduction in continually deeper terms. We can think of the epoché as adopting a critical stance towards scientific theories, knowledge, explanations, personal views, and experiences. The taken-for-granted perspectives which must be interrogated and brought into awareness – paradoxically – before we can discover them.

Husserl's reduction becomes increasingly radical beyond the *epoché*. The *eidetic* reduction takes place as consciousness penetrates the essence of a phenomenon. It is difficult to describe, as such essences are usually beyond the capacity of descriptive language to capture, grasp, and contain. Unfortunately for Husserl, the project to establish a linguistically constituted *eidetic* reduction began before Wittgenstein's philosophy of language. When we understand language to be constitutive, how can we speak of a universal or essential consciousness? How do I establish that my intuitions about my conscious states can be shared – in a universalising way – with you?

Language gets in the way if we see it as a derivative phenomenon, something reduced to verbalised expression. There can be no irreducible symbols to mediate between my experiences and your experiences, and as Wittgenstein reminds us, there are limits to what can be said – talking to others about our internal states comes perilously close to talking to ourselves. Thinking becomes trapped not inside the human mind, but within language.

The Husserlian project sought to manage pre-understandings by bracketing them. In contrast, Heidegger, Merleau-Ponty, and Gadamer understood that meanings can never be fixed or described once and for all. They are forever emergent, contextual, and historical, which means that the therapist can never escape their givenness to presuppositions, prejudices, and foregrounding. The preface to Merleau-Ponty's *Phenomenology of Perception* is a tempering critique of the ambitions of transcendental phenomenology. It is clear to Merleau-Ponty that the most important thing we can learn from Husserl is that a complete reduction is impossible (1962: xiv). Since our reflections are performed in the temporal flux of a world we are attempting to seize, there can be no thought which embraces all our thoughts.

As Gadamer reminds us: "the fundamental prejudice of the Enlightenment is the prejudice against prejudice itself" (Gadamer, 2013: 282–283). The therapist who seeks to understand themselves and their client must be prepared to be told something. This is where Wittgenstein's notion of the Language Game helps. The psychotherapist, like the chemist, biologist, or physicist, similarly seeks to obtain what is essential about their subject of attention, while differentiating or bracketing those matters which seem accidental to the enterprise – such as the passing of the seasons (Section 1.3). It is unnecessary to aspire to the transcendental aspirations of Husserl because holding our empirical and speculative theories lightly is all that is required (Zahavi, 2021).

We finally encounter the *transcendental* reduction, which can be thought of as an escape from empirical subjectivity, its suspension, into the radical realm of transcendental intersubjectivity: dismantling the binary categories of object and subject, outside and inside. If words struggle to capture the *eidetic* reduction, then prose becomes even less useful in the almost ineffable transcendental realm. This is not to say that efforts to convey this experience – through poetry for example – should be abandoned (Taylor, 2024).

Husserl's transcendental reduction, and the practices of yoga and Buddhism are often compared, which is not surprising as they are seen to have similar effects on the practitioner. Interest in mindfulness represents the latest move to repurpose ideas and practices derived from Eastern contemplative traditions for Western therapeutic purposes. Mindfulness is often understood as invoking a sort of non-judgemental, present-centred awareness, which orients the practitioner in a more direct relation to what appears to their experience. The therapeutic benefits of being released from entrenched, psychologically unhelpful feelings and behaviours are obvious. However, Buddhist scholars and philosophers complain that too often Buddhism gets reduced to mindfulness, and mindfulness to the non-judgemental observation of present-moment experience (Hanna et al., 2017; Stone & Zahavi, 2021).

Philosophers agree that while there is an exciting future for a phenomenology *of* mindfulness – or other forms of meditation – they are adamant that phenomenology is not a sort of meditative practice or technique. One of Husserl's decisive contributions was to highlight the extent to which experience involves relational time – all three temporal modes of the present, past, and future. The most ordinary perceptions involve the commingling of not-now, now, and not-yet-now: a retaining of what has just happened, an openness to what is currently happening, and an anticipation of what is about to occur. *How do we reconcile this with the claim that mindfulness is exclusively concerned with the present moment, and what presents itself as flatly here and now?*

*In conclusion*, the fact that phenomenology is relevant to so many non-philosophical activities and continues to be a powerful source of inspiration for counselling and psychotherapy is a testament to its value. However, the approaches which afford the most innovative and influential outcomes are not those adhering to a liturgical exegesis of Husserl's reduction. *They are those which prize the unprejudiced description of, and a fidelity to, experience as lived through and made sense of.*

## 9.3   Experience as Field

Kurt Lewin, having been influenced by the Berlin School of Gestalt Psychology, developed the idiom of the *life space,* a metaphorical force field (i.e., mimicking the physical fields of gravity or magnetism) for rendering intelligible the psychological relatedness of our wider social and psychological milieu. The ephemeral nature of the field becomes for practitioners of both psychoanalytic and Gestalt traditions alike, the means for overcoming the realist or naturalist ontology of positivism and the metaphysics of substance. A psychology based on field theory became for Lewin the *Method* for conceiving what seems unrepresentable about the underlying dynamic properties of the psyche, and a turn towards what is involuntary, pre-reflexive, and passive about consciousness. However, Lewin differed from the Gestalt psychologists in that he conceived of the psychic field as granting – albeit passively – its own existence, rather than being something co-created by mental states or indeed any physical substrates (Bazzi, 2022).

Wilfred Bion extended the physical metaphor of the *field* to the dynamics of therapeutic groups in the thrall of shared dreamlike phantasies. By merely bringing two or more minds together – as Bion saw it – a field is created in which waking dreams and reveries take place in the mind of the analyst who becomes the *magical filter* through which patient experience is transformed into narrative form for the analyst to interpret. In what has become known as Bion–Field Theory, the mystical and the meteorological combine, and as Bion puts it (Mazzacane, 2022):

> I imagine that between me and the patient a cloud begins to form, almost little by little in the way that, on a summer's day, clouds are sometimes seen forming above a hot spot.

For some, *Gestalt* is a near-synonym for the field and is considered relational insofar that there is a connection between all parts of the continual dynamic. When I look on the face of a friend for example, the complex arrangement of "experience data" – such as eyes, nose, skin colour, hair, lips – do not *possess* Gestalt; their face *is* Gestalt. It explains the jolt I experience when I encounter your face in an unfamiliar context. It is within the meaningful whole of their face that the parts receive their value and meaning.

Gestalt psychology saw itself as a protest movement against the atomising assumptions of positivism. On the matter of perception, positivism holds that a point-for-point correspondence exists between stimulation and sensation. For example, a single photon stimulates a single retinal cone, which corresponds to a single sensation. The prevailing positivist paradigm excludes meaning from explanations of behaviour, which build on *Gestalten* or forms, as the building blocks of how the world is perceived.

Gestalt psychologists argued that if perception follows such a "mosaic" model, then how do we have contrast, the illusion of time flowing as in McTaggart's A-series, geometrical illusions (rabbit-duck), or the perception of motion? Indeed, all perceptual phenomena which lead to insight often involve seeing relations between events as things embedded within other things.

Merleau-Ponty found value in Gestalt psychology's efforts to overturn positivist perspectives of behaviour which embraced the value-laden world of meaning and therefore the symbolic value of phenomena. By adopting the *Gestalt* attitude of reflection, he acknowledged the originality of phenomena in relation to the objective world *out there*, since it is through phenomena that the world becomes known to us. The science of the laboratory becomes more like a collaboration between people, instruments, and the objects they work with (i.e., particles, molecules, or microbes), rather than the revelation of some hidden reality.

The idea that inanimate tools imply no less than the animate subjects who use them corresponds with the agential realism of Barad encountered earlier. Yet Merleau-Ponty went further than the Gestaltists in his opposition to the atomising sensations, claiming that positivists misunderstood not only physical forms, but the domain of physics itself. Because causality presumes unidirectional relations between isolated events, there cannot be laws of causation since there are no such isolated physical events. To think in any other way requires two significant positivistic errors (Sheredos, 2017).

The first is to presume that an experiment could verify a single law. It must be seen that the law is already embedded in a network of complementary laws which are at stake in any experiment. A system of laws is itself a form in which each law – as a part – has no independent standing, just as no object can exist by itself but must be encountered by a perceiving consciousness. A *body* of scientific knowledge can only have empirical significance as a Gestalt.

The second is to treat objects in a law's scope as independently existing, stable entities, rather than dependent parts of transiently stable whole. Only a family of laws held in unison can confront the discontinuous flow of physical forms which arise and dissolve in the flow of entropy. There is always some idealising and approximating involved in applying laws because they presume that we apprehend "moments" as a totality, as if they were isolable temporal atoms in McTaggart's A-Series.

This line of argument led Merleau-Ponty to cleave from Gestalt and by implication psychoanalysis, with its physicalist notions of *resonance* and other force field claims about how perception and behaviour are related (Casement, 2014: 82–84). While Gestaltists in particular are critical of the role of positivism in psychology, they fail to perform a genuine phenomenological reduction to see how Gestalt is rooted in physics itself. This blind spot is perhaps unsurprising, given the context of its founders in Berlin during the early twentieth century: Kurt Koffka and Wolfgang Köhler were both physicists, and Max Wertheimer had a long-standing interest in Einstein's theories of relativity. In the language of physics, forces such as magnetism, gravity, pressure, and friction (as manifest in the meteorologically relevant Coriolis effect, and Bion's clouds) are *field* concepts used to explain and even predict, to a degree, the weather.

Both Gestaltists and psychoanalysts are beguiled by the analogy between the chaotic motion of atoms in a physical field, and how an active consciousness – for which the body is the instrument – engages with the world and strives to achieve the best grip on its environment. If this thinking is correct, it would be possible to understand perception and action in terms of explicable laws governing fields, with disturbances or movements in those field "causing" corresponding changes in behaviour.

The implication of field theories which encompass physical reductionism is that the natural laws of perception authorise a psychological account of human behaviour which is both perfectly qualitative, yet brazenly quantitative. Be it Caesar crossing the Rubicon, or the behaviour of an atom, both are guided through the void by a set of forces which orient the object at an optimum position with respect to the background field.

Perception and behaviour in this view thus become explained through physical forms; what we perceive as a meaningful figure in our environment of forms becomes a function of how our environment and nervous system interact in a physical sense. Merleau-Ponty points out the circularity of this thinking, and its fatal grounding in the ontology of physics: the building blocks of Gestalt psychology are thus unwittingly borrowed from an object of perception. It is a fundamental error – Merleau-Ponty concludes – *to believe that the constitution of a "thing" within human perception is necessarily a characteristic of the universe more generally.*

Embodied Relational Ontology. Maurice Merleau-Ponty cleaved from the Roman Catholic Church in his late twenties; early exposure to scholastic theology and a dubious "Christian Socialism" would seem to account for his rejection of organised religion as a whole. Though by no means a Christian, his long formation in the Catholic imagination nevertheless shaped his logic of *incarnation* – a supposed union of opposites (Edgar, 2016). Merleau-Ponty sought to reconfigure our understanding of consciousness as a relationship of bodies with their environment – a process through which we react and interact along with other beings in a field that is not reducible to the sum of its parts. The field is instituted or established *through* the openness of a body – in the flesh as it were – to its environment.

His iconic ontology of "flesh" – a term of art (French – *chair*) deployed to express the meeting point of all things visible and invisible – represents a communion of opposites in the way the body relates to other bodies through their immediate contact (1968: 136–149). Merleau-Ponty's recommendation is that we see nature in terms of flesh rather than as a fixed system of ahistorical physical laws. Perception thus becomes the basis of knowledge, and the body the vehicle for being in the world: "I am conscious of the world through the medium of my body" (1962: 82).

The defining character of flesh is its reflexivity and reversibility, the intertwining of intelligible and sensible such that one cannot easily distinguish subjects and objects, inside and outside; the connection between them isolates each as a separate body and yet holds them together in one world. A typical example of this reflexivity is when one hand touches the other. Neither hand is both purely active and touching or passive and touched. The concept of flesh is an attempt to establish an ontology of mobility between bodies which are dynamically constitutive. So, when I talk of being "in the flesh" I refer both to my body as the medium through which I live my life, and the relations that organise my life.

I provide a phenomenological account of flesh as I live in relation to other things, and an ontological account of flesh in terms of the relations that constitute my body as a medium. Conceiving the body as the "vehicle" of meaning emphasises space, time, and movement as radically relational processes. Reconceiving the human relationship to nature as Merleau-Ponty does opens the way to an entirely different conception of ethics; one that circles less around principles of moral obligation and one that is instead concerned with our dwelling within the world.

Flesh also has an ecological appeal; it radically decentres humanity. It conceives perception not as a human act but as something with transpersonal and indeed transhuman dimensions. To attribute interiority to other beings with whom I share flesh does not require the attribution of consciousness or even sentience to non-humans: what is important is the ontological continuity between all beings, since each being *is* its field. Since all living bodies share a common nature, human ontological continuity with nature is preserved. Given our ecological crisis, rather than proceed into the future informed by a nostalgia for a world without humans, an embodied relational ontology gestures towards a world where humanity becomes a "better citizen" within its worldly community. The earth does not belong to us; we belong to the earth.

The specific ways of being in the world are also preserved as different bodies are open to different dimensions of their environment and therefore capable of different behaviours, some of which seem intelligible, and others which seem not. If I go on and say that "my body is made of the same flesh as the world", I mean to say that my body participates in the same kinds of natural relations as those that happen between all other things within my field: my world, in turn, is the product of these relations. The flesh of the world, then, is the radical Gestalt formed by the contact between beings in the field.

Nature becomes the largest field of flesh that constitutes my own lived spatial-temporal context where I exist and in which I actively participate, where *becoming* replaces *being*, because I adopt an attitude of openness to the process of interacting with other fields. Perception is just one form of relation which requires neither intelligibility nor reduction of all beings to their appearance to human observers. Horses, cats, and dogs engage in their own process of spatialising and temporalising relations with the world of flesh irrespective of what humans have in mind for their fellow beings, whether it is sitting on a horse, eating a cow, stroking a cat, or walking a dog.

The fullest expression of Merleau-Ponty's ontology of flesh understands the perceiver not as abstract consciousness, but as a subject-body; engaged, interested, and indeed hungry insofar that those sorts of things perceived – foregrounded – are also the sort of things desired. The perceiver mediates desire and flesh, self and world, things and thought, and is both shaper and shaped by the world. The Enlightenment privileged the eye above all other sensing organs. The ontology of flesh requires a more apt metaphor than that of "scientific" *vision* because the significance of our seeing is not something we superimpose on the world – it arises from our involvement in the world. It is our radical involvement in the world of Others that we turn to next.

## 9.4 Empathy, Sympathy, and Intersubjectivity

Enactment and Mimicry. Philosophers consider emotional contagion – enactment – to be the most rudimentary form of empathy (Darwall, 1998). It refers to the feelings or emotional states we seem to "catch" from others, not by imaginative projection, but more directly. Yawns, coughs, smiles, and frowns are examples of the embodied expressivity we borrow from others. Joining a group of people full of laughter and frivolous conversation, for example, conveys quite a different feeling to one where the mood of the crowd is marked by frowns, averted eye contact, and other embodied expressions of tension. I "take on" these impressions, but not because I project myself into the standpoint of one who smiles and imagines what it would be like to see the world from their perspective.

Being in the company of the anxious initiates anxiety even for those who are unaware of anxiety in others. What marks out emotional contagion as primitive is that it does not involve seeing myself from your standpoint. It does not even require an awareness of the other as a distinct self. The sympathetic care of which I spoke earlier has done no work as yet.

Relational approaches to psychotherapy are often defined by their attention to such "weird" dynamics (Casement, 2014: x). Psychotherapists have long recognised that borrowed emotions can be informative to the person who experiences them. They are a source of insight into oneself and what may be going on for others in a diffuse and non-specific manner. When we pick up fear, anxiety, anger, or happiness, there is usually some awareness and understanding of how the emotion was obtained. We may realise immediately, or perhaps later through the filter of reflection, that we have borrowed strong emotions from others.

What matters here is that such insights can be useful for helping us understand what belongs to whom. It is the hope that therapists hold for their clients – that they may become better acquainted with the ebb and swirl of emotional contagion and develop confidence in navigating their affective world.

There are times when I am unaware of having interpreted an encounter as harmful or threatening. Such moments are accompanied by taking on difficult emotions, either because those around me are defensive, or relationships are fragile and ambiguous. Here, my lack of awareness of borrowed emotions is viscerally felt, a flutter in my "guts", or a yawn – arguably a release of tension. More dramatically, my experience of such a phenomenon is accompanied by an elevated awareness of my heart beating, blushing, or breathlessness.

Emotional contagion is relatively passive, unintentional, and pre-verbal. It seems to work through automatic mimicry where we synchronise facial expressions, vocalisations, postures, and movements so that we converge emotionally. Many of us are oblivious to the importance of mimicry/synchrony in our social encounters. The trigger can emerge from one individual and be perceived and interpreted by others, to yield corresponding or complementary embodied experiences (i.e., facial, vocal, postural expression) and gross emotional behavioural responses in others.

Our borrowed emotions are distinguishable from first-person experiences – they are a pale imitation of the real thing, which are more intense and belong elsewhere. Some of the emotions we catch can evoke the same feelings, while others trigger complementary or even contrary feelings. An angry face can trigger fear and confusion as well as anger itself, bringing anger to the encounter on some occasions. Our own self-referential concerns can overlap with the emotions we catch. For example, a therapist who starts to drift and think about lunch can – after monitoring the sensation – become curious instead about being physically present yet emotionally absent.

There will be those in whose presence we feel calm, secure, and reflective, indicating the therapeutic advantages of taking on other people's emotions. Inviting mimicry can be socially useful, such as when I want to distract a child from pestering their sibling, or when rushing to hospital in an ambulance with a loved one and remaining outwardly calm though feeling the opposite within. We habitually seek to dominate interpersonal encounters, and this is often the crux of psychotherapy with its attention to embodied micro skills: conveying sympathetic care by leaning in, smiling at the right moment, and nodding our heads periodically.

Projective Empathy and Simulation. It is the gap between me and you, which is both necessary and productive when it comes to empathic relationality. Empathy as a perceptual experience becomes a higher-order relational act when it is "other-related". Given the insistence on a difference between my empathic understanding of your experiencing, and having that experience myself, it comes as no surprise that phenomenologists reject the suggestion that projective empathy offers a unique sort of insight, or anything particularly profound or deep about my understanding of you.

Projective empathy differs from emotional contagion in that we imaginatively place ourselves in the situation of the other and suppose what we ourselves would feel or do in their situation. Attention is focused, not on the other, but on the *situation* as we imagine they would see it, or as we think they ought to see it. Again, the work of sympathetic care has yet to be done as it is the *Other*, and the relevance of their situation *for them* that has yet to come into focus.

We are still responding to the Other's situation *as if* from their standpoint, rather than from their actual perspective of their situation. Empathy of this sort – which simulates being you – is centrally involved in attributing mental states to others. Here, someone doing the projecting works out what you would do, or think, or want, or feel *as if* "I was you". The thinking involved is not explicitly first personal and self-conscious: "If I were they, I would feel terribly disappointed, so they probably feel that too". Instead, we unreflectively project ourselves into the other's standpoint, responding imaginatively from their perspective, and attributing the result to them.

Projective empathy leads to well-intentioned collisions with others. For example, as I cycle along the path I see before me, in the middle of the lane, a pedestrian. They are unaware of my existence because they face away from me. As I approach, I ring my bell to bring myself to their attention. Looking over their shoulder, the pedestrian communicates their intention to move to one side. The confusing dance of parallel projections and second-guessing begins; they pull left then right in an attempt to anticipate me. I too, change my speed and swerve from right to left, then back again. We painfully collide – with best intentions.

In emotionally charged environments, projective empathy tires us out and burns us up. The imagined distress thus causes some level of physical distress in projective empathisers. It is understood that feeling responsible for "rescuing" others for example, is an expression of our sense of propriety towards the feelings of others, whether we think it warranted or not. In his autobiography, Arthur Miller explained how he fell in love with Marilyn Monroe, in part because she was so trusting, vulnerable, and needy. Yet it was her fear to which he responded, thinking he could rescue her because, after all, that is what he would want for himself, in her situation (Hatfield et al., 1994: 195).

This is the stuff of Stephen Karpman's *rescuer–persecutor–victim* drama triangle. When we are unable to "enter into" the sense of vulnerability a person's feels in a given situation, we adjudge their response to be somehow inappropriate, improper, or unwarranted. If I cannot see features of your situation as providing justification for how you feel, then I cannot share in them. Alternatively, if I can share your feelings – because through my own first-person experience of your situation, I can vicariously feel for you, on my account, then I affirm those feelings. This moves closer towards empathic sympathy, and the compassion of the winner's triangle: I care, rather than rescue (Costello, 2020: 81–84).

It is important to recognise that projective empathy is not just about cloning the feelings or thought processes of others as we imagine them. Rather, we place ourselves in the other's situation, and work out what to feel, as though we are they. When we projectively mirror the feelings of another, we not only *show* them how they feel, but we also show them that we condone *how* they should feel. We inadvertently validate those responses which we approve and consider appropriate or disapprove of those feelings we consider unwarranted in the context.

The therapist who views their client as "depressed like I was" typifies the client rather than communicates genuine care, because it is inferred that we fall under the same type of "depression": your experience is my experience, and we therefore have and know the same kinds of experience. Therapeutic emotional sharing must encompass the idea that you participate with me in the experience of that which we hold in joint attention. The otherness necessary for caring is undermined when we assume a fusion of two abstracted selves. What is central to empathy is recognising and collaborating with the phenomenological differences between you and me and our respective identities in difference. You are not alone, insofar that there is one common world in which we all share; *this is the steadying anchor for all this empathy talk.*

While it may seem inglorious to have tried to understand your experience but concede defeat: "I really cannot imagine what it must be like for you", at least I have acknowledged that there is a difference between us, one that I cannot comprehend. The greater failure of care is to communicate my infallibility, my inability to see or recognise the difference between us. The possibility of entering into *your* experience, imagining what it may be like for *you* to see the world as *you* do, is not even entertained. As therapists, we may shy away from the uglier emotions of our clients, because in fact it is the projected emotions of the therapist that are being avoided as we steer clients to more positive emotional states. Problematically, projective empathy is central to the formation of normative communities: like-minded groups who can agree on what is acceptable to feel and when it is acceptable to feel it. This is again therapy as sedation, a place to be calmed, relaxed, and subdued – to be comfortably numb (Section 1.4).

Proto-Sympathetic Empathy. Projective empathy offers a unique sort of insight, but it does not amount to anything particularly profound or deep about my understanding of you. I need not have a depression-like experience myself to empathise with your experience. What is central to proto-sympathetic empathy – which is necessary but not yet sufficient for care and compassion for the other – is recognising and collaborating with the phenomenological differences between you and me, our respective identities in difference.

When we genuinely care it is the other and the relevance of their situation for them that we really focus on. Proto-sympathetic empathy brings this into view. It is the difference between imagining what a client would feel like if their partner left them (projective empathy); yet it goes further and imagines what it would be like for *you* – the client – to feel that way. The latter requires simulation, not simply a person *with* those feelings, but a person conscious of their feelings, along with the phenomenological textures, and relevance for *their* life. It is on the way to genuine sympathetic empathy, as it brings the other's relationship to *their* situation into view in a way that allows *me* – the therapist – to engage care and compassion on *your* behalf.

Empathic distress – that which comes about through projection – has the self (therapist) as an object and can give rise to efforts to comfort or relieve oneself. Proto-sympathetic distress, on the other hand, has another's distress as the object of attention. When you make the effort to imagine what *my* grief is like for *me* – the client – you focus on *me*. This means that the distress you feel vicariously by projective identification may find a new target, namely my distress, which potentially gives rise to authentic sympathy.

This distress might be supported by its association with the therapist's own similar experiences, say the recollection of your own grief at losing someone. So while proto-sympathetic empathy can give rise to sympathy, it is not necessarily so. If you felt resentful towards me for some reason (i.e., there is envy or some prior sense of feeling wronged), then you may take delight in a vivid appreciation of my pain, by imagining how awful it must be like for me. In such cases, sympathy is corrupted and empathy goes astray in some wider concern involving ill will – such as revenge or a vendetta.

Authentic sympathy – acceptance or unconditional positive regard as Rogers called it – is characterised by a non-possessive, other-directed caring attitude towards a person's good and involves concern for *them*, and thus for their well-being, for their sake alone. To the degree that the therapist can provide this climate of care, Rogers was undoubtedly correct in proposing that "significant learning is likely to take place" (Rogers, 1967: 284).

The Second-Person Perspective – Intersubjectivity. We are by now familiar with distinctions between first- and third-person perspectives – with the latter being seen as the achievement of the former. They differentiate how we situate our attention, either through subjective or "objective" experiencing, respectively. While we all perceive the world diversely, the world is not *my world*, one given to me alone – *solus ipse*. It is a world made real through intersubjective relating and collective achievement. You and I are far more than points of self-referential activity and interest, but sources of meaning to which I must respond, outside first- or third-person lived experience.

The second-person perspective – the feeling of togetherness – is an apt term for joint attention, which is more than two people simultaneously focussing on the same thing. In a way, that is different from having some experience on my own; it requires attending jointly to the same object, which in turn becomes mutually manifest. I am not referring to two or more people triangulating their attention on some external object, but something which has developmental precursors. It requires more than experiencing the wonder – alongside my wife – of her simultaneous breastfeeding of our twin daughters. It goes beyond moments when one of these infants fixes their gaze on the spectacle of her sibling feeding.

The second-person perspective in this context involves a proto-conversational social exchange, through the rhythmic turn-taking of the mutual gaze between mother–daughter, sister–sister, and back again to mother–daughter dyads. Sensations of hunger, satisfaction, and comfort take place throughout such reciprocal interactions, providing the foundation of a social world not from the perspective of "you" as seen dispassionately from "over here", but "you" with whom I join in a collaborative activity with shared goals and attention.

What is required then is to elaborate this second-person perspective, the subject–subject (me–you) relation, where I hold you in mind while simultaneously am aware of myself as being held in mind by you. The subjective me–you relation encompasses the dance between similar–different and connectedness–differentiation.

To illustrate the relevance of the second-person perspective in psychotherapy, I differentiate between belonging in an observing sense and belonging from within "we". Through the accident of birth, I am thrown into groups (gender, family, socio-economic class, nationality, ethnicity, etc.) irrespective of whether I am committed to, or even aware of them. Though there is often the surreptitious influence of interpellation, such group membership does not necessarily amount to a "we" as a distinct way of being with and relating to non-group members.

In both one-to-one and group processes, the notion of a working alliance is crucial to the psychotherapeutic process. To become a part of a "we" in this sense my relationship with you, the therapist, or you the group, must transcend something I observe from without to become something experienced from within. By understanding – in the context of attachment theory – how the strength of the pack is the wolf, and the strength of the wolf is the pack, we need not abandon the first-person point of view but exchange its singular form to its plural one.

To belong to the "we" of the group, prospective members must identify with the group. It is the attitude of lone "wolves" towards each other – and towards themselves – that is important. It is not to say that interpellation happens voluntarily, but that in important ways, individuals must bypass some degree of self-understanding and first-person perspective to belong to the group. I become aware of myself as a wolf as "one of us" – of the pack. It is when our pre-reflective experience of interlocking individual consciousness with others occurs to the extent that our perspectives are co-produced through mutual involvement, that we come into being-with-one-another on the shared project of therapy.

In an exploration of the second-person perspective, Niall Keane begins with something both obvious yet fundamental: the other whom I encounter is similar to me, but also distinct (2022). My experience of you begins from the experience of myself as a centre of interest, orientation, and activity. I then perceive you as I would perceive myself *as if* I were to go over to where you are and be where you are. You "over there" seeming similar to me does not mean that you live as I do, but rather that you are subjectively *analogous* to me, a term of art claimed by Husserl to mean that this subjective *you* can see the world "like me" but from "over there".

When I encounter this subjective you, what I experience is the lived body of someone else, and not just an indication of someone else as if I could mistake you for a mannequin. While lounging on a bench just inside the door of a local shop, I witnessed the "shock" of apprehension by a stranger walking past me who had taken my form to be inanimate – a mannequin. In realising that I was *not* the inert figure I had been taken to be – I was in fact *alive* – the person "jumped" with the shock of my *being* suddenly materialising and entering her awareness as analogous to her.

Perceiving you as distinctly akin to me, yet over there, means I can consider the possibility of a perception of the world analogous to mine. This alerts me to the objectivity of the world and reassures me that the same world is somehow accessible for others to perceive too; the world becomes objective and transcendent and not merely a figment revealed to me alone.

Reflecting on my experience of solo travelling, with all I needed in a shabby rucksack, it struck me that memories of such times were distinct from those shared with cherished others. The impactful appearance of a partner in a treasured experience does more than furnish a second perspective of say, a moon-lit trip along lake Nicaragua. Their subjective perspective was more than just another perspective; it is another mode of the world's appearance where my world became one of shared horizons in an intersubjective world. The fact that she "over there" is analogous to me meant that she acts on a basis of motivations and intentions I can understand and share.

Furthermore, in our encounter, my time and your time become something shared and yet uniquely experienced. In my encounter with you, I realise that I am no longer the sole source of the *present*: a living present becomes established. Your impact on me indicates nothing other than a present that is both there for me, and for others; you have a unique lived present of your own. This multiplication of lived presents transforms me from self as a "point" into self as existing in a second-personal and horizontal relational plane. The appearance of you as simply me "over there" makes no sense because the existence of other temporal streams prevents me from being simultaneously "here" *and* "there" and thus there can be no fusion of perspectives.

The therapeutic encounter between the client and therapist becomes similarly, the relation between two distinct temporal and historical streams of experience that meet without merging. To the degree to which you are constituted by me, I am constituted by you by the act of relating; what was my "here and now" ceases to be privileged because it commingles with the "here and now" of your experience, touching upon it and being touched by it but without merging into it.

When I enter into relation with you – the client – my time transforms your time and your time transforms my time; you bring about a transformative expansion of who I am. The fact that your living body appears in my temporal stream reminds me that I can never constitute myself perfectly as an analogous version of you. Contrary to what "empaths" might think about themselves, I cannot apprehend your experience as my experience. To argue a kind of first-person acquaintance with your consciousness in the same way that I have with my own, is tantamount to claiming that I am capable of inhabiting your conscious life, or of fusing with it. The fact that my experiential access to your mind is different from my first-person acquaintance with my own is not an imperfection or shortcoming of empathy. It is precisely because of this asymmetric difference that I can claim that the minds I experience are not an extension of my own mind but are other minds.

Now, we must avoid any confusion between access to our own minds and fantasising about access to the minds and emotional world of others. If I claim to have the same access to your consciousness as you, you will cease to be different. You would instead become a part of me, or worse a mere variant of me. To claim that I can only have a real experience of you if I experienced your feelings or thoughts in the same way as you makes little sense; it fails to respect what is distinct and unique about you. It would lead to an abolition of the difference between you and me, and without embodied self-differentiation, there can be no talk of radical relationality since it is only made possible by the gap between me and you.

Although a strong commitment to the essential individuation of experiential life is a necessary requirement for any account of intersubjectivity, the inaccessible parts of me – which come from delays and limitations of my self-reflection – inserts itself into the inaccessibility of you. On this basis emerges – both within and without – a unique *I–Thou* relation in which the idea of *we* can be founded – where every person is determined reciprocally. To *en*counter someone in this sense means to stand "counter" to someone and be moved by you, "over there".

It is in the presence of you, someone over whom I have no control and no fundamental psychological access, that there emerges for me a being that looks me in the face, baffles me, cares for me, misunderstands me, listens, or fails to listen to me, and in so doing causes me to question myself and understand myself differently. This gives rise to a self-altering differentiation within myself, a newly self-understood distinction between your experience of me and the experience of me that I can never have, namely, your experience of me as a reciprocating, ego-altering someone from "over there".

In constituting who I am by drawing me out, you are not only a necessary condition for my experience of a valid world that precedes and exceeds me, but you free me from my internal universe, making me more than myself. It is you who awakens me to my motivations and interests, revealing their meaning as conditions of individuation and self-conscious life.

Radical relationality sees therapy as more than simply understanding; it is also not-understanding, of being on the way to understanding differently. It is not just support and facilitation; it is demand and challenge. In a word, confrontation is an essential part of therapy because it signals what must be bridged. Consequently, the task of the therapist is to be open to the timeless flow of experiencing the self along with the other. Through self-awareness, the therapist becomes conscious of their flow of experiences, which is why personal development and the capacity to bridle the natural attitude is fundamental to therapist practice and development (Schmid & Mearns, 2006).

What do we learn from Husserl's analyses is that *even though our first-person lived experiences are individuated and indexed back to some primal "I", it does not make me who I am*. It is only when I enter into social relations and become vulnerable to my encounter with an altering and enlarging you, that I become rich and increasingly concrete, purged of anonymity and emptiness.

## 9.5   Implications for Practice

The Phenomenon of Therapy. Linda Finlay differentiates between the lone philosopher undergoing the reflective process of reduction and the reflexivity of the therapist adopting a phenomenological attitude (Finlay, 2008: 11, 2011: 75). The therapist must perform a necessarily limited reduction from within the hurly-burly of the encounter. In this context, it is perhaps better to talk not of reduction but a "bridling" of the therapists' pre-understanding, personal beliefs, theories, and other assumptions that might otherwise deflect them from experiencing the client. Otherwise, there is something suspect about a therapeutic attitude whose utility and plausibility depend on the practitioner undergoing some esoteric, stupor-like experience as suggested when "working at relational depth" (Mearns, & Cooper, 2005: 40–41).

The therapist cannot transcend or forget their fore-conceptions but must remain open to the constitutive experience of shared temporalities when we encounter an analogous consciousness "over there". Using reflective practices, such as nurturing the psychoanalytic "internal supervisor", a therapist can hover between disinterested attentiveness and vulnerable engagement with the other (Casement, 2014: Chapter 2). It is a condition which requires a continual, layered, and ephemeral process of reflection and improvised movement between the phenomenon that draws our attention as a figure, and the way it is interpreted.

Winnicott takes us into the world of *potential space* where the therapist learns to remain close enough to what the client is experiencing while preserving sufficient distance for them to function as a therapist. Psychotherapy in this sense resembles a field once again: an activity which takes place in the overlapping realms of a client and therapist's capacity for playfulness.

By *play*, Winnicott means going beyond the boundaries of mere calculative or deductive reasoning and being open to intuitive, embodied and nonrational – as opposed to irrational – subjective processing. If the therapist cannot play, then they are not cut out for the work; if the client cannot play, then something needs to be done to facilitate the process before therapy can begin. The internal supervisor is Casement's term for the capacity of a therapist to slip into the first-person realm of free-floating present-moment flow – to play among the swishing trees of experience – momentarily leaving behind third-person active self-monitoring.

Like art, therapy is understood in interpretation, and so it follows that the therapeutic encounter is becoming – never complete, never finished. There is no definitive interpretation of what we create – especially in therapy – so it remains open to the play of interpretation. It is not a sealed, static item, but a dynamic outcome of a process that integrates the horizon of our past and the future of its creators.

The relationally oriented therapist wants nothing more than to understand your experience, filled as it is with lived meanings, intentions, and feelings, which are an expression of your subjectivity. No matter how distraught and "messed-up" you may feel as a client, you are believed. You are the intentional co-creator of your world, and you are living as best you can in the here and now. You are understood through an exploration of the meanings which are sensually made available to you.

The first major review of people's lived experience of depression tells us that it is accompanied by an existential shift in how we find ourselves in the world (Ratcliffe, 2008; Fusar-Poli et al., 2023). It is a different world, an isolated world, an alien realm that is indifferent to others, painfully cut off from other people. Depression is thus an expression not only of emotions, body, self, or time but changes in the structure of interpersonal experience, which brings with it an overarching feeling of being disconnected from others. People report struggling with communication, loneliness, and estrangement, and perceiving stigma and stereotypes; these features lead to an overall loss of dynamism and openness to life.

An openness to first-person experiences urges the relational therapist not to see depressive disorders as an intra-individual state, localisable within the psyche or the brain. It involves desynchronisation, the failure of embodied attunement to the shared world of emotions. The relational therapist sees depression then as a de-tunement from the present moment, and not the converse, where a person's past is the cause of present difficulties. *The real problems are the present problems, and so it is in the present that the therapist must seek contact – involvement – with the client.*

Addressing relational experiences of the past and expectations of the future can only be understood and changed in the encounter now, in the living present. It is the co-created world of therapist and client in the present that becomes the place for change. It is within the experience of therapy – literally but hopefully not always within four walls of a room – that all of the life of the client can be brought into play. It is in the present that awareness of what sectors of a client's world need be recovered for healthy living come to the fore. If the therapist is to offer the level of integration that the client seeks, then the role of phenomenology in the training of the psychotherapist is critical. I come to this shortly.

A source of frustration for the trainee therapist is that the conclusion of therapy is rarely an arrival at a neat destination but an open dynamic sense of coming into being. Becoming open to relationships and searching for who I am are not two separate problems but an open dialectical process leading to a confident vulnerability in my encounter with you. Successful therapy returns the client to themselves, as co-creators of life, as people with emotional and intersubjective rights, who can be truly present to other people. When therapy succeeds, it is a dialectical, creative, playful, attuned, and responsive process that touches both client and therapist with "wonder and force" (Becker, 1992: 237). *Becoming* then is something never realised. Like love, it is rarely perfect and requires constant practice to realise something that goes beyond the need to possess.

Rogerian Phenomenology. Merleau-Ponty was critical of philosophy's juxtaposition of experience in terms of either a discontinuous static *being* or a more fluid and dynamic *becoming*. The former suggests completion, permanence, unity, and is allied with structuralism and system-building, which seek to master the uncertainties of life. Perception becomes directed towards truth in itself, a thing waiting to be found behind appearances – it is a perspective which downgrades the world we inhabit in favour of a construct.

Whether it is positioned in the person of the client, or a certain dilemma or situation, there is an implied promise that *truth* can be uncovered. The being/ becoming antimony is not remote from traditional psychological therapies, which see themselves groping for *methods* to reveal the *truth* of the matter, the thing which pre-exists for a distressed person. While appearing indeterminate, *truth* – it is believed – *can* be determined with more knowledge, which in this context means more therapy.

*Becoming* finds itself positioned in opposition to being – something incomplete, impermanent, nebulous, and suffused with ambiguity in a world of inexhaustible meaning. It is by definition, indefinable, and stands for change, flux, and the unmotivated upsurge of the world as it presents itself. Becoming requires we discard "being" as an abstraction because there is nothing beneath or beyond the world of phenomena. It is consistent with how Merleau-Ponty saw our hold on the present, as elusive and never entirely comprehensible: "what I understand never quite tallies with my living experience … I am never quite at one with myself" (1962: 346–347).

This has implications for therapeutic practice because what we "bridle" shapes our practice: a priori notions – whether spiritual, scientific, or psychological – are the ground into which we plant our therapeutic *methods*. Though the term was ubiquitous in his writings and deployed interchangeably with *personality* and *self*, "person" was never defined by Rogers, leaving the way open to the play of interpretation. This gestures to the fluidity of the person-centred approach wherein the self is neither discarded nor indulged but gently examined in its ongoing unfolding. What we call "I" becomes a relational instrument – and the therapist the facilitator of healing.

Rogers was clearly inspired by phenomenology although his approach was not consistently phenomenological. The "authentic" enough relationship characteristic of Rogerian phenomenology lies beyond the natural attitude ordinarily encountered by the client. It renders for the therapist all manner of theoretical constructs beyond value in the cultivation of what Rogers called "presence" (1992: 832). It is held in the pragmatic frame of psychological contact, which precedes the therapist communicating their own experience of "bridling" their attitudes towards the client. The therapist endeavours to communicate their experience to the client through a realness or fidelity to the phenomenon of the encounter.

The capacity to observe one's continually unfolding first-person feelings and thoughts, screening them for attribution and thoughtfully disclosing them helps the therapist become more aware of what may be of therapeutic use to the client. Contemporary person-centred theorists seek to articulate this momentary transcendence of the epoché – from the therapist perspective at least – with Mearns emphasising even a commitment to the phenomenological bracketing of any possible "lust" for contact itself (Mearns & Cooper, 2005: 113–135).

The Rogerian approach is grounded in empirical observation and an ongoing fidelity to a phenomenal engagement with the other. As such it is tentative, descriptive, non-dogmatic, and non-prescriptive. Empiricism in this sense does not refer to "things" but "states of things" – neither unities nor totalities but multiplicities. Hence the therapeutic attitude deals with the dynamic process of becoming rather than static notions such as being a "person".

Paradoxically, in *On Becoming a Person*, Rogers sees people as immanent and organismic, attributing to them a fundamental and seemingly self-evident essence, and a "drive toward self-actualisation, or a forward moving directional tendency" (1961: 35). Rogers implies that the essence of a person "dwells" within *being*. For those who believe in a Humanistic immanent universe as opposed to a transcendent relational field of phenomena, the Rogerian encounter with the *natural spirit* of a person contrasts with the transcendent encounter described in the Torah (Exodus 3:1–4). Moses thought it a strange sight that flames could appear within a bush without being consumed. As it turned out, Moses saw the encounter with the bush as something which transcended the bush. The bush itself was purely situational and ephemeral. The Rogerian therapist in their encounter would see something no-less extraordinary: a burning bush with an indwelling spirit – much like the *naturans* power within a person that causes them to thrive and flourish. The practitioner pursuing *relational depth* is similarly committed to the illusion of an essence, of a situated "being", or burning bush with an indwelling *naturans* power.

The radically relational practitioner eschews such notions of an illusory indwelling essence, depth, an unconscious, and so forth. There can be no depth to becoming, only surface, only phenomena, only the world-fully expressive, endowed with intrinsic, pre-cognitive meaning. There is no "inner Man"; we are in the world and only in the world can we know ourselves (Merleau-Ponty, 1962: xi). When we live in a universe of becoming, one without a situated being, we live as an examined ongoing process of transformation, and not as a final product striving – yet never quite being – at one with ourselves.

Trauma, Dementia, and the Self that Observes. The boundary between traditional verbal and body-oriented psychotherapies must be traversed when addressing somatic experiences such as post-traumatic stress disorder. As Babette Rothschild points out, the body that remembers trauma is a body adrift in the temporal flow of experience (2000). Traumatic experiences can inscribe themselves into embodied memory, which later, through some trigger, awakens them often in the form of an intense recurrence in the present, as if the event were happening once again, that is, flashback memories.

The ultimate goal of therapy here is to relegate the effects of trauma from the present experience to its rightful place, which is in the client's past. For that to occur, good therapy must resolve the perceptual Cartesian split between first- and third-person experiencing an event, which subjectively feels real in the present, despite belonging to the past. The client must be secure in the belief that the trauma is over, past, done and survived.

It is an example of how therapy can transcend first recalling then theorising about how the past has caused the present in order to loosen its grip on the future. Indeed, overemphasising the past as a causative factor may prevent the client from imagining and creating alternatives for the future: *the purpose of remembering the past is to re-imagine it*. When we decentre ourselves and shift our focus from what happened to imagine new alternatives, we change the possibilities for our existence.

Synonyms used to describe this splitting of experience are drawn from a range of traditions and include core–witness, Child–Adult, and internal–external reality. Rothschild, however, prefers the unfussy terms, *experiencing* and *observing* selves. The phenomenological response to trauma begins with bringing into awareness aspects of the experiencing and observing self (Merleau-Ponty, 1962:143):

> The blind man's stick has ceased to be an object for him and is no longer perceived for itself; its point has become an area of sensitivity, extending the scope and active radius of touch, and providing a parallel to sight.

Eliding between bracketed pre-understandings while simultaneously exploiting them as a source of therapeutic insight exposes the therapist and client – once again – to the paradoxical experience of involvement with and detachment from experience. In reconciling the split between an observing self that is unable to make sense of the body, Rothschild recommends a range of techniques for dissipating experiences which intrude from the past through a communion of the seen (the *presented* affect) and unseen (the *re-presented* emotion).

The process of communion infers Merleau-Ponty's idea of being in "the flesh", which integrates the biological aspects of affect with the conscious awareness of emotions. Our emotional experiences are inseparably commingled with changes in our body: there is no fear without a pounding heart, no joy without an expansion of the chest, and no shame without blushing, holding my hands to my face, or turning my eyes downward. It is no mistake that I speak of "choking-up" as I reflect on the embodied experience of having a lump in my throat when taken by feelings of sadness.

Without a biological body, there cannot be feelings – which is what distinguishes a human from an AI system. It is vital we recognise how sensations are like a gauge – they inform us when we are tired, hungry, uncomfortable, happy, and so on. Life becomes hazardous when we ignore the sensations and the emotions they communicate. When we become more familiar with our embodied sensations – it is argued – the less frightening and overwhelming these experiences become. And because sensing our bodies is a current time activity, through body awareness we become sensorially anchored in the present. This is because while I can remember a sensation, I can only *feel* a remembered sensation *now*.

What is at stake here is the peculiar human capacity for stepping out of my body and taking a virtual perspective of myself, which is simultaneously the perspective that others may take. It requires the capacity to rise above the here-and-now of current experience to locate myself in an objective spatial and temporal context, much like what happens when reading a map or calendar. It requires abilities such as reflective thinking, taking a view towards myself and the situation I am in and anticipating and deliberating on what I will do next.

With dementia, it is this capacity to step out of my bodily experience and take a virtual view of myself that becomes unmoored. While the unique personal orientation framed by the lived body remains in dementia, it is the vantage point from which we observe ourselves which seems dislocated. It is why those experiencing memory loss implicitly seek stability in safe and familiar surroundings; they offer coherence and dependability against the disruption of spatial and temporal orientation.

So even when dementia cheats me of my explicit memories, I retain my corporeal memory – the familiarity with my environment, my habits, and sensual recollections. So rather than relying on rationality – which brings with it frustration for carers – I may still be regarded as embodied with the capacity for inter-corporeal experiencing despite the progress of the illness. A hand massage, a favourite food, familiar music, sounds, or old habits like rolling a cigarette promises access to inter-corporeal personhood, submerged histories, and sensual experiences. This is something understood by those who have cared for a loved one with dementia: "the fundamental continuity of a person exists in the unified connection of their life, and in the uninterrupted temporality of their body" (Fuchs, 2021: 213).

Implications for Training. Moving away from the fantasy of a unified, solid self has implications for training the radically relational therapist. The terrain of phenomenology – which rejects the possibility of final and totalising theories – points to the irreducibly incomplete and evanescent character of any framework seeking to encapsulate being a "person". A commitment to intersubjectivity is not a theory but a realisation that comes about through phenomenological bridling. Orientation towards the encounter with others is therefore a firmer foundation for training therapists compared to alternative approaches grounded primarily on theories, or at worst, driven by atomised and atomising "topics".

Theoretical constructs invite at best the fallacy of integration to address human particularity, or worse they reify and universalise attitudes about how "best" to understand people. A "topic"-driven approach to training equally undermines any sense of relatedness and continuity; its well-meaning commitment to particularity reduces to a form of positivism. Like Caesars decison to cross the Rubicon, no amount of atomising detail about a person will uncover the necessarily wider context of their actions..

The practice of therapy is after all just that: an *activity* whose pioneers firstly experienced, reflected, abstracted, then actively experimented with their concepts. Gadamer reminds us there can be no neutral standpoint from which to bracket the implicit influences exerted on our orientation towards phenomena. There can be no argument against trainees – or any person doing emotionally complex work – engaging in therapy, reflexive activities, professional mentoring, or supervision.

Training and personal development in the practice of therapy are not so much about imparting explicit knowledge, although trainees in the thrall of neoliberalism sometimes see themselves as "customers" in a wisdom-for-sale transaction. This was something understood by Plato: "when the soul is searching, not for what something is like, but what it is", then wisdom is more properly imparted and acquired rather than taught by instruction.

The point I wish to make is that while it may be possible to describe the necessary and sufficient conditions for the achievement of all kinds of expertise, this is not possible in the search for wisdom. Implicit knowledge requires direct insight illuminated by the spark of dialogue between those compelled by goodwill to search for wisdom. The closest we can come to understanding this "spark" of relationality is phenomenological attunement (Politis, 2020).

Our private monologues, or the inner forum of continuous internal conversation between our sociocultural, embodied interpellated selves is different from the performative external speech of our secondary encounters with the external world. The therapeutic encounter then is primarily one where the intrapersonal domains of the client and the therapist come into contact through this secondary interpersonal exchange. The practise of externalising this symbolic self-talk is an experiential, affective process achieved in training through both classic and radical triad methods, the practice of interpersonal process recall, the encounter group experience, one-to-one and group supervision, and of course personal therapy (Pedersen, 2000; Mearns & Cooper, 2005: 136–157).

Our involvement in the world is what must be understood and to grasp the paradox of the world we must challenge and perhaps even break our familiar acceptance of it. The reduction, for Merleau-Ponty, becomes a process and not an end in itself because we are too tightly held in the world to be able to know it at the moment of our involvement (1962: xv). It is why in the training of psychological therapists much emphasis is rightly placed on group processes which activate hermeneutic reflexivity: a process of continual dialogic and radical reflection on the interpretations of bodily emotional intersubjective intuitions, experience, as well as the phenomenon disclosed to the therapist.

The Balint group for example invites participants to share their experience of an encounter before the group are then asked to engage phenomenologically, that is to focus on their own experience, feelings, behaviours thoughts, and impulses in relation to what is presented. Although bewildering at first, an openness to the Husserlian reduction can offer clues to support the therapist encounter the experience of the client who is not physically present but whose phenomenal presence may be felt and amplified (Leggatt & Marwardel, 2004; Rüth, 2009).

Our embodied expressivity is more complex than language allows and when linguistic constructs do not fit with the experience of being human, then we need alternative approaches which challenge our reliance on what can be uttered. There are reasons, of course, for our continued emphasis on verbal therapies: the intellectual influence of psychoanalysis and cognitive therapies, the ready access to accounts of the past, categorising what we feel and do, and the ambiguity of interpreting nonverbal communication.

Yet the myth remains that body psychotherapy eschews language, seeing it as superfluous, when in fact it is clear that language, in the way words are formed, is entwined with sensations (Westland, 2009). The *how* of the words we utter can be more important than *what* is actually said, because words can deceive, but their mode of expression rarely does.

Our deepest, spiritual connectedness with others is often silent and beyond words. Winnicott was attuned to this, and aware of the importance of silence especially in our earliest relationships, where we learn to have: "… the experience of being alone in the presence of someone" (Winnicott, 1958/ 1984: 36). A well-meaning carer (or therapist) who impinges on the play of an infant (or client), intrudes on the development of silent processing and self-talk by disrupting the evolution of *me* who observes and makes intelligible the *me* of experience.

*To conclude*, without a developed observing *me*, it becomes difficult to decouple from the flow of experience. The therapist attending to embodied experience communicates care without impinging or depriving the client of space for self-talk. You – the client – must trust that you are free from the need to be alertly watching me and my moods to feel cared for; you can simply *be* with your emerging experience.

## References

Bazzi, D. (2022). Approaches to a Contemporary Psychoanalytic Field Theory: from Kurt Lewin, Georges Politzer, and José Bleger to Antonino Ferro and Giuseppe Civitarese. *International Journal of Psychoanalysis*. 103 (1), 46–70.

Becker, C.S. (1992). *Living and Relating – An Introduction to Phenomenology*. Sage.

Casement, P. (2014). *On Learning from the Patient*. 2nd edition. Routledge.

Costello, J. (2020). *Workplace Wellbeing: A Relational Approach*. Routledge.

Darwall, S. (1998). Empathy, Sympathy, Care. *Philosophical Studies*. 89(2/3), 261–282.

Edgar, O. (2016). *Things Seen and Unseen: The Logic of Incarnation in Merleau-Ponty's Metaphysics of Flesh*. Cascade Books.

Finlay, L. (2008). A Dance Between the Reduction and Reflexivity: Explicating the 'Phenomenological Psychological Attitude'. *Journal of Phenomenological Psychology*. 39(1), 1–32.

Finlay, L. (2011). *Phenomenology for Therapists: Researching the Lived World*. Wiley-Blackwell.

Fuchs, T. (2021). *In Defense of the Human Being – Foundational Questions of an Embodied Anthropology*. Oxford University Press.

Fusar-Poli, P. et al. (2023). The Lived Experience of Depression: A Bottom-Up Review Co-Written by Experts by Experience and Academics. *World Psychiatry*. 22(3), 352–365.

Gadamer, H.-G. (2013). *Truth and Method*. (Tr. Revised by J. Weinsheimer & D.G. Marshall), Bloomsbury.

Hanna, F.J, Wilkinson, B.D., & Givens, J. (2017). Recovering the Original Phenomenological Research Method: An Exploration of Husserl, Yoga, Buddhism, and New Frontiers in Humanistic Counseling. *Journal of Humanistic Counseling*. 56(2), 144–162.

Hatfield, E. et al. (1994). *Emotional Contagion*. Cambridge University Press.

Husserl, E. (1991). *On the Phenomenology of the Consciousness of Internal Time* (1893–1917) (J.B. Brough, Trans). Kluwer Academic.

Keane, N. (2022). "Empathy, intersubjectivity, and the world-orienting other", In *Empathy, Intersubjectivity, and the Social World* (Eds. Anna Bortolan & Elisa Magrì), De Gruyter.

Leggatt, C. & Marwardel, S. (2004). First Encounters with Psychotherapy: experiences from a Balint Group. *Psychodynamic Practice*. 10(2), 195–206.

Mazzacane, F. (2022). The Bion-Field Theory (BFT): Theory, Clinical Tools, Controversial Points. *European Journal of Psychotherapy & Counselling*. 24(1), 15–36.

Mearns, D. & Cooper, M. (2005). *Working at Relational Depth in Counselling and Psychotherapy*. Sage Publications.

Merleau-Ponty, M. (1962). *Phenomenology of Perception* (Tr. Colin Smith). Routledge & Kegan Paul.

Merleau-Ponty, M. (1968). *The Visible and the Invisible* – followed by working notes. (Tr. A Lingis). Northwestern University Press.

Moran, D. (2000). *Introduction to Phenomenology*. Routledge.

Pedersen, P. (2000). *Hidden Messages in Culture-centered Counselling: a Triad Training Model*. SAGE.

Politis, V. (2020). Plato's Seventh Letter: A Close and Dispassionate Reading of the Philosophical Section. *Classics Ireland*. 27, 56–77.

Ratcliffe, M. (2008). *Feelings of Being: Phenomenology, Psychiatry, and the Sense of Reality*. Oxford University Press.

Rogers, C.R. (1967). *On Becoming a Person*. Constable.

Rogers, C.R. (1992). The Necessary and Sufficient Conditions of Therapeutic Personality Change. *Journal of Consulting and Clinical Psychology*. 60(6), 827–832.

Rothschild, B. (2000). *The Body Remembers: The Psychophysiology of Trauma and Trauma Treatment*. W. W. Norton.

Rüth, U. (2009). Classic Balint Groupwork and the Thinking of WR Bion: How Balint Work Increases the Ability to Think One's Own Thoughts. *Group Analysis*. 42(4), 380–391.

Sabar, S. (2013). What's Gestalt? *Gestalt Review.* 17(1), 6–34.

Schmid, P.F. & Mearns, D. (2006). Being-With and Being-Counter: Person-centered Psychotherapy as an In-depth Co-creative Process of Personalization. *Person-Centered & Experiential Psychotherapies.* 5(3), 174–190.

Sheredos, B. (2017). Merleau-Ponty's Immanent Critique of Gestalt Theory. *Human Studies.* 40(2), 191–215.

Stone, O. & Zahavi, D. (2021). Phenomenology and Mindfulness. *Journal of Consciousness Studies.* 28 (3–4), 158–185.

Taylor, C. (2024). *Cosmic Connections: Poetry in the Age of Disenchantment.* Harvard University Press.

Westland, G. (2009). Considerations of Verbal and Non-verbal Communication in Body Psychotherapy. *Body, Movement and Dance in Psychotherapy.* 4(2), 121–134.

Winnicott, D. W. (1984). The Capacity to be Alone (1958), in *The Maturational Processes and the Facilitating Environment.* 1st edition. Routledge. pp. 29–36.

Zahavi, D. (2021). Applied Phenomenology: Why It Is Safe to Ignore the Epoché. *Continental Philosophy Review.* 54(2), 259–273.

# EPILOGUE

*A Personal Understanding of Radical Relationality.*
This part considers the reader pressed for time who seeks to review the salient –
for me at least – characteristics of radical relationality, before either passing on
or choosing to return to the beginning and take a closer look at what I have to
say. For you, there is something more recognisable as a summary of the book in
Section 1.4. Then, there is the reader who, having read the book – *thank you* –
would appreciate a more personal and compact overview of radical relationality.
To make it easier for both, I refer you to the origins of these statements in
the main body of the text. In the spirit of radical relationality, it would not be
fitting to extrapolate too much from these isolated statements without gaining
some prior understanding of the context from which they emerged.

*So, to begin* – I understand that truth is not something revealed through
therapeutic methods, because truth is not like an object "within" waiting to
be discovered. Some pristine, preexisting consciousness has not been led astray
by the traditions that shape my understanding; I am entangled with them.
Because there are no facts in this regard – only interpretations – all that I can
do is seek to grasp what lies "between" me and the world (Section 1.1).

At heart lies a profound sense of care towards the client, their wellbeing,
and their good. This is not a first-person point of view of what might be good
for you if I were in your shoes. It is the third-person perspective of one who
cares – for the sake of the greater good. In this way, the practice of therapy is
deeply ethical, and not limited in the sense that I must only avoid the *red flags*
found in various codes of practice (Section 1.2).

While all approaches to therapy accept the value of relationships, I make a
distinction between radical relationality and a shallower, *ethereal* sort which
sees relationships as the inert medium through which the data of therapeutic

methods are transmitted. I am alert to modernity's beguiling tendency to render abstractions from an intertwined, intuitive prior whole. Taking things apart and separating them has led to dazzling technological achievements, and I value this approach when trying to make the world a better place. But if I am to avoid "technology" supplanting "wisdom" and the ancient concerns with life and living well, I must remain wary of what dissection demands (Section 1.3).

To the extent that there can be things that discipline the way I am in the world, I declare a commitment to the most compelling of these, namely: what I notice about the world as it presents itself for inspection. The idea that therapy could be disciplined by one method, or one philosophical tradition, whether it be analytical reasoning or phenomenological descriptions or whatever, misunderstands that I am an unending dynamic process of unfolding orientation to my co-created, disciplining context (Section 1.3).

Beyond the context of my relationships – so Aristotle argued – I am but an inert block of wood whose true meaning only comes about through my place on the checkerboard of life. A sense of transcendence is vital to me because it suggests a movement out in the first place to give meaning to the polarities of "me" and "not me", which ultimately needs to be bridged. It is only when I enter into social relations and am vulnerable to my encounter with an altering and enlarging you, that I am purged of emptiness and anonymity (Section 2.1).

Therapeutic Socratic questioning can connect the lives of clients with their context: understanding the way that I am situated in time and place is thus an important undertaking synonymous with responsiveness. I am claimed by a question, word, or experience to which I am called to respond with understanding in a way which leads to further experiencing. I try to maintain a genuine "not knowing" so that I may accept that I do not know how to live in the world in which you exist (Section 2.2).

I align with the belief that the being of a person is to be found neither in *individualism* – which sees us only in relation to ourselves, nor in *collectivism* – which fails to see us at all, as it only sees society. The intimate unity of inner and outer life is something inseparable from knowing myself as part of a greater whole (Section 3.4). This has profound implications for understanding my place in the order of things. The totality of objects in Nature is not just the finite individual products of Nature. Though it was necessary for humans to separate from Nature to understand themselves, I nevertheless stand in relation to the *whole* (Section 4.4).

The morally neutral therapist sees themselves as an abstracted thing. Instead, I am aware that I am enmeshed in the ethical flow: like braider and braided, bound by the common cord of the plait there is no alternative to being entangled in the tangle of it all. Thus, I acknowledge that it is necessary to articulate not only the goals but the ethical assumptions of the goals of therapy (Section 5.2). I only move towards an authentic ethical self when I understand myself in terms of my cares and projects when I am powered by a higher way of being. Moving along this path is not better insofar that I will feel better; it is a better way to be (Section 5.3).

I am not prior to my environment but am codetermined with my environment. While I did not begin my time here on earth aware of the metaphoric structures into which I was born – which includes on a larger human scale imperial rule, racism, colonialisation, and misogyny – I believe that generally speaking, seeing better and doing better tend to go hand in hand (Section 6.3).

The implications for therapy are clear. Undifferentiated, diffuse, unrefined responses to an unusual – or persistent – relational context are open to re-valuing, re-interpretation, and re-articulation in relation to my social and ethical context. To be in therapy, to understand therapy, to do therapy without appreciating its linguistically constructed ethical dimension is to overlook what is central to the social practice of living well. Making therapy more transparent requires that I be clearer about the values, ethics, or ideologies to which I may uncritically subscribe (Section 6.4).

The power of the narrative turn is that it embraces the interlocking nature of philosophy, ethics, and practice as something which transcends methods; it is an attitude to living, a political project, and an alternative to prevailing, pragmatic, empiricist, instrumental approaches to therapy. It forces a re-evaluation of the unquestioned or unquestionable truths of traditional psychological discourses. But only when I reject its naïve relativism, and sterile deconstructionism, can I accept it as radically relational (Section 7.3).

Telling and re-telling stories rests at the heart of therapy and indeed autoethnography. It implies the discipline of observing myself observing, interrogating what I believe, feel, and think in a way that challenges my assumptions (Section 7.3). I am alert to the ways in which my attempts to ameliorate distress can inadvertently oppress the people I want to support. Well-meaning, benevolent, helping professionals armed with individualising psychological interventions risk perpetuating civilising colonial attitudes towards trainees, supervisees, and clients (Section 7.4).

I appreciate the inescapable, culturally bound, and often contradictory linguistic expressions that characterise the experience of slipping in and out of lived time. But however important it may seem, separating the world into binary perspectives is just one (i.e., modernism) amongst other possible views to take of the world (Section 8.3). I reject the durationless present: I have an intuitive sense of the presentness of the future because actions in the present are already oriented towards the future in terms of my dreams, expectations, hopes, anticipations, and goals of a future yet to unfurl. The bridge of causality is unnecessary for me because past and future cannot be understood without the other. Recollection without meaning, and a meaning without recollection is experientially irrelevant, if not implausible. Temporal relationality allows for the past to be a meaningful influence in the present without the present being a mere effect of the past (Section 8.4).

When I speak of being "in the flesh", I am referring to both my body as the medium through which I live my life, and the relations that organise my life. The intertwining of intelligible and sensible – where I cannot easily distinguish subjects and objects, inside and outside – decentres *me* from the world. It conceives perception not as a human act, but as something with transpersonal and indeed transhuman dimensions. Given our ecological crisis, an embodied human becomes a "better citizen" of their worldly community, because the earth does not belong to me; it is I who belong to it (Section 9.3).

I do not confuse access to my own mind with fantasies about accessing the minds of others. If I claim to have the same access to your consciousness as you, then you cease to be different. This fails to respect what is distinct and unique about you. Without embodied self-differentiation there can be no talk of radical relationality since this is only made possible by the gap that separates us. Therapy is more than simply understanding; it is also not-understanding, of being on the way to understanding differently. It is not just support and facilitation; it is demand and challenge. In a word, *confrontation* (*L. – Face the Other*) is an essential part of therapy because it signals different ethical world views being brought together, made visible, understood, and transcended (Section 9.4).

While valuing what a therapeutic method offers, what matters is the process of stepping back from the psycho-mundane and appreciating that I do not encounter an individual in therapy, but the temporal nexus of histories, including my own. It means adopting a critical stance towards scientific theories, knowledge, explanations, personal views, and experiences. These are the taken-for-granted perspectives which must be interrogated and brought into awareness – paradoxically – before I can discover them. This has implications for training: when the soul searches – not for what something might be *like*, but what it *is* – then wisdom is more properly imparted and acquired, rather than taught through instruction (Section 9.5).

# INDEX

ABC model and cognitive behavioural therapy 49

Abraham: ethics of parental sacrifice in *Fear and Trembling* 64–5; Kierkegaard and paragon of faith 58, 115

addiction recovery: alignment with neoliberal and humanistic self-mastery 134

agential realism: social media entwined with social behaviour 179–82; *see also* Barad

alexithymia: language games as constitutive of flourishing 145; *see also* Wittgenstein

alternate possibilities: cognitive behavioural therapy and moral responsibility 50; existentialism 109

Althusser, L.: constitutive role of language 131; disciplines of the Self 19; ideology as cultural superstructures (*Subject*) 130–7; therapeutic interpellations 134–5

Anscombe, E.: against emotivism 117; attack on secular ethics 112; ethics of intentionality 57 (*see also* Wittgenstein); human flourishing 120

anthropocentrism 79, 193; climate change 93–5

antidepressants (SSRI's) 70

antihumanism 80, 87–92

Aristotle 5, 14, 46; the good life and *Nicomachean Ethics* 32–3; life comes to fruition at its end 48; *see also* virtue

Armstrong, K.: *A History of God* 60

artificial systems: agential cut 181; agential realism 182; attachment theory 139; embodiment 209–13; rabbit-duck 145–6, 220; therapeutic 7

Athens: symbol of disengaged reason 65–70; *see also* Jerusalem

attachment theory 139; affect regulation 50; interpellation 228; intersubjectivity 140; nonhumanism 92; structuralist internal working models 139

Aurelius, M.: *Meditations* 34; stoicism 139–40

authenticity: humanism 127; ideal self 116; instrumental reason 86; manufactured sameness 28

Bakhtin, M. 137

Balint group 238

Barad, K.: post humanism 179–82

base and superstructure metaphor 126

Beck, A.: therapeutic ideologies 134

being and becoming: Freud 157; Heidegger 200; infinite 96–7; Kierkegaard 115; Nature 222; Rogerian phenomenology 233–5; therapy 232–3

belief and faith: definition 62

beneficence 81–4, 105

Bion field theory (BFT) 219

Bohr, N.: anticipates the *differend* 180

boredom: existentialism 115;
phenomenology and therapy 186,
213–14
Boyd, J. OODA loops 21
Buber, M.: temporal *thou* (*Other
becomes It*) 73–4; eternal *Thou* 86
Burckhardt, J.: relationship with
Nietzsche 87; renaissance man 82–3
bureaucracy: instrument of colonialism
128; instrumental reason 47

Campbell, J.: hero's journey 152
care 9–11; empathy 223–7; pastoral
71–4; Rogers and unconditional
positive regard 227; self and
Foucault 174–7
categorical imperative: secularised
Protestantism 107–8; *see also* Kant
Catholicism: conflict between Judeo-
Christian theology and rationalism
6; cradle 62; Epicureanism 42;
Protestant work ethic 75–6; relational
ontology 221
causality: Merleau-Ponty and the
positivist error 220; relic of a bygone
age 51; therapeutic hazard of a linear
view of time 196, 202, 244
Christianity: alignment with stoicism
65; apparatuses of interpellation
131; counselling 72; Descartes 67;
Epicureanism denies immortality
of the soul 42; Freud 72, 156–8;
humanism 79, 83–5, 93; Paul's address
to Stoics and Epicureans 48
chronocentrism: flat earth distortion 6
cognitive (and rational emotive) therapy:
Beck's therapeutic interpellations
134; British imperialism 45; ethical
plasticity 47, 51; evolution of 49;
fatalism and morality 50–1;
75–7; philosophical paradox 51;
philosophical roots 24, 45–6; problem
in the patient 168, 171; purposeful
reason (*logos*) 45 (*see also* Christianity);
stoicism language and folk causality
51–2; *see also* ABC model
colonialism: English language 44–5;
Franz Fanon and psychotherapy
176–7; humanism 81; modernity 175;
structuralism 128
Columbo and Socrates 37–9
compassion: care 11, 28; (existentialism)
109; Nietzsche and its disreputable

motivations 88; towards others for
their lack of enlightenment (stoicism)
51; unconditional positive regard 227;
untangling humane from humanism
81–4; winner's triangle 226
constructivism 209
COVID-19: dignity of work 14;
disembodied therapy 182; global
racialised oppression and injustice
175; the greater good 10; rescuing
capitalism from itself 89
Crates and Hipparchia: defying
established authority 41–3
Crenshaw, K.: differend 166;
intersectionality 173
criterionless choice: against 26,
114–17; delusion of ethically neutral
therapy 122
Cynic: Diogenes of Sinope and acts of
personal liberation 41

Dasein 211–12
De Montaigne, M. 39, 48, 83; Metrocles
and shame 46; *see also* scepticism
de Saussure, F.: I do not speak I am
spoken 127
death: Aristotle 47–8; Descartes and the
soul 67; Epicurus 42; existentialism
47, 110–11; fatalism 50; Freud 158–9;
of God 88, 108; Jung and Kierkegaard
116; life after 41, 81; liminality of
children 113–14; providence 74;
rejection as human drive 72; Seneca's
consolation to Marcia 43;
of Socrates 36–7
dementia: phenomenology 29, 211,
235–7
depression: decoupling from temporal
flow 204–5; lived experience of 57,
186, 232–5; material explanations 68
(*see also* phenomenology); typifying
the client 226
Derrida, J.: destructive nihilism 129,
171 (*see also* structuralism); the play
of meaning 126; sterility of
deconstruction 129–30, 168;
*Structure, Sign and Play* 128; waking
from the structuralist dream 128–30
Descartes, R.: body as *extensa* 67; *cogito*
66–7; cures for the disembodied mind
68–70; *Discourse on the Method* 93;
humanistic epistemology 141; I think
therefore I am 66; loss of perceptual

faith 65–9; ontological argument 67; transcendent animal 79

determinism: attachment theory 139–40; empiricism and existentialism 42; relational temporality 201–7; Sapir-Whorf theory 198; therapeutic 50–2

differend 165–6; agential realism 180; Foucault 170

diversity: anti-oppressive practices 178–9; linguistic 45, 148; models of flourishing 105; psychic colonialisation 139

dodo bird conjecture 7

drama triangle 225

dualism: avoiding theological discontinuities 58; cartesian 67–70; dissolving 122, 209; humans and Nature 96; ontological bifurcation of reality 159; *see also* emergentism; Wittgenstein

durationless present moment: against 190–3

Dussel, E. D.: non-European culture which lies beyond and prior to the colonising structures of the modern Occident 160

ecology: shallow 93; deep 95

Einstein, A.: corroboration does not imply universality 91

Elias, N.: apparatus of colonialism 127–8; emotionally curbed self 127

Ellis, A.: philosophical origins of REBT 46–9; principle of alternate possibilities 50

embodiment: artificial intelligence 209–10; emotivism and therapeutic distortions 119–20 (*see also* phenomenology); language and ventriloquism 140; space-time mappings 111, 198

emergent phenomena 69–71, 94, 217; providential ontology 76

emotions: borrowed 223–6; Cartesian notions of 24, 85; communion with affect 236; embodied attunement 233; emotivism 117; frozen 206; language 147–9, 162, 168, 198; reasoning with 46–50, 163; Romanticism 93–4, 134; therapy as sedation 25, 226

emotivism: against 117–20; Humes distinction between facts and values 117; MacIntyre's *After Virtue* 119

empathy 223–1; artificial 182; intersubjectivity 227–31; mimicry and enactment 223–4; projective 224–6; proto-sympathetic 226–7

empiricism 234; the scandal of philosophy 90–2, 163

environment and climate change 24, 33, 93–4, 128

Epictetus: CBT 46; live alongside your difficult colleagues and annoying friends *Discourses* 32–4; therapeutic arguments *Enchiridion* 34

Epicurus: eudaimonia 43; existentialism and empiricism 40–2

epistemology: bias 90; Cartesian 66; definition 3; epistēmē 5; humanistic 141; modernity 160

epoché: Husserl's reduction 215–17; person-centred therapy 234

ethics and morals: aretaic 121; a coherent framework to help therapists understand how to engage ethically with the world 101; difference between 99; dilemmas 101–2; in a meaningless universe 112–13, 123; life goods 122–3; moral sources 123; myth of therapist neutrality 101–6, 120, 170, 174; pluralism 101, 108, 112, 104; realness 121–4; red flags in therapeutic practice 26, 102, 242

eudaimonia: definition 40; the greatest good 43

existentialism: choice 109–17; beyond false consciousness 130; as ideology 133

experience: Carl Rogers 234; fidelity to185–8; plane of 138, 210

faith: attachment theory 140; leap of 64, 95, 111, 116; loss of perceptual 65–7; scientism 59; in statistics 163

Fanon, F.: curing the institution of psychotherapy 176–7

fatalism free will and morality 50–1, 130

faux individualism 135

field theories 20; Bion 219; gestalt 203, 219–21; Lewin 219; Merleau-Ponty 192, 221–5

flesh (Fr. Chair) 209, 221–3, 236, 245; *see also* Merleau-Ponty

Foster Wallace, D.: choosing a transcendent thing to worship 63; what the heck is water? 59

Foucault, M.: against humanism 86, 127; changing institutions 174; differend in psychiatry 165, 170; emancipation 169; enlightenment 182; ethics 160, 175; narrative therapy 167; polemics and problematisation in therapy 169–70; power 167, 177; resistance 172

frailty of narratives created in the bubble of therapy 174

Frankenstein: complex and antihumanism 80; objective-subjective split 193

Frankfurt school 109

Frankfurt, H.: against economic egalitarianism 43; equality of therapeutic provision 44

freedom and autonomy: romantic delusions 130–7

Freud, S.: atheistic science 71; better Christian there never was 158; most humans are trash 158; physical thermodynamics and the ontology of psychic energy 126, 157; Plato and tripartite division of self 156; positivism 65; postmodernism 155; profession of lay curers of souls 159; radical epistemological break through 157; relationship with Oskar Pfister 77, 158, 166; secular pastoral care 71–4; unknowable mind undermines human claim to autonomy 92; walled-off punctuated self 155–7; we now expect to find hidden meanings 63

fundamentalism 60

Gadamer, H-G.: fullness of time 192; prejudice against prejudice 217; reflexivity in therapy 238; therapy as socially recognised healing 5, 13; tradition 59, 136, 202; *Truth and Method* 4, 216

gatekeeper ethics 26, 104

gestalt: humanism 81–4; Husserl 187; mindfulness 218; Perls F. 87, 203, 210; Perls L. 203; phenomenality 210; phenomenology 212; present moment 206, 218, 232–3 (see also time); psychology and Berlin School 219–22; therapy 203–10

God: disembodied transcendence 48, 57, 65; *A History* (*see* Armstrong); humanism 83; inward lies the road 60–3; death of-Hegel 108; Descartes 108; Kant 106; Martin Buber 73; moral enforcer 67, 106–13; Nature 96; Nietzsche 88; ontological arguments-Anselm 59; Paul and the Athenians 58; perspective 193; Popper and metaphysics 91; providential ontology 74–7; Tertullian 58; therapy 172–3

golden rule 64, 105, 157

good: common 10–1, 14–15, 37–40, 111, 117, 168; creative therapeutic practice 11–16; and evil 55, 60–1; of therapy 7–16

habitus: embodied disposition habits and skills 9

Hall, S.: there can be no reassuring foundation 132

healing: art of 13–15; souls 216; therapist as facilitator 234

hedonism: stoicism and pleasure principle 43

Hegel, G.: radical relationality of the Geist 56, 108

Heidegger, M. D.: asein 211; Mitsein 212; unity of time 200

Heisenberg: cut 180–1; Epicurus 42

hermeneutics 57, 127, 201, 212; bifurcation of 129

holism: bracketing as an open-ended striving for 217; cosmic interconnection 24, 40, 45–8; denies the individual 96; Gaia 95–6; inner unity 61, 108; Nature as eternity 96; unimaginable perfection 20, 216; von Schellinginfinite becoming 96–7

hope: analytical credo 57; Kafka-but not for us 94; and therapy 7–8, 16, 21, 200, 203, 224

Horkheimer, M.: *Eclipse of Reason* 46; ethical plasticity of cognitive therapies 47; instrumental *vs.* platonic reasoning 88–90

Hughes, T.: *Wodwo* 97

human nature: climate catastrophe 92–7; Foucault 169; Freud 57; as something created 81, 92; spirituality 72; stoicism 41

humane *vs.* humanistic 81–7

humanism 79–87; antihumanism 87–92; mastery of the cosmos 93; nonhumanism and radical relationality 92–7; Pauline 84; posthumanism 175–83

Hume, D.: Hume's problem 90; moral relativism 106, 108, 117

Husserl, E.: bridling in therapy 231–5; eidetic reduction 217; extended now 185–7; intersubjectivity 229; mindfulness yoga and Buddhism 218; natural attitude 215; objectivity of subjective experience 193; protension and retention 187, 207; reduction 215–19; things in themselves 213

idealism and realism 188–9

integrative/eclectic models, problems of 18, 104, 164, 237

interpellation: constitutive of emotional language 147–51; ideological (*Subject*) 131–9; individuals (subjects) 131; narrative resistance 169–70; phenomenology 216; therapeutic 134; training 144–5; transactional analysis 139

intersubjectivity: the second person perspective and radical relationality 227–31

intuition 213–18

irony (eirōneía) 37–8, 88

Jerusalem: spirituality and transcendence 60–5; *see also* Athens

Jung, C.: apolitical child archetype 13; hero's journey 152, 177; shadow 116; uroboros 1, 22–3, 155

justice: days 113–14; the good life 43–4; injustice and the differend 165–6, 176; morality 99, 107

Kant, I.: he abolished *God* and made *humans* in *Gods* stead 112; Isaac Newton of morality 106–8

Keane, N.: phenomenology of second person perspective 229

Kierkegaard, S.: ethics of living *Enten-Eller* (Either/Or) 114; Jung and the shadow 116; leap of faith in *Fear and Trembling* 64; myth of the criterionless choice 114–17; not what we believebut the way in which we believe 115; social media 86; therapeutic change 136; transcendent love 73

Klein, M.: emotional and cognitive synthesis required for human flourishing 61

language: anger 122, 149–50; bilingualism and time 198–9; Taylor-*The Language Animal* 141; discovery and invention of emotion 146–51; embodied 140–1; emergence of meaning 140–53; enframes 141; implications for therapy 150–1 (*see also* Wittgenstein); spoken English and inequality 44–5; time 185; unsayable and the surrounding sayable 111, 143

language game: changing our relationship with what is spoken 145; differend 165; intersubjective communion 144–4; therapy 170, 218

Larkin, P.: existentialism 110; separation of body-mind 66

liberal individualism: as naïve freedom 112; woven into the fabric of therapy 99–108

living present: ethnography 129; intersubjectivity 229–33; in practice 202–4; radical relationality 28–30; transference 30, 182

love: heart not head 54; human condition 72–3; humanistic therapy 84; I-thou 86; rarely perfect 233

luck: determinism and free will 51; fate and stoicism 40, 45, 50; providential ontology 74–7; social classand therapy 13–15

Lyotard, J-F: authority of stories 160–1; crisis of legitimacy 161–4; *The Postmodern Condition* 161; universality without consensus 164–7

Manchester screwdriver: blunt end as a hammer 164

Marx, K.: metaphor of base and superstructure 126; stoicism and freedom from suffering 130–1

MacIntyre, A.: *After Virtue* 119; emotivism 119–20; faith in psychotherapy 63; therapists as characters 162

Maslow, A.: existentialism as high I.Q. whimpering 111

materialism: d'Holbach *Systéme de la nature* 68; only matter matters 90

Matrix: Descartes-my existence may just be a dream 66

McTaggart, J.: *A* and *B* series of time 189; flaw of the durationless present

190–2; gestalt psychology 220; narrative structure 201; *The Unreality of Time* 188

Menopause 29, 136

Merleau-Ponty, M.: embodied relational ontology 221–3; fidelity to experience 185–8; gestalt psychology 220–1; *Phenomenology of Perception* 211, 217; relational entwinement 199, 204–7; Rogerian phenomenology 233–5 (*see also* phenomenology); time 192–6; trauma 236

metaphors: alternate modes of truth 59, 65, 88; that disembody 29, 57, 162; Freud 156–7; hazards in therapy 193–4, 196–8; making sense of theworld 6, 27, 30; myths 151–3; therapy 135, 150

Midgley, M.: masculine idea of emancipation 87; Nature 92

mitsein: being with Others 212

modernity: Cartesian epistemology of science 66; decolonial theory 175; defined 159–60; divergence of reason 46; existentialism as reaction toward 109; Freud 157; grand narratives 172; secularity 65; weakness 2–3

monism 42, 48, 68; *see also* emergentism

narrative: intersubjective time 199–202; radical relationality 28, 244; structure of a life 133, 161–3; turn in therapy 167–74

natural attitude: curtain of the ordinary 215–7; Rogerian self-awareness 234 (*see also* Husserl); therapist development 231

Neural plasticity and free will (Libet) 51–2

Nietzsche, F.: antihumanism 87–8; narrative turn 163

Næss, A.: relational ecology 93–6

nonhumanism 92–7

ontology: defined 3, 110–11; dualist 157; bifurcation (dualism) 160; embodied relational 179, 221–3; Freuds psychic energy 157–9; of mind 70; providential 74–7; Socratic 37

OODA loops 21

orientation 22–30

others 175–83; anti-oppressive practice 178–9 (*see also* colonialism); colour blindness 177; COVID-19 175;

Māori and Samoan cultural attitudes to therapy 178; racism 121, 127–8; 173–7

Pavlenko, A.: cross-cultural miscommunication 147–8

perception: phenomenality 210 (*see also* phenomenology)

Perls, F. *see* gestalt

person-centred therapy: congruence and incongruence 20; fluidity 234; Gloria linguistic manipulations 85, 134; Pauline humanism 84; Rogerian phenomenology 233–5; teleological predisposition toward actualisation 72; therapist as liberator 168; unconditional positive regard 227

Pfister, O. *see* Freud

phenomenology: anger 213, 224; anxiety 9, 38, 223 (*see also* Barad); body therapy 239; Buddhism and mindfulness 218; critique of gestalt and positivism 221; definition 210–12; dementia 212, 235–7; depression 9, 57, 68, 144, 204–5, 226, 232–3; embodied relational ontology (flesh) and ecological crisis 221–3; Husserl's reduction 215–17; implications for training 237–9; intersubjectivity 227–3; Heisenberg cut 180 (*see also* Merleau-Ponty; time); trauma 235–7

placebo and therapy 16

Plato: *Apology* 35, 37–8

play of meaning 126–30

Plotinus: elusive inner world *The Six Enneads* 56, 67, 144

Popper, K.: physics metaphysics and pseudoscience 90–1

postmodern condition 159–67; Freud shatters modernist dream 155; limitations of theoretical integration in therapy 18, 164, 237; materialistic and discursive 162, 167, 179–82; morality as a matter of power 117; ontological bifurcation of reality (dualism) 159–60; poststructuralism 129; radical relationality rejects naïve relativism 244 (*see also* post structuralism); relativism 170; therapeutic methodological nihilism 171; universality without consensus 164–7

praxis 2

presence: contact 214; emotional contagion 224; involvement-detachment in therapy 230–4, 239; limit and limitlessness of being human 97; radical reflexivity 61; spiritual 64; synchronising with Others 204–7; temporal flow 186, 192 (*see also* time); *vorhandenheit* 21

property dualism: anomalous monism, emergentism, or supervenience theory 70

Protestant reformation and the ethic of self-mastery and self-control 75–6

psychic colonialisation 139

psychoanalysis: Freud's metapsychology 157–9; physicalist notions 220; secular pastoral care 71–2

quantum mechanics 135; Epicurus 42; Libet 52

radical relationality: characteristics of 22–30

rational mysticism: will of Godor universal Nature 48

reason: Athens as metaphor 65–70; Augustine of Hippo 60; Cartesian *cogito* 67; disengaged calculating external stance 55; *ego* as disengaged agents of instrumental 156; Freudian *ego* 156 (*see also* Jerusalem); instrumental 28, 86–9, 106–9; CBT 47; modernity 46, 159; Nietzsche laments the demise of truth in all its forms 88; Platonic 156; subjective 144

relational depth: esoteric stupor-like experience 231; indwelling *naturans* power 235; transcends method 202

relationship: æthereal (shallow) 16–18, 28, 109, 114, 226, 242; comfortably numb 226; mundane 33, 216, 245; radicalising the client-therapist 168–70; therapy as mediocre 25

relativism 26–8, 117, 129; against 135, 166, 167, 170–4; attachment theory 92; existentialism 109; humanistic therapy 87–9, 120; interpretive circularity in therapy 170–2

renaissance Man 82

Rogers, C.: *On Becoming a Person* 235; *see also* person-centred therapy

Romanticism: defined by more than disengaged rational reasoning 134; the importance of emotion, feeling, and a nostalgia for loving Nature 93

Rorty, R.: against relativism 117; Feud and Plato 156

Rothschild, B.: body remembers 235; ontic bifurcation 236

Russell, B.: analytical/continental split 56; nothing properly understood as a cause or effect 51 (*see also* causality); time 188

Sapir-Whorf hypothesis: are we thinking differently when we talk differently about time 196–9

Sartre, J-P.: condemned to be free 116–17; critique of heroic individual freedom 87; our *projet fundamental* 206; the past is gone the future is unknown 200–1

scepticism: CBT 48–9; Descartes 66; moral realism 139; Nietzsche 88; rejection of 35, 168; therapeutic 39; *see also* Montaigne

school based therapy: questionable wisdom of humanistic approach 81–2

scientific positivism: Freud's metapsychology 157; gestalt psychology 219–20; rueful Wittgenstein 143; topic-driven approach in training 237

scientism: conflict with Indigenous knowledge 161–2; faith in science 11; ignores transcendence 71; replaces religious belief 24, 59; structuralism and 161; time and causation 196; value free therapy 26, 99

secularism: *paraphylum*-paraphernalia left over when we remove all the things that are obviously religious 71; secular piety and pastoral care 71–7; self-mastery and merit 76; the moral vacuum left by 100

self: atomised 79–97; Augustine question to myself 61; care of 9–11; emotionally curbed 127; more than a point of self-referential activity 227–31; orientation 16–22; punctuated 17–20, 60, 155; radical relationality 22–30; splitting the human atom 155–9 (*see also* Freud); when falling asleep I retire to myself 203

Seneca: consolation to Marcia 43; Rogerian actualising tendency (*oikeiosis*) 43; stoics and the Roman Empire 40

sex: asceticism and stoicism 41; discrimination 168

shame: colonial relations of dependence 177; embodied 236; emotional language 148–9; Metrocles 46; shameless Diogenes 41

silence: benign ideologies which 170, colour blindness 177; differend 165; ethics of *omerta* 107; Kierkegaard-talkativeness afraid of 86; language not reducible to words inserting themselves into 211; oppression of those who seek the services of a therapist 171; Sartre-monstrous 116; Winnicott-experience of being alone in the presence of someone 239

sleep 203

social class and humanistic therapy 13–14

Socrates: Columbo 38; death 36–7; elenchus or induced perplexity 36; from the celestial to the terrestrial 34–40; Husserl's reduction 215; irony (eirōneía) 38; therapeutic dialogue 35–40, 58, 110, 243

spirituality 60–5; *see also* secularism

splitting the human atom 155–9

St Augustine: *Confessions* I have become a question to myself 60–1; contemplative now 191–2; Husserl 187; Klein–inner unity 61; phenomenology 212; time 186–7; why be good? 101

St Paul/Sauland humanism 84

stoicism: alignment with Christian thought 58, 64; British imperialism 45; cognitive therapy 45–52; fatalism 50–1, 130; Kant-sovereign rational individual adhering to a set of universal rules 112; language and causality 51–2; no definitive account of ethics 47; passive matter subjected to divine and purposeful reason (*logos*) 45; self-interested self-preservation 42; self-mastery of feelings 45–50; temporality 189

stories 155–83; *see also* narrative

Strawson, G.: narrative and ethics 201

structuralism 126–37; becoming *vs.* being (Rogerian phenomenology) 233–5; language identity and therapy 137–40 (*see also* Bakhtin); prioritises impersonal systems of relations that downplay rational subjectivity 214

super structures of culture *see* interpellation

sympathy: empathy and intersubjectivity 223–30; implications for practice 231–9; regard *for* someone for their own sake because *their* good matters 10–11

Szasz, T.: risks of stigmatising people through medical categorisation 172

Taylor, C.: language 141–9; moral sources and life goods 122–3

technē: Aristotle and the craft of practical wisdom 5; the good therapist 55

telos: Abraham goes beyond utilitarian reciprocity 64; higher purpose 8, 10; inherent moral justifications or motives 120; non-structuralist therapy 138

temporal experience: desynchronization 199, 204–7, 233; retention and protention 187, 207; *see* time

Tertullian: prestige affords scientism dignity 58–9

Thatcher, M.: capitalised on a grand narrative of progress 164

theodicy: the paradox that God allows evil in the world 60

therapists as characters: the ideal of being right 119, 162

therapy: art of 2, 13, 161; beyond the bubble of 170; body 239; colour blindness 177; comfortably numb 25; data of 4, 16, 242; good of 4, 7–16; guided discovery in 36; interpretative circularity 170; as moral practice 101–8; shifting narratives of identity 138–9

time (temporality): consciousness 187; contemplative now 187; dance between explicit and implicit 204–6; durationless present (against) 190–3; fidelity to experience 185–8; figure-ground reversals 193–8; gestalt therapy 203–6; hazardous metaphors 193–4; intersubjective 199–207; language 196–9 (*see also* MacTaggart A/B-series); relational and practice 202–4; schizophrenic auditory hallucinations 207; synchronising with others–depression grief anxiety 204–7; thinking differently when talking differently 197–9

transactional analysis 139; drama triangle 225–6

transcended animal 79–80

transcendence: Aristotle 243; beyond the sayable 110, 116; Freud 59; God 57; humanistic and religious 80; Jerusalem 60–3; Nietzsche's heroic 88; person-centred theory 234; radical relationality 99; scientific piety 70; stoic 48

transference 194–6

trauma embodiment 235–6

truth: idiographic and nomothetic truth in therapy 172–3 (*see also* narrative turn and relativism); truthfulness and therapeutic methods 4, 36

*Truth and Method*: implications for therapy 4–8, 36, 44–50, 62, 102–5, 163–7, 202 (*see also* Gadamer)

unconditional positive regard: non-possessive other-directed caring 227; universal altruism 88; *see also* person-centred therapy; sympathy

universality: dissolves particularities 106–7; ethics in counselling and psychotherapy 113; without consensus 164–7

uroboros: Freud 155; hungry for more sophisticated hungers 3; Jung 22; radical relationality 23; unity of the material and spiritual 1, 179

*vergegnung*: Buber and relational mismeeting 73

vital beings 209–13

virtue 117–20; beneficence 105; a good life 41; justice 107; and moral realism 117–24; MacIntyre's *After Virtue* 119–21; making correct ideological choices 133–4; moderation 39; the moral high ground 112; Protestant work ethic 76; retrieving 120–1; stoicism 40–2; therapy 5, 45, 101

von Schelling F.: radical relationality and Nature 96–7

Wald, A.: differend 165

Weber, M.: *The Protestant Ethic and the Spirit of Capitalism* 132

Winnicott, D. 232, 239

wisdom: Plato 238; practical (phronesis) 2, 5, 32, 161; Sinatra 172; Socrates 36; super ego 156; training 245

Wittgenstein, L.: aspect perception-rabbit-duck image 145–6, 181, 220; get the life of a speaker into view 143, 199; *Essay on Logic and Philosophy (Tractatus Logico-Philosophicus)* 142; homosocialisation in therapy training 144–5; implications for therapy 146–52; listen to what I mean not what I say 142; metaphor and myth 151–2; Monk's biography 142; old problems discarded with the old garment of expression 145; *Philosophical Investigations* 143 (*see also* language and language games); the liberating word 147; translation and interpretation not the same 143

Zeno of Citium and psychotherapy 45–53

Zeno of Elea: arrow paradox and durationless present moment 190